The Health of Dairy Cattle

Edited by

Anthony H. Andrews BVetMed, PhD, MRCVS

Independent Veterinary Consultant
Specialist in Cattle Health and Production

**Blackwell
Science**

© 2000 by
Blackwell Science Ltd
Editorial Offices:
Osney Mead, Oxford OX2 0EL
25 John Street, London WC1N 2BL
23 Ainslie Place, Edinburgh EH3 6AJ
350 Main Street, Malden
　MA 02148 5018, USA
54 University Street, Carlton
　Victoria 3053, Australia
10, rue Casimir Delavigne
　75006 Paris, France

Other Editorial Offices:

Blackwell Wissenschafts-Verlag GmbH
Kurfürstendamm 57
10707 Berlin, Germany

Blackwell Science KK
MG Kodenmacho Building
7-10 Kodenmacho Nihombashi
Chuo-ku, Tokyo 104, Japan

First published 2000

Set in 10/12.5 pt Times
by Best-set Typesetter Ltd., Hong Kong
Printed and bound in Great Britain by
MPG Books, Bodmin, Cornwall

The Blackwell Science logo is a
trade mark of Blackwell Science Ltd,
registered at the United Kingdom
Trade Marks Registry

DISTRIBUTORS
Marston Book Services Ltd
PO Box 269
Abingdon
Oxon OX14 4YN
(*Orders:* Tel: 01235 465500
　　　　　Fax: 01235 465555)

USA
Blackwell Science, Inc.
Commerce Place
350 Main Street
Malden, MA 02148 5018
(*Orders:* Tel: 800 759 6102
　　　　　　　781 388 8250
　　　　　Fax: 781 388 8255)

Canada
Login Brothers Book Company
324 Saulteaux Crescent
Winnipeg, Manitoba R3J 3T2
(*Orders:* Tel: 204 837 2987
　　　　　Fax: 204 837 3116)

Australia
Blackwell Science Pty Ltd
54 University Street
Carlton, Victoria 3053
(*Orders:* Tel: 03 9347 0300
　　　　　Fax: 03 9347 5001)

A catalogue record for this title
is available from the British Library

ISBN 0-632-04103-X

Library of Congress
Cataloging-in-Publication Data
is available

For further information on
Blackwell Science, visit our website:
www.blackwell-science.com

Contents

Contributors

Anthony H. Andrews BVetMed, PhD, MRCVS   Independent Veterinary Consultant, RCVS Recognised Specialist in Cattle and Health Production, Welwyn, Hertfordshire

Roger W. Blowey BSc, BVSc, FRCVS   Veterinary practitioner, Wood Veterinary Group, Gloucester

James M. Booth BVM&S, MRCVS   Veterinary Consultant, Worcester

Frank H. Dodd BSc, PhD, FIBiol   Formerly Head of the Animal Science Division, The National Institute for Research in Dairying, University of Reading

Dick Esslemont BSc, PhD, NDA, CertEd, CBiol, FIBiol, FIAgrm, FRAgS, Hon Assoc RCVS, FBIAC   Senior Lecturer, University of Reading

Laurence A. S. Gibson MA, VetMB, MRCVS   Veterinary Adviser, Ministry of Agriculture, Fisheries and Food, State Veterinary Service, Veterinary Notifiable Diseases Team (Endemic Animal Diseases and Zoonoses)

John Hughes MIBiol, CIBiol, NDD, CDD, Hon Assoc RCVS   Independent Dairy Consultant, Whitchurch, Shropshire

Jim Kelly BVM&S, MRCVS   Senior Lecturer, Easter Bush Veterinary Centre, University of Edinburgh

Chris H. Knight BSc, PhD   Head, Animal Physiology Group, Hannah Research Institute, Ayr

Mohamed A. Kossaibati BSc, DipAg, MSc, PhD   Senior Research Fellow, Department of Agriculture, University of Reading

David Noakes BVetMed, PhD, FRCVS, DVRep   Professor of Veterinary Obstetrics and Diseases of Reproduction, Royal Veterinary College, University of London

Roger Spooner OBE, MA, BVetMed, PhD, MRCVS   Consultant and Honorary Professor, Centre for Tropical Veterinary Medicine, University of Edinburgh

A. David Weaver BSc, DrMedVet (Hanover), PhD, Dr.hc (Warsaw), FRCVS Professor Emeritus, Veterinary Consultant and Lecturer, Glasgow

David A. Whitaker MA, VetMB, MVSc, MRCVS   Senior Research Fellow, Easter Bush Veterinary Centre, University of Edinburgh

Preface

In most parts of Europe, as well as other parts of the world, milk production has been suffering from economic pressures. This makes it imperative that producers become increasingly efficient in their management. In particular it means that the cattle used to produce milk must be kept as productive and healthy as possible. This veterinary area is not as exciting as treating disease and often does not involve the latest molecular technology, but it is the fundamental basis for health and welfare of the cattle. Much is simply the application or basic principles and common sense to the management of the animals. However, it will become increasingly important over the next few years as more and more pressures are placed on the use of treatment for disease.

The aim of this book is to provide a practical guide to maintaining or improving the health of dairy cattle from birth until they leave the dairy herd. The book looks at the ways to reduce and overcome the many problems, both of production and disease, which can afflict the animal during its life on a farm. Thus, information is provided to try to ensure that the calf and heifer are reared correctly. Some points here are perhaps not exclusively concerned with welfare, as some of the old-fashioned principles of disease control do appear to work on many farms and involve the maxim 'The enemy of one animal is another of the same species'.

The book then goes on to discuss the main problems that face the dairy herd, such as nutrition, lameness, fertility and mastitis. Many other factors influence the cow's production and so chapters on mammary development, genetics, housing and production are also included. Finally, some health schemes are outlined.

This book does not aim to be comprehensive, but it does allow the veterinary surgeon to initiate some suitable preventive strategies. The contents are based on the wide range of experience of the contributors who are all experts in their particular fields, but is obviously biased towards the United Kingdom dairy system. However, the principles the book contains are relevant to all systems of dairy production whatever the country or however extensive or intensive the management involved.

Anthony H. Andrews

Disclaimer

While every effort has gone into checking the ideas, facts and figures presented in this book, the authors, editor and publishers cannot accept responsibility for any errors or omissions.

When using the book, readers should check the product information currently provided by the manufacturer of each drug in the country concerned. A product may not be licensed for use in dairy cattle or for the indication or dose used, but nevertheless in the opinion of the veterinary surgeon it may be the drug of choice. It is the responsibility of those administering and prescribing for farm use, relying on their professional skill and experience, to determine the best treatment and dosage, and whether the benefits of a specific drug justify the attendant risk. However, prescribing must be within the bounds of the law.

Chapter 1
Calf Health

Anthony H. Andrews

Managing calf health

In all dairy herds the essential raw material is the production of strong healthy calves which can be grown at a satisfactory level to produce cows with acceptable milk yields, good fertility and extended longevity. Despite continued veterinary inputs to fertility (Chapters 2, 5 and 11) and attempts to reduce dystocia, the only large surveys available indicate that the number of live calves produced per 100 cows calving is nearer 90 than 100 (Table 1.1).

The birth period is critical and many calves will die during or at parturition from dystocia, congenital problems or poor management. The first day or so is also critical in ensuring adequate hygiene for the newborn calf and that sufficient colostrum is provided to ensure adequate passive protection to infection during the first few weeks of life.

Navel treatment

As soon after birth as possible the navel should be dressed with a suitable preparation. Ideally it is best to use a strong iodine-based solution in alcohol and in some cases phenolic disinfectants and also added to assist with desiccation and antimicrobial activity. This will help to prevent infected navels, septicaemia and joint ill (p. 192). It is better to dip the navel using a receptacle such as a teat cup rather than to spray as it allows a complete covering of the navel. However, spraying is better than nothing. Antibiotics are not as effective as disinfectants because of their usually lower spectrum of antimicrobial activity and reduced desiccant effect.

Colostrum

As the placenta is impermeable to protein the calf is born with little immunity to disease. The sucking of colostrum after birth provides passive protection in the period before the animal mounts its own immune response to organisms. The constituents of colostrum and milk are very different (Table 1.2). Heifer's colostrum tends to be less concentrated and lack of exposure to potential pathogens often means that specific immunity is reduced. Non-specific antimicrobial activity

Table 1.1   Estimates (%) of normal parturition and loss at birth.

	Great Britain (Dairy and beef*)	Ireland (Dairy **)
Abortion	2.1	2.1
Stillbirth	3.3	5.9
Died or sold unfed	5.0	—
Live gestation up to 270 days	2.8 } 89.6	92.0
Live gestation over 270 days	86.8	—

* Leech *et al.* (1968); ** Bakheit & Greene (1981).

Table 1.2   The main constituents (%) of cattle colostrum and milk.

	Casein	Albumin/ globulin	Fat	Lactose	Ash	Total solids
Colostrum						
At birth	2.7	16.0	3.5	3.0	1.2	27.0
24 hours	4.5	6.3	4.7	2.9	1.0	19.4
48 hours	3.3	3.9	4.2	4.4	0.8	16.6
Milk	3.4	Minimal	3.8	4.9	0.7	12.9

includes lactoperoxidase, lysozyme and lactoferrin. Besides being high in immunoglobulins, colostrum has high concentrations of calcium, phosphorus, magnesium, vitamins A ($10 \times$ milk) and D ($3\times$), iron ($10–17\times$) and copper.

The passive immunity produced by colostrum has two important roles, one in the circulation, to prevent septicaemias, bacteraemias and viraemias, and the other, a local role, at the gut surface (Table 1.3) to deter alimentary pathogens.

The amount of colostrum absorbed depends on various factors:

(1)   Constituents of colostrum (cow/calf/farmer factor)
(2)   Volume of colostrum ingested (cow/calf/farmer factor)
(3)   The absorptive capacity of the calf (calf/farmer factor)
(4)   Management practices (farmer factor)

Constituents of colostrum

The gammaglobulin quantity and its specific immunity depends on the individual cow, its breed and breeding. Parity is important as heifers' colostrum is less concentrated. Amounts alter if there is a short dry period, poor general nutrition or if there is any milking before calving, a big flush of milk occurring at calving or induction of parturition by long-acting corticosteroids. Infection in the dam prior to calving will reflect in less immunity, as does mastitis, etc.

Volume of colostrum ingested

Maximum protection is provided by 3–5 litres of colostrum and the optimum amount is 5% or more of the body weight in the first 24 hours. If the calf is

Table 1.3 Some features of colostrum activity in the calf.

	Parental (absorbed) immunity
Septicaemias	*Escherichia coli*
Bacteraemias	*Salmonella* spp.
	Listeria monocytogenes
	Pasteurella sp.
	Streptococcus sp.
	Haemophilus somnus
	Navel ill/joint ill
Pneumonia	Various causes
	IBR
Viraemia	BVD/mucosal
	Oral (local) immunity
Enteritis (scour)	*Escherichia coli*
	Salmonella spp.
	Clostridium perfringens types A, B and C
	Rotavirus
	Coronavirus
	Other enteric viruses
	Cryptosporidia

sucking, then it is difficult to determine the quantity taken, but hard sucking for at least 20 minutes should be allowed. It is possible to estimate the amount of globulins absorbed by plasma or seen by the direct or indirect methods including zinc sulphate turbidity test, refractometer, sodium sulphite precipitation, radial immunodiffusion and electrophoresis. The ability of the calf to feed depends on how active it is following parturition as well as the physical shape of the udder and teats. Feeding is hampered by large, pendulous udders as well as teats which are badly positioned or overwide. Recumbency of the dam is also unhelpful.

Absorptive capacity of the calf

The absorptive capacity of the calf depends on the colostrum concentration as well as how active the calf is after birth. Maximum amounts of immunoglobulin are able to be absorbed soon after birth (first 6–8 hours) and this then declines so that absorption is little, or none, after 24–36 hours.

Management practices

Generally, the more natural the situation at calving the higher the absorbed immunoglobulin by the calf. Thus, calves born outside have higher values than those born indoors. Lower plasma values occur in calves born in byres than those born in calving boxes. Calves left in loose boxes with their dams for more than 24 hours have a higher blood immunoglobulin level than those removed at birth or immediately after sucking. Cows fed colostrum by bucket in the presence of the mother also have higher levels than those similarly fed away from the dam. In temperate climates, there is variation in immunoglobulin uptake with decreased absorption in the winter period.

Despite all the knowledge available about the importance of colostrum, much of which has been known for over 25 years, blood immunoglobulin levels in calves are often inadequate, and on many farms over half will not have received adequate colostrum early enough in life. This contributes considerably to disease on these farms. Provision of colostrum frozen in half-litre or litre packs can be of use in emergencies to ensure that the calf obtains about 3 litres in the first 6 hours of life. When problems have arisen it is always best to ensure that calves are physically fed colostrum, preferably from a teated bottle. If frozen colostrum is used it can be thawed by surrounding its container with a warm water bath or by thawing at the dethawing setting of the microwave. The latter will reduce immunoglobulin levels more than in a water bath. The use of colostrum substitutes is widely practised, but these are not as satisfactory as the natural product. Colostrum should continue to be fed in small quantities of 1–3 litres daily after gut closure to ensure adequate continued levels of IgA in the intestines. This will help prevent enteric infections. Colostrum can be stored in plastic containers and allowed to sour. It is best to put the colostrum in bins according to how long it has been produced after calving. The soured colostrum retains most of its globulin content and can be heated up in water baths if necessary. Dilution with water may reduce its clotting properties.

Calf pens

Calves need to be managed well and often this is neglected. They require clean dry plentiful bedding, for insulation, and they should not be exposed to draughts or chilling. Only small numbers should be kept in the one air space, preferably a maximum of 30. The house should be cleaned and disinfected after each batch and then left empty for at least 2 weeks. The pens should be dismantled and stored outside after disinfection. The calves should ideally be single penned and all calves, whatever the feeding system used, need to be seen at least twice daily.

There are advantages and disadvantages to single and group penning (Table 1.4). The former is usually associated with bucket feeding whereas the latter normally involves some form of mechanical or group feeding system, which again have their pros and cons (Table 1.5). It is essential that calves are readily identifiable particularly when penned in groups. Records should be kept of date of birth, any illnesses, their treatment and the result, routine procedures undertaken, date of death/weaning and sample or postmortem results. This can assist with future preventative procedures.

Calf feeding

Calf feeding is critical in helping to prevent or control alimentary problems. In almost all instances the degree to which clinical signs of disease occur depends

Table 1.4   Advantages and disadvantages of single and group penning.

Single penning	Group penning
Reduces risk of infectious disease	More likelihood of infection
Allows maximum individual attention	Needs improved stockmanship
Allows early disease identification	Hard to identify early signs of disease
Assists in preventing navel sucking	Allows navel sucking
Removes bullying	Allows bullying
Allows individual recording	Recording is less accurate
Unable to huddle	Able to huddle
Higher critical temperature	Lower critical temperature
Unable to avoid draughts	Can avoid draughts
Calf size not important	Calves must be same size in group
Sometimes unable to groom	Can groom
Routine procedures take less time	More time required to catch calves
Individual identity easy	Must be able to identify calves
More expensive per calf place	Less expensive per calf place
Fewer calves in a given area	More calves in a given area
Labour input greater as necessitates regular inspection	Less labour except in early stages
	Tendency to neglect regular inspection
Higher costs	Lower costs

Table 1.5   Advantages and disadvantages of bucket and machine or group feeding.

Bucket (individual) feeding	Machine (group) feeding
Milk intake restricted	Allows greater milk intake
If bucket, less natural	If teat, more natural feeding
Can affect oesophageal groove reflex	If teats positioned well oesophageal groove reflex works
May need to train to drink from bucket	Need to train to drink from machine
Lower growth rates	Higher growth rates on milk
More dry feed consumption	Less dry feed consumption
Smaller check at weaning	Larger check at weaning
Less affected by power cuts	Mechanical failure can occur
Milk powder mixed by stockman	Milk powder mixed by machine and may clog
Easier to control feed consumption	Difficult to control feed intake

on management and feeding. It is essential that any system used is simple and a suitable regime is adopted for the calf to grow and remain healthy. Usually the quantity fed is determined by the number of feeds per day and the type of feeding system. Any feed supplying more than 1.5–2 litres of milk or milk substitute in a feeding is likely to be greater than the abomasal capacity, so digestive upsets can occur such as bloat or enteritis. The concentration of the milk substitute is normally similar to cows' milk unless once-a-day feeding is practised. Too low or too high a concentrate can interfere with the normal clotting mechanisms and digestion of the milk. Milk substitutes are normally fed warm and, if so, it is critical to maintain a constant temperature at each feed. Cold milk feeding can work, but often consumption is reduced at environmental temperatures under 10°C and it may cease completely below 5°C. It often seems that the best people to feed

Table 1.6 Important points in calf feeding.

Read the instructions about the food and how to prepare it.
The feed must be mixed as directed.
The feed must be fed at the correct temperature.
The calves must be fed in the same order.
Feeding should be at the same times daily, including weekends.
Do not alter the amount fed quickly.
The correct quality should be fed.
If fed by bucket raise these above the floor.
Milk pails and machine teats and tubes must be cleaned out properly at least once a day.
Ideally use one bucket per calf all the time (number buckets).
Ideally keep number of calves per teat on machine low.
Pelleted feeds should be rationed initially to prevent overfeeding.
Coarse feeds can be fed *ad libitum*.
Dusty and mouldy feeds should be avoided.
Stale feeds should be cleaned out at least twice a week.
Water should be available unless milk substitute is fed to appetite when access can be
    less.
Water buckets should be cleaned daily.
Long fibre roughage should be available from the second week.
Ideally calves should be weighed every 2 weeks to monitor progress.

calves are female particularly where it is considered to be the person's major job. Problems often arise where it is undertaken by heavily pressured stockmen with many other responsibilities, e.g. cowmen.

Whatever feeding system is used it should be conducive to good digestion with production of a good abomasal clot, the extrusion of whey and subsequent efficient digestion during the rest of its passage through the gut. The only exception to the need for good abomasal clot formation is in substitutes without casein, i.e. whey-based production. The main rules for feeding are provided in Table 1.6.

Deficiency diseases can occur in calves but are commonly the result of the nutritional inadequacies of the dam. However, predominantly milk feeding without other feeds or adequate supplementation can lead to hypomagnesaemia, zinc, selenium, iron and copper deficiencies, and vitamin A or E deficiency. Problems can develop in individual animals as a result of disease processes or malabsorption syndromes, one of the most common of which is diarrhoea.

Usually as the animal grows it will become more interested in consumption of roughage and dry feeds. This allows the rumen and other parts of the alimentary tract to develop so that the calf can adapt to its subsequent role as a ruminant. Weaning from milk substitute to solid feeds is a critical time as it can result in an animal which is stressed and so less able to counteract infectious agents.

Access to roughage and other solid feeds should occur at least from the first week. Very small quantities should initially be offered to ensure little wastage. If pelleted feed or prills are used and it is not restricted some calves can engorge on them and develop digestive upsets. Many recommend the use of coarse mix. This requires to be eaten more slowly and results in more mastication and induces extra salivation. This ensures the feed is not overeaten and does not have to be restricted.

Weaning

Weaning should be done on a feed intake basis rather than on age, ideally when birth weight is doubled. In the single-penned Holstein/Friesian calf it can be safely undertaken when the calf has consumed at least 0.7 kg daily of concentrate for 3 days. This rises to at least 1 kg daily for the same or a greater period when in groups. If calves are fed by machine it is best to cut off the access for increasing periods starting from about 2 weeks before intended weaning, initially 1 hour twice daily and increasing these periods daily. When doing this there must be access to water and it us useful to have a trough of creep food next to the feeding teat. Thus, the disappointed calf comes away from the teat and can find some comfort from mouthing the creep feed.

Any routine procedures should be undertaken at times that are not going to compromise the health of the animal. Thus, disbudding, feed changes, vaccination, etc., should not take place for about 10–14 days before or after weaning.

After weaning the most common problems which present are respiratory in nature. Much can be done to reduce these by ensuring good management and adequate housing and ventilation. Most of the organisms involved in such cases are normally present in the respiratory tract of calves and only cause disease when the animal is compromised by stress, its environment or climatic changes. The main factors in good housing are included in Tables 1.7, 1.8.

Bovine respiratory disease (see also p. 20)

The term bovine respiratory disease (BRD) was first used in North America to describe a group respiratory disease problem of uncertain aetiology. Currently, the definition is often confined to a condition synonymous with shipping fever. It is used in this review as the respiratory problems in young growing cattle. Most of these conditions can be further subdivided according to the two main management systems involved (Fig. 1.1). The first involves young housed calves reared as dairy replacements. As described, they are usually weaned off their dam at a few days old and then fed milk, or milk substitute, until subsequent weaning onto a solid diet, often between 5 and 8 weeks old. This system predominates in most of the USA, Europe and Britain. Under such conditions the calves can suffer two main problems: a chronic or cuffing pneumonia, or an acute pneumonia also known as calf or enzootic pneumonia which may result from various infectious agents and is often commonly described, sometimes erroneously, as viral pneumonia without any supporting aetiological evidence.

The second form involves weaned suckled heifers usually 6 months to 2 years old and initially reared outside. The problem involves stress and is often precipitated following transport and housing and results in a condition often described as transit or shipping fever or pasteurellosis. This is the predominant problem in North America, but it occurs in Europe to a lesser extent. In Britain the syndrome is seen particularly in Scotland.

Table 1.7   Housing factors for calves.

Ensure as few calves as possible in one air space (30 or less).
Ensure adequate air space (see Table 1.8).
Minimum space per calf 6 m³/calf (212 ft³/calf) in climatic house.
Ventilation ideally natural.
Number of air changes per hour probably about 10 in climatic house.
Minimum ventilation rate 35 m³/hour (0.15 ft³/min/lb BW).
Maximum ventilation rate 105 m³/hour (0.5 ft³/min/lb BW) but can be increased.
Inlets 1 m (3 ft) above calf.
Inlet 1.5–2.5 m (5–8 ft) below outlet.
Inlet 0.045 m²/calf (0.5 ft²/calf).
Outlet 0.04 m²/calf (0.4 ft²/calf).
Usually there is no need for extra heating.
Infrared heaters should be available for sick calves.
Sidewalls need to be insulated.
No need for insulated roof.
Bedding ideally should be straw, dry and deep.
If uninsulated concrete floor, at least 30-cm (1-ft) deep bedding at calf entry.
Floor should have sufficient drainage gradient of 1 in 20 in pens.
Gradient in gulley outside pen 1 in 60.
Ideally feed from outside pen.
Good drainage must be beneath feed points or water troughs.
All walls impervious and capable of easy cleaning.
Central passages at least 1.2 m (4 ft) wide.
Trough frontage in group pen at least 350 mm (1 ft 2 in) per calf.
At frequent intervals (ideally after each calf) clean out, disinfect, dismantle pen and
  leave outside.
Leave building empty as long as possible (at least 2 weeks between batches).
Do not keep older and younger animals in the same air space.
Ensure all changes in feed, management, etc., are introduced slowly.
Routine procedures should not be undertaken at times when other stresses are
  occurring.
Mix calves from single pens to groups by removing pens.

Table 1.8   Adequate space for housed calves.

	Area		Length*		Width*	
	m²	ft²	m	ft	m	ft
Single up to 1 month	1.13	12.5	1.5	5.0	0.75	2.6
Single up to 2 months	1.8	19.5	1.8	6.0	1	3.3
Group up to 2 months	1.5	16.5	3.1	10.2	0.35	1.2
Group up to 3 months	1.7	19.0	4.3	14.1	0.35	1.2

* Legislation now defines width equivalent to height at withers and length from tip of nose to caudal edge of tuber ischii × 1.1.

Cuffing pneumonia

The term cuffing pneumonia reflects the lymphocytic peribronchial cuffing which occurs with this condition. It is considered to be mainly the result of mycoplasmal involvement with infections such as *Mycoplasma dispar* and *Ureaplasma* spp.

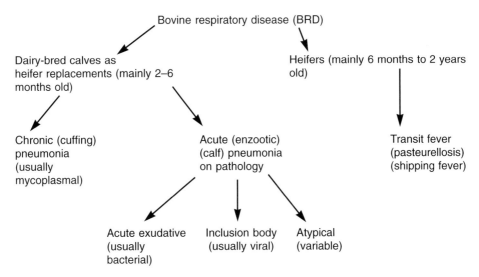

Fig. 1.1 Schematic diagram of the bovine respiratory disease complex.

The problem is often initiated by environmental, management, animal or stress factors. Treatment is not usually undertaken, but, when it is, it involves antimicrobial agents. It is very difficult to determine an incidence of cuffing pneumonia as most calves are not treated and do not die. Residual damage is minimal by the time animals reach maturity. It is probable that the majority of dairy calves initially reared indoors are affected.

Enzootic pneumonia (see also pp. 21–3)

The aetiology of enzootic pneumonia, an acute condition, is very complex and as such it is best described as multifactorial. A large number of different agents are involved (Fig. 1.2), many of which inhabit the respiratory tract of healthy animals, and disease is precipitated by management, environmental or stress factors.

    The purchase or rearing of a large number of calves for dairy production and then keeping them in the same housing allows the easy spread of potential respiratory pathogens between animals often stressed and in close contact. The most common viruses causing enzootic pneumonia are bovine respiratory syncytial virus (BRSV), parainfluenza III (PI3), infectious bovine rhinotracheitis (IBR) and, to a lesser extent, bovine viral diarrhoea (BVD) virus. Obviously these are unaffected by antibacterial agents. BRSV is now a prominent pathogen in Britain. The main mycoplasma involved are particularly *M. bovis, M. dispar* and *Ureaplasma* spp. *Pasteurella haemolytica, P. multocida* and *Haemophilus somnus* are the main bacterial causes of infection together with *Actinomyces pyogenes* and *Fusobacterium necrophorum*. Antibiotic activity against both mycoplasma and bacteria is possible.

    There is limited information about the incidence of the disease in dairy calves. However, Thomas (1978) obtained health records from 12 beef units in 11 British

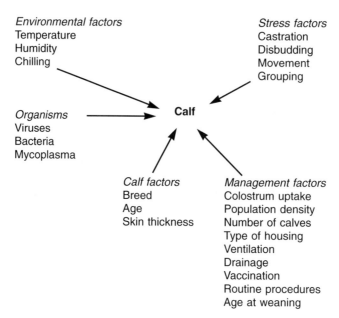

Fig. 1.2 Infectious agents and other factors involved in enzootic pneumonia.

counties involving 10 955 animals between 1970 and 1977 and found the overall proportion treated was 32.6% and ranged from 3.1 to 52%. Morbidity is variable according to the rearing system, but the average mortality in bought-in beef animals is about 5.5% of which about half the deaths are due to enzootic pneumonia. The percentage of animals requiring a repeat treatment is not known but thought to be about 10%, with a level of 8.9% present in a study involving 2040 animals over 5 years in which 22% had initially been ill and 3.6% were culled following treatment and before ready for slaughter. Weight gain after respiratory disease was reduced by 2.6% on one farm from 1970 to 1972. In Ireland it has been suggested that there is an increasing incidence of respiratory disease and it is estimated to cost millions of pounds annually.

Pasteurellosis

The aetiology of pasteurellosis is still open to some disagreement. It is usually considered to be a stress- or management-induced problem in which infectious agents then participate. In severe respiratory disease the cause of the outbreak may not be conclusively determined. The most common organism isolated is *Pasteurella haemolytica* and has given rise to the name pasteurellosis. However, some consider the problem to be primarily viral, mainly due to PI3 or IBR infection, followed by secondary bacterial invasion. *Pasteurella haemolytica* biotype A1 is considered to be the most common isolate and produces a heat labile cytotoxin that is ruminant specific, destroying leukocytes. *P. multicida* is occasionally isolated. Experimentally most infection has been initiated by

PI3 aerosol infection followed by *P. haemolytica.* However, recently *P. haemolytica* biotype A1 has been shown to produce disease as a primary agent in non-immune calves, but this depends on administering the bacteria intratracheally or intrathoracically.

Small numbers of *P. haemolytica* can be isolated from the nasal passages of healthy unstressed calves, and can be found in the trachea although they are not considered to be normal lung inhabitants. Usually the problem is considered to be stress induced and occurs within 1 month of moving and most cases are seen about 10 days after housing. Outbreaks can occur outdoors. The number of *P. haemolytica* biotype A1 tends to increase in the nasal tract, tracheal air and lungs following transport, or move to market or the entry to housing. A sudden change of diet to one containing largish amounts of cereals may make the cattle more prone to respiratory disease depending on the season of the year. Fluctuations in daily ambient temperature and relative humidity influence the problem. Spread of infection from individual cases can occur and is optimised by crowded conditions, probably resulting in increased organism virulence through passage. Generally, the stress of movement plus mixing with other calves (or bought in), the introduction to housing and a new diet are sufficient to initiate disease. As the problem is usually primarily bacterial, early antibacterial therapy is usually successful.

Transit fever

Transit fever is the most important respiratory problem in older calves following stress such as housing or transport (Fig. 1.3). The condition is common in North America, Europe and Scotland. Mortality and morbidity rates vary considerably and are based on beef animals, but after travelling levels of up to 35% morbidity and 5–10% mortality of those affected or 0.75–1% of the susceptible population are often quoted.

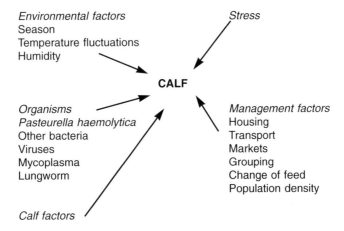

Fig. 1.3 Infectious agents and other factors involved in transit fever.

Other post-weaning problems

Most other post-weaning problems are dietary in nature and can follow sudden changes in feed, resulting in digestive upset or acidosis. Most problems are prevented by ensuring that adequate good quality feed is available and any changes are made gradually. Feed should be provided in receptacles that help avoids faecal contamination as this will assist in preventing coccidiosis, salmonellosis and other infectious causes. (See also Chapter 2.)

Vaccination

In most instances good management will prevent the need for vaccination against disease, particularly as most herds rear their replacements rather than buying in calves and the ensuing problems which can occur from mixing animals from different sources are thus avoided.

Enteric disease

Vaccination against any enteric problem, to be successful, requires confirmation of its presence in the herd and that it is the cause of the problem. In most instances local immunity is more important than systemic and, as these infections are often encountered early in life, the only effective method of control is to vaccinate the dam and thereby supply passive protection to the calf. One successful vaccine making use of these principles has been that for protection of calves against rotavirus and *E. coli* K99 antigen. Following vaccination before calving, the dam's colostrum needs to be fed to the calf for at least 2 weeks. Coronavirus vaccination is possible in some countries, including Britain.

Vaccination of the dam can also be used to provide protection for the calf against *Salmonella dublin*, *S. typhimurium* and some serotypes of *E. coli* using killed adjuvenated vaccines. The same products can be used for calves, but active immunisation involves the use of the vaccine at an interval of 14–21 days. This will not be satisfactory if disease occurs at a younger age. In some countries and in the past in Britain, live salmonella vaccines have been used which will allow more rapid development of immunity. Hyperimmunised serum, usually derived from horses, can also overcome the problems of protecting calves not receiving sufficient passive immunity from their dam. Successful vaccination against *E. coli* often depends on the specific serotypes present on the farm being in the vaccine. While there is some crossover in protection between various salmonella species following vaccination it is far from complete. Clostridial vaccines are available for those few farms that have problems with tetanus, blackleg and *Cl. perfringens* infections. If problems occur in the young calf, passive protection can be gained by injecting the dams, otherwise the calf can be vaccinated.

Vaccination of cattle against BVD has been undertaken with a dead vaccine in Britain and should provide the calf with immunity. At present it is not marketed for calves. In other countries live and dead vaccines are used for both dams and calves with varying degrees of success. Live vaccines can provide good anti-genicity, but some have produced systemic reactions in those vaccinated and, on occasions, disease. Some of the modified live virus vaccines have been fetopath-ogenic and should not be used in pregnant cows. At present there are no vac-cines commercially available for other viruses that can cause calf diarrhoea, coccidiosis and cryptosporidiosis.

Respiratory problems

The other main group of vaccines available for calves help protect against some of the various pathogens that are involved in calf pneumonia (see also p. 23). Several of the most effective vaccines are live, including ones for IBR, PI3 and RSV, and some of these are given intranasally to allow the production of high levels of IgA locally in the respiratory tract. One vaccine for use in IBR and another for PI3 are temperature-sensitive variants which will only multiply in the upper parts of the respiratory tract which have a lower temperature than distally. These vaccines can provide protection when maternal antibody is present. Where immunity is required in calves with uncertain levels of maternal-acquired anti-body, dead vaccines can also be used. Vaccination with live vaccine intranasally has produced effective control of calf pneumonia when used in unaffected calves at the start of a disease outbreak. In recent years a live IBR depleted vaccine has been used; this is a so-called marker vaccine in that antibodies generated can be distinguished from those produced by the field infection. This can enable the eradication of IBR from a herd while still allowing the animals protection against disease.

Dead vaccines are available for immunisation against *P. haemolytica* and *P. multocida* and can at times be useful. Some also target leukotoxins. Hyperim-mune serum is also marketed. In other countries, such as the USA, a killed bac-terin of *Haemophilus somnus* in aluminium hydroxide has produced good results experimentally and in field trials when given as two doses 2–3 weeks apart. Exper-imentally, mycoplasmal vaccines have been used with some success but are not available commercially. In North America a formalised *Moraxella bovis* vaccine gives good protection against experimental infection. An irradicated third-stage larval vaccine of *Dictyocaulus viviparus* has been available for over 30 years and when given as two doses before turnout can help to control parasitic bronchitis once calves are at pasture.

Other vaccines

A live attenuated *Trichophyton verrucosum* vaccine initially developed in Russia has been very successful in controlling ringworm in calves in many countries and is available in Britain. This vaccine has assisted in eradication of the disease in some countries. A vaccine made from the sonicated pili of *Moraxella bovis* may induce passive protection against some cases of New Forest eye but is not used in Britain.

Prophylactic antibiotics

In some herds with severe calf scour, problems are sometimes treated by the use of prophylactic antibiotics, usually administered orally. This should only be used as a last resort and is not a substitute for good husbandry. When the conditions are right, the affected housing should be thoroughly cleaned, disinfected and rested. Continued use of antibiotics is likely to lead to the emergence of antibiotic-resistant strains. When an outbreak of virulent *E. coli* or *Salmonella* spp. occurs it can be of use to undertake antibiotic treatment of the in-contact animals as this may help prevent the establishment of the infection.

The same reservations hold for antibiotic preventive use in calves for respiratory disease such as for enteritis. However, prophylactic antibiotics can be considered useful in cases where there is an established infection within the calf group and where about 30% of the calves are ill at time of first antibiotic treatment. Injection of in-contacts at this time can be beneficial in reducing the likelihood of further cases occurring. This is often termed metaphylaxis. It is based on the principle that the infection is rapidly spreading and the in-contact animals are probably infected but not at present showing signs. If the problem is only slowly spreading, the metaphylaxis is not worth undertaking. It also does not always work when used under the correct criteria.

References

Bakheit, H. A. & Greene, H. J. (1981) Control of bovine neonatal diarrhoea by management techniques. *Veterinary Record* **108**, 455–8.

Leech, F. B., Macrae, W. D. & Menzies, D. W. (1968) *Calf Wastage and Husbandry in Britain 1962–63*. Animal Disease Surveys. Report No. 5. Ministry of Agriculture, Fisheries and Food, London, pp. 1–59.

Thomas, L. H. (1978) Disease incidence and epidemiology – the situation in the UK. In: *Respiratory Diseases in Cattle* (ed. W. B. Martin). A seminar in the EEC Programme of Coordination of Research on Beef Production, Edinburgh, 8–10 November 1997, pp. 57–65. Martinus Nijhoff, The Hague.

Chapter 2
Rearing the Dairy Heifer

Roger W. Blowey

Introduction

This chapter follows the calf at weaning through its development to a down-calving heifer. Its intended emphasis is on the promotion of positive health, but, in so doing, it is often necessary to describe disease syndromes in some detail. Only when the cause of a problem is understood can its prevention and control measures be fully appreciated.

The chapter is divided into four sections: the post-weaned calf and the early housing period; preparation for turnout and first season at grass; second winter housing; and, finally, second summer at grass and the precalving period. Therefore, the emphasis is on autumn-born calves leading to calving at approximately 2 years old. There are, of course, many other systems, for example spring-born calves rearing to calve at 2.5–3 years old. It would be tedious for the reader to have each system described in detail, since there are many similarities in aspects of disease and management which would lead to endless repetition. The autumn-born calf, reared for a 2-year-old calving, is therefore taken as the 'typical case' and only where important differences exist in relation to promoting health will the other systems be discussed.

Targets for growth

Rearing dairy heifers is generally considered to be a low profitability exercise, resulting in a high cost at first calving. Even so, it has been estimated that almost 40% of all heifer calves born alive fail to calve for a second time. The wastage of an already expensive product – and yet one with an enormous potential – is therefore considerable. Much of this could be avoided by more detailed attention to feeding, management and disease control. Regular weighing of heifers is essential if growth targets are to be maintained and errors corrected. Table 2.1 indicates approximate weights according to age and expected growth rates for Friesian-Holstein heifers calving at 2 years old. Clearly, Jersey or Guernsey replacements or animals fed to calve at 2.5–3 years old would have lower growth rates.

Table 2.1 Target weights and daily liveweight gains for heifers calving at 2 years old. (Adapted from Blowey, 1988.)

	Target weight (kg)	Liveweight gain (kg)
Birthweight	40	
5 weeks	55	0.5
12 weeks	85	0.55
6 months	150	0.7
12 months	270	0.67
Service	330	0.7
18 months	375	0.7
Immediately precalving	510	0.5
Immediately post-calving	455	

An alternative guide is that for 2-year calving only the daily weight gain in grams per day should be numerically equal to the mature body weight in kilograms (see Fig. 2.1). For example, Holstein cows with a mature body weight of 700 kg should grow at 700 g per day during their rearing period. The achievement of this depends on adequate nutrition, good management and the avoidance of disease.

Excessive growth rates in the early rearing period, particularly prior to puberty, can be detrimental. In the normal animal, just prior to puberty, the parenchymal (secretory) portion of the mammary gland begins to grow at a rate considerably faster than the rest of the body (Tucker, 1987). This is maintained for the first few oestrous cycles after puberty, but then returns to a normal rate of body growth. There is then a second phase of rapid udder tissue development after conception, this time maintained until parturition and beyond. Overfeeding of heifers during the prepubertal growth period leads to the earlier onset of puberty, but also to depressed milk production due to excessive deposition of fat in the mammary gland. This lowering of milk production is associated with change in udder development and not simply serving and calving at an earlier age (Little & Kay, 1979).

These findings were emphasised by Harrison and others (1983), who reared heifers at high (1.1 kg liveweight gain per day) and conventional (0.74 kg liveweight gain per day) rates of gain until 11 months old and then further subdivided the groups into low, medium and high planes of nutrition. The mammary glands of conventionally reared heifers weighed 39% more and contained 68% more secretory tissue than those grown rapidly during the prepubertal period. However, there was no impairment of mammary development in heifers with higher growth rates during later pregnancy. Problems occur only with excess feeding around puberty. The deposition of excess mammary fat is probably associated with changes in growth hormone secretion in response to a high energy diet. However, inadequate feeding during pregnancy, leading to low weights at calving, will depress yields. In a survey of Friesian-Holstein heifers calving at 2 years old, Drew (1988) showed that heavier heifers at calving gave significantly higher yields (Table 2.2). This relationship persisted in both high and low pro-

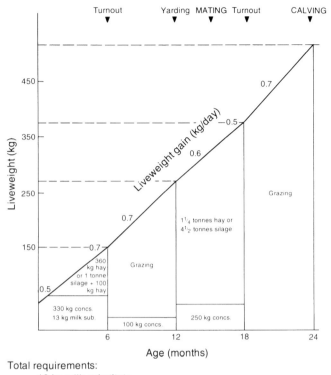

Total requirements:
    13 kg milk substitute
    680 kg concentrations
    5.5 tonnes silage + 100 kg hay, or 1.9 tonnes hay
Note: Feed quantities are approximate.

Fig. 2.1 Growth patterns for autumn-born heifers due to calve at 2 years old (Stansfield, 1983; data from MMB/MLC).

Table 2.2 Effect of weight at calving on subsequent yield for heifers calving at 2 years old. (From Drew, 1988.)

Weight of heifer at calving (kg)	First lactation 305-day milk yield (l)
<480	4278
480–520	4578
>520	4770

duction herds, and was not influenced by management (viz. it was not that those farms which were poor at rearing heifers were also poor at feeding cows). Heifers that are served at an early age and therefore well below target weight will of course calve lighter and hence yield less. However, this is no reason for delaying calving to 2.5–3 years. Numerous trials have shown that, although the 3-year calver produces more milk in her lactation, her total lifetime production, fertility and longevity are all reduced. Table 2.3 shows that milk production per day

Table 2.3   Effect of age at first calving on lifetime performance. (From MMB data.)

	Age of heifer at first calving (months)				
	23–25	26–28	29–31	32–34	35–37
Herd life (lactations)	4.0	4.0	3.8	3.8	3.8
Lifetime yield (kg)	18747	18730	17964	17991	17657
Yield per day in herd once lactating (kg)	13.1	13.2	13.1	13.1	13.1
Yield per day of life (kg)	8.8	8.4	7.9	7.5	7.3

of life is 20% higher in the 2-year calver compared with her counterpart at 3 years old. Older heifers, particularly 3 years plus, also tend to become overfat before calving.

Weaning and the post-weaning housing period

Feeding

Although traditionally weaned at 8–10 weeks old, with the advent of improved diets calves are now often weaned at 5–6 weeks, or when they are eating sufficient quantities (1.5–2 kg/day) of concentrate. Some calves are abruptly weaned, but it is more common to change from twice to once daily milk feeding, probably gradually reducing the amounts fed, before total withdrawal. This helps the rumen to adapt to its changing function, rather than expecting it to cope with a sudden increase in concentrate intake. Inadequate rumen development and especially oesophageal groove closure problems leading to milk spillage into the rumen can lead to many post-weaning digestive problems, with bloat and post-weaning scour being the most common.

At weaning, the rumen is not fully mature, being more acid (i.e. lower pH) than in the adult and unable to synthesise sufficient microbial protein, relative to energy, to meet the calf's high requirements for growth. Preweaning, milk passed directly into the abomasum and this source of undegradable protein must be replaced by high quality undegradable rations containing foods such as fish meal or linseed, to give an overall diet of 17–18% CP and 12.5–13.0 MJ ME. The higher the growth rate required, the higher will be the requirement for additional undegradable protein. As feed conversion is much more efficient at a younger age and therefore lighter weight (see Table 2.4) it is still cost-effective to feed expensive nutritious diets to freshly weaned calves.

Digestive disorders

Post-weaning bloat

Rumen development consists of the expansion of rumen *size*, reaching a maximum of 80% of the total volume of the four stomachs by 12 weeks old, and

Table 2.4 Variation in feed conversion ratio (FCR) according to body weight. (Adapted from Blowey, 1988.)

Bodyweight (kg)	FCR
50	2:1
100	3:1
300	5.5:1
500	8.5:1

the development of rumen *papillae*. These small finger-like projections from the rumen wall increase the absorptive surface area and therefore improve function. Diets with inadequate long fibre or a high starch content can lead to poor rumen development. The young calf is particularly susceptible to acidosis and, if fed excessive amounts of highly fermentable concentrate, ruminal acidosis develops. This in turn leads to ruminal atony (i.e. the rumen stops contracting and the calf is no longer seen to be cudding), depressed food intake, poor development of ruminal papillae and, in severe cases, bloat. Often the addition of 10–15% chopped straw to high starch concentrates will improve rumen function, thereby increasing overall digestibility of the ration, at the same time as improving feed intake. Any type of long fibre may be used, viz. hay, straw or silage, but straw alone is becoming increasingly popular. It is probably best not to offer silage to young calves until they are 8 weeks old and, even initially, only up to 50% of their forage ration.

It has been suggested that concentrate intake in heifer calves being reared for dairy replacements should be restricted, as this will encourage greater consumption of forage and the development of a larger rumen, capable of sustaining greater intakes later in life. There is evidence that bouts of acidosis at weaning can leave the rumen wall permanently scarred, thus reducing its absorptive capacity. Ruminal bloat in the post-weaned calf is therefore a 'gassy' bloat (not 'frothy') and is associated with failure of rumen contractions resulting from poor rumen development. Affected calves may develop a pasty scour. They have poor appetites and often remain severely stunted, with little hope of reaching the 2-year-old calving target.

Pot-bellied calves

It has been stated already that the calf requires a highly nutritious post-weaning diet to cope with the loss of milk nutrients. If concentrate intake is restricted to significantly less than 1.0 kg per day and the calf is allowed access to a palatable but poorly digestible forage (typically hay), then it will eat the hay because it is hungry. However, because its underdeveloped rumen cannot digest it properly, the hay accumulates and a pot-bellied appearance (i.e. bilateral ventral abdominal enlargement and poor ruminal contractions) develops. Inadequate access to a good supply of fresh clean water will also depress intakes and can exacerbate the problem.

Post-weaning scour

Post-weaning scour is a less well-defined syndrome, but is considered to be of dietary origin. Calves 2–6 weeks after weaning may develop a pasty yellow–brown or grey scour. Some are not affected, while others become severely stunted and, in neglected cases, may even die. The aetiology is unknown and it is probable that no one single factor is involved. Suggested causes include poor ruminal development preweaning and the use of inappropriate concentrates post-weaning. Examples of the latter include adult dairy rations containing high levels of allergenic vegetable protein and/or inadequate undegradable protein, feeding finely ground high starch cereals leading to acidosis and chronic rumenitis, or sudden feed changes. Maize gluten is quite acidic and is best not fed in large quantities to a freshly weaned calf which has an immature and already acid rumen. This author has seen outbreaks of post-weaning scour associated with the withdrawal of sugarbeet from a 1:1 sugarbeet: maize gluten mix fed to weaned calves at 2.5 kg per day. Replacing the sugarbeet resolved the condition in all but the worst affected calves. These needed to be returned to milk feeding for 2–3 weeks and then weaned again.

In some cases dietary management can prevent the problem by ensuring adequate dry matter intake before weaning, continuing milk substitute longer than usual if the other feed intake is insufficient.

Coccidiosis

Although not a digestive disorder, coccidiosis has been included in this section because in the chronic form it can resemble post-weaning scour. Coccidiosis is also common in preweaned calves. The cause, a protozoan parasite, particularly the species *Eimeria zurnii* and *E. bovis*, originates from the dam and may be carried in otherwise healthy calves without producing any adverse effects. Disease (scouring, straining and, classically, the presence of high blood in the faeces) occurs typically where hygiene is poor and there is thus a greater risk of faecal–oral contamination. Overstocking, humid buildings, inadequate bedding and fouling of feed and/or water troughs are all potentiating factors. The oocyst stage of the protozoan is extremely resistant to environmental and standard disinfectants. Infected pens should therefore be thoroughly cleaned of all faecal material, washed and then soaked with an ammonia-based or other proprietary anticoccidial disinfectant, before a new batch of calves is introduced.

Housing and pneumonia (see also p. 7)

If reared in individual pens, calves should be left in situ until 2–3 weeks after weaning. Moving into loose housing immediately after weaning is a stress factor at a time when the calf's defences are already compromised by a reduction in its nutritional status. In addition, withdrawal of milk encourages calves to suck one another, a risk that is much less when they are eating well 2–3 weeks after weaning. It has also been suggested that cross-sucking as calves can lead to similar problems in lactating cows later in life.

Environment is of paramount importance during the post-weaning period in the prevention of calf pneumonia. Loose housing is almost universal and should consist of a light airy shed with generous stocking density in terms of both floor area and volume of building. For calves 6–12 weeks old suggested figures (Blowey, 1988) are:

1.5–2.0 m² of floor area;
8.0–9.0 m³ of air space.

In a calf house that provides only 2.4 m³ of air space, pneumonia is almost a certainty. Even though the importance of adequate ventilation is well accepted, it is surprising how many farmers feel the need to 'keep calves warm', by housing them in small enclosed buildings. Provided that the animal has a dry bed (and this is vital) and can lie somewhere within the shed away from draughts, then temperature is not important for the weaned calf. (A draught is defined as a wind speed just detectable on the face = approximately 0.2 m/s.) Yards with an inside, lean-to bedded area and at least part of the feeding area outside are ideal, for example a round feeder standing on a concrete pad. Provided with this facility, it is surprising how many calves prefer to lie outside on bare concrete, even on a frosty day. Only when it is wet and cold will all calves go inside.

To understand the importance of environment and pneumonia, it is necessary to review its causes, the defence mechanisms of the young calf and the factors likely to overcome those defences.

Causes of pneumonia

Calf pneumonia is a syndrome of multiple aetiology, that is, it is caused by one or more of a whole range of organisms, including bacteria, viruses, mycoplasmas and fungi, plus poor environmental management. Some of the more important organisms are listed in Table 2.5. All calves on every farm will be carrying some of these infectious agents, but disease only occurs when their natural defences are low, or when there is an excessively high load of infection in the environment. The latter is known as the *atmospheric load*. (See also pp. 8–11.)

Table 2.5 Important infectious causes of calf pneumonia.

Viruses	Bacteria	Others
Respiratory syncytial virus (RSV)	*Pasteurella multocida*	Moulds
Parainfluenza type 3 (PI3)	*Pasteurella haemolytica*	*Mycoplasma*
Bovine viral diarrhoea (BVD)	*Haemophilus somnus*	*Acholeplasma*
Infectious bovine rhinotracheitis (IBR)	*Actinomyces pyogenes*	*Ureaplasma*
Coronaviruses		

Natural defence mechanisms

Preformed antibodies to pneumonia organisms are received via the colostrum (i.e. passive immunity) and calves receiving inadequate colostrum are therefore more susceptible to disease. In early life, as the passive immunity wanes, the calf should remain unaffected, as it produces its own antibodies (i.e. active immunity) in response to exposure to a low dose of infection. This is the ideal situation. Thus the calf becomes *infected* by the organism and produces protective antibodies against further attacks, but because it is able to withstand the challenge it is not *affected* by disease.

In addition to antibody defences, the calf has a number of physical barriers against infection: (1) in the nasal cavities, a mesh of hairs and a layer of mucus lining the turbinate bones trap the large- and medium-sized particles in the incoming air; (2) in the trachea and bronchi, glands within the walls produce a layer of sticky mucus which lines the air passages, thus trapping further particles. Contaminated mucus is propelled up towards the mouth (and either swallowed or voided) by the action of *cilia*, small hair-like projections which move in a wave motion. Bronchioles and trachea macrophages and other white blood cells engulf any small particles that may have escaped the earlier defences. The particles are either destroyed by the cell or carried to a lymph node where they are simply 'dumped'. (These are the points where accumulations of 'soot' can be seen in smokers!).

Atmospheric load

Atmospheric load is a general term describing the amount of particulate matter carried in the air. Probably 99% of the different bacteria, moulds, viruses and dust could not cause disease on their own. However, if present at a sufficiently high dose they may overload and thus compromise the calf's defences, thereby allowing pneumonia-causing infections to become established in sufficient quantity to cause disease. A good example of this is respiratory syncytial virus (RSV). It is difficult to produce pneumonia experimentally with RSV alone, even with quite high doses, but if calves are first exposed to a high level of dust, then pneumonia develops. Typically, 'fresh air' outdoors contains 150–200 particles per m^3 of air, whereas in a enclosed calf house this may rise to 4000000 per m^3. Where does all this material come from? There are several sources:

- Bedding, especially if the straw is mouldy due to poor harvesting or storage. Sometimes excessively dry straw disintegrates to produce dust.
- The calf's skin.
- Exhaled air. The mucus and ciliary mechanisms are a very efficient filtering system, however, and probably 95% of all inhaled particles are removed.

Surprisingly, the disease-causing organisms which the calf breathes out do not live for very long. For example, RSV survives for only 40–60 s. This short survival time has two important consequences:

(1) Calves have to be in very close contact to pass infection from one to another. (Licking is thought to be an important means of transfer.)
(2) Once a building has been depopulated, all RSV infection has gone and it can be restocked almost immediately. (However, other pneumonia agents, e.g. *Pasteurella*, can survive for longer.)

Control measures

Many of the control measures for pneumonia are features affecting the calf's defences and the atmospheric load. For example:

- Provide a warm, dry bed. Chilling is a stress factor which reduces cilial activity and the efficiency of the calf's immune system generally.
- Provide adequate drainage and reduce humidity levels in the house. Humidity is a very important factor, in that if humidity levels rise:
  - more infection is given off by the bedding;
  - the survival rate of organisms in the atmospheric load increases;
  - high ammonia, often associated with humidity, reduces the activity of cilia.

Increasing humidity from 60 to 90% is said to lead to a ten-fold increase in the atmospheric load. This is why more pneumonia is seen in damp, foggy weather.

- Keep stocking density within acceptable limits. Because the calves themselves, their bedding and faeces are a source of atmospheric load, it is possible to reach a situation in a heavily stocked calf house where no amount of ventilation can reduce the atmospheric load. Conversely, halving the stocking density is equivalent to increasing ventilation rate by twenty times!
- Avoid mixing calves of different age-groups and especially from different sources, as they are likely to have a different immune status and be carrying different organisms. A common fault is that the calf yard shares the same area (air-space) as the collecting or dispersal yards for the dairy herd. This means that twice each day the calves are subjected to a very high stocking density and therefore a heavy atmospheric load.
- Vaccination. Good, effective vaccines are now available against the major viral causes of calf pneumonia, namely RSV, IBR and PI3. Vaccines are available in Europe for *Pasteurella* infections. IBR and PI3 vaccines are temperature-attenuated, that is they will only grow at the lower temperature of the calf's nose. They are administered as an intranasal spray, whereas RSV and *Pasteurella* vaccines are given by injection. The major problem with vaccination is the timing of administration. If live vaccine is given too early, colostral antibodies interface with vaccine 'take' and poor immunity results. If given too late, colostral antibodies may have totally waned, leaving a susceptible calf which has already developed pneumonia before the vaccine has been administered. The manufacturer's instructions should be carefully consulted therefore before usage. (See p. 13.)

Other common diseases of housed calves

It is not the intention of this text to give a full catalogue of all the possible disease states that can occur in cattle, but rather to describe those that are primarily affected by management, housing and nutrition. Into this category must come skin diseases such as lice, mange and ringworm; and deficiency diseases such as rickets, cerebrocortical necrosis (CCN) and white muscle disease (vitamin E/selenium deficiency).

Skin diseases

Lice, mange and ringworm are most commonly seen in heavily stocked, poorly ventilated housing systems, where the level of nutrition and overall performance are often less than optimal. Conversely, calves that are affected by lice, mange and ringworm will suffer depressed liveweight gains and performance, all of which will detract from the target of a 2-year calving heifer.

Lice: there are two separate types of louse – the sucking louse (*Haematopinus eurysternus*, *Linognathus vituli*) and the biting louse (*Bovicola bovis*). Both live on the surface of the skin and can just be seen with the naked eye. They are dark grey/brown in colour and approximately the size of a flattened pin-head. Eggs are seen as small white dots, glued to the lower hair shafts. Clinical signs include biting, rubbing and scratching and, in advanced cases, quite severe anaemia. The shoulders, neck and back are the worst affected areas and often the coat over the neck is arranged in vertical lines, due to rubbing. Areas of hair loss over the shoulders may occur from biting.

Lice are so common in calves in winter housing that routine preventive treatment is a sensible precaution, for example, in January and February for September-/October-born calves. Traditional louse powder (0.6–1.0% gamma benzene hexachloride) is no longer available, having been replaced by various pyrethroid and organophosphorus pour-on preparations (now being phased out). These may be combined warble (use at half strength for lice) or fly repellent preparations and have the advantage of being absorbed through the skin, to pass to all parts of the body. Ivermectin and other avermectins and bambermycin compounds can also be used by subcutaneous injection and some by pour-on. The new endectoparasiticides and the pour-on warble preparations have the advantage of persisting for 2–3 weeks and are therefore able to kill lice hatching from eggs (incubation takes 2 weeks). A second dose of warble dressing should be given 2 weeks after the first for most organophosphorus preparations. (See also p. 40.)

Mange: mange can occur in calves, young stock and adult cattle. It is caused by a small family of mites which also produce canker in dogs, scabies in man and scab in sheep. However, mites from cattle are host-specific and not transmissible to other species, nor vice versa. Whereas lice live on the surface of the skin, mange mites burrow into the epidermis, producing thick, white, crusty scabs and causing intense irritation. Chorioptic mange typically occurs at the base of the tail and is seen as thick, white, crusty scabs, sometimes with a moist exudate. Sarcoptic mange is seen in both adults and calves and can affect the whole body. Psoroptic mange primarily affects the perineal region, extending from the anus, down the hind legs to the udder or scrotum.

Organophosphorus pour-on preparations (e.g. warble dressing) are very effective, but a second treatment needs to be given 2–3 weeks after the first, to kill mites recently emerged from their eggs. Avermectin and bambermycin injections have sufficient persistency for only a single treatment to be necessary. (See also page 40.)

Ringworm: this fungal infection of the skin and hair shaft is caused by *Trichophyton verrucosum*, although occasionally other species of ringworm (e.g. *Microsporum* spp.) may be involved. Affected hairs become very brittle, breaking off at the surface of the skin, to leave the typical circular bald patches which expand from the periphery. The head and neck are most commonly affected, probably because these are the areas most likely to be in contact with adjacent cattle and other infected objects. Lesions are not very irritant, but affected calves often rub themselves on posts and food troughs, thereby spreading infection. The spores of ringworm are very resistant and may persist for up to 4 years if they are in a dry place, e.g. a crevice in the wall. Cresosote, 4% sodium carbonate and flame guns are traditionally used to eliminate infection from a building, but even these are not 100% successful. Many farms seem to have affected calves for 3–4 years, then the problem largely disappears (presumably because the progeny of infected calves have some immunity), only to reappear as an outbreak a few years later. There are two main types of treatment. Griseofulvin is a fungistatic antibiotic which, when given orally, is incorporated into the growing hair and prevents any further fungal growth. The ringworm is then destroyed by the calf's own defence mechanisms. Natamycin is a topical preparation, administered as a spray. Troughs and fittings can also be treated. Whichever treatment is used, it is best to administer it to the whole group, rather than only the affected calves.

As the incubation period is 3 weeks or more, if only clinically affected animals are treated, there are likely to be further calves in the group which are acting as a reservoir to reinfect those currently recovering. Vaccination has been found to provide good protection.

Deficiency diseases

A wide range of deficiency diseases are possible in weaned calves, for example cobalt deficiency causing pine, copper deficiency producing lameness, poor growth and loss of coat colour, and many others. This section deals only with the more commonly occurring conditions.

White muscle disease or vitamin E/selenium deficiency: although they are two totally unrelated substances chemically, vitamin E and selenium act on similar metabolic mechanisms within the animal, namely in the removal of peroxides

Table 2.6   Dietary sources of vitamin E.

Good	Average	Poor
Grass and dried grass	Cereal grains	Poor hay
Grass silage	Maize silage	Straw
Kale	Good hay	Root crops
	Brewer's grains	

Total dietary selenium requirement = 0.1 ppm in dry matter.

formed during the oxidisation of fat to produce energy. Calves deficient in vitamin E and selenium may therefore have an excess of peroxides in their muscles. This leads to muscle damage, calcification and subsequent necrosis, seen on gross post-mortem as large white areas in the muscles. By no means are all muscles affected and often a thorough search has to be made to find lesions in the heart, diaphragm or skeletal muscles. Some soils, and hence the forage crops grown on them, are inherently low in selenium and this can be an exacerbating factor. Vitamin E levels in feed are related to the type of plant, its stage of growth and method of conservation (see Table 2.6). For example, hay badly weathered during drying will be low in vitamin E.

Typically, disease is seen in late winter or following turnout. Affected calves will either be stiff (skeletal muscle degeneration), breathing with difficulty (diaphragm and chest muscles) or simply found dead (heart muscle failure). Calves turned out to spring grazing experience two additional stress factors which can precipitate the onset of clinical disease. Sudden exercise can precipitate muscle degeneration and the relatively high level of polyunsaturated fatty acids (PUFAs) in spring grazing considerably increases the vitamin E requirement in a calf whose vitamin E status is already marginal. Sometimes disease is seen in housed animals that are fed unusually high levels of PUFAs in their concentrate. Treatment of affected calves and prevention of further cases depend solely on provision of the deficient vitamin E and/or selenium. This can be given by injection, oral dosing, e.g. using intrareticular 'bullets', or supplementation of feed or drinking water with selenium or vitamin E. However, white muscle disease induced by high dietary PUFAs can only be corrected by vitamin E supplementation. (See also pp. 64, 101.)

Rickets: this condition is rare in cattle; calcium accounts for one third of the total composition of teeth and bones and in fact 99% of all the calcium in the body is found in the animal's skeleton. If young growing calves are affected by a combined calcium and vitamin D deficiency, then clinical signs of stunting, poor growth, lameness, stiffness, abnormal bending and swelling of the legs and other clinical signs of rickets may be seen. This can occur in the winter, with calves that are on diets of poor quality hay and unmineralised barley and is exacerbated if they are totally housed in dimly lit buildings, because ultraviolet light from the sun is required to synthesise vitamin D in the skin. Treatment is by improving both diet and housing and providing oral and parenteral supplementation with calcium and vitamin D. (See also pp. 65, 197.)

Cerebrocortical necrosis (CCN): the name simply means degeneration of the grey matter of the brain. It is not a true dietary deficiency disease, but rather an induced deficiency caused by proliferation of thiaminase-producing bacteria such as *Bacillus thiaminolyticus* and *Clostridium sporogenes*. Disease is most commonly seen in calves between 3 and 9 months old, in calves on high concentrate: low fibre diets, and may be precipitated by an outbreak of scouring or some other digestive upset.

Clinically, affected calves are blind and wander around the pen with their heads held high and noses forward. Advanced cases become recumbent and eventually die, following fits of extensor spasm. Provided it is administered early, treatment with large doses of intravenous thiamine is surprisingly effective, even in severely affected calves. Further cases can be prevented by altering the ration (e.g. reducing starch, increasing digestible fibre or adding 1.5–2% sodium bicarbonate to concentrate), or by supplementing the diet with an external source of thiamine, e.g. brewer's yeast. (See also p. 65.)

Preparation for turnout and first season at grass

Nutrient requirements and vaccinations

Preparation for turnout must start at the end of February and certainly by early March. Oral lungworm vaccine should be ordered and administered, two doses being given at an interval of 4 weeks apart, the second dose at 2 weeks prior to turnout. This means that the first dose is given 6 weeks prior to turnout and must therefore be ordered 8 weeks prior to turnout – in other words, in late February for a late April turnout. Depending on local needs, calves may also be vaccinated against clostridial infections such as tetanus and blackleg, once again two doses being required at an interval of 4 weeks. If lungworm or blackleg vaccinations have been overlooked, then it is better to give the second dose after turnout, rather than to neglect vaccination altogether. Although the calves will not be fully protected initially against either disease, the risk during the early grazing season is relatively low, particularly from lungworm.

If specific mineral or trace element deficiencies are known to be a problem on a particular farm (e.g. copper, cobalt or vitamin E/selenium) then specific supplementation should be given.

Ideally, calves should be well grown and between 150 and 200 kg in weight before turnout and the timing of turnout should be planned to coincide with a reasonable quantity of lush, leafy (not stemmy) grass and clement weather conditions. Often this is almost impossible to achieve and provision of some form of shelter can be highly beneficial. Whatever the feeding system, calves invariably 'lose their bloom' and reduce in weight to a certain extent immediately after turnout. However, this can be minimised by continuing with supplementary concentrates (1.0–1.5 kg) for the first 3–4 weeks, depending on pasture growth, stocking density, weather, etc. It may also be worth offering conserved forage (hay or silage) for as long as the calves will eat it. Numerous grazing systems, stocking densities and nitrogen applications have been proposed, details of which are outside the scope of this book. The leader–follower system, in which young calves graze each paddock ahead of older heifers or cows, was once popular, but it does involve careful planning and management and many farms now seem to rely on the strategic use of anthelmintics for worm control.

As pasture availability wanes during July or August, calves must be carefully monitored (i.e. weighed) to ensure that growth targets are being maintained. Supplementary feeding may be needed at this stage. A further flush of grass is produced in September, but by the end of that month, and certainly into October, sward nutrient quality is falling and supplementary feeding with high energy concentrates may again be needed, or even housing. By far the best way of assessing the heifers' requirement is by monitoring weight change and growth rates, yet this is little performed.

The major factors restricting growth during the first grazing season are undernutrition and parasitism. Grazing management is of vital importance and on a continuous grazing system the stocking rate should be adjusted to match grass availability, aiming for a sward height of 5–6 cm in spring, 7–8 cm in mid-summer and 9–10 cm in the autumn (Drew, 1990). This often involves grazing a limited area in May and June, then expanding onto silage aftermaths in July.

Parasite control

Although there are some 18 known species of stomach and intestinal worms in cattle in the UK, the parasite posing the greatest risk is the stomach worm *Ostertagia ostertagi*. Other parasites such as lungworms, liver fluke and ticks may also be a problem in certain areas and could seriously depress growth and production.

Ostertagiasis

A full understanding of the life cycle and epidemiology of *Ostertagia ostertagi* is essential if control measures are to be successful. Figure 2.2 depicts the life cycle. Third stage larvae (L_3), overwintered on pasture or passed earlier in the season, are ingested with grazing. They burrow into the wall of the abomasum where they develop into the L_4 stage, then L_5 and finally emerge into the lumen as egg-laying females. The period between eating the L_3 on pasture and eggs appearing in the faeces of the calf is 3 weeks. However, the rate of development and hatching of the worm eggs passed in faeces depends on temperature, so that eggs deposited in April and May take several weeks to develop, while those passed in the warmer weather of June complete the transition to infective L_3 in only 2–3 weeks. The net effect of this is that all the worm eggs passed by calves 3 weeks after turnout onwards (3 weeks for the ingested L_3 to become egg-laying females) become infective L_3 at approximately the same time, namely in early July. This presents a massive challenge to the young heifers, whose weight gains drop, or even reverse. The pattern of infection is shown diagrammatically in Fig. 2.3. Clinical disease is the result of damage to the gastric glands in the abomasum. Pepsino-

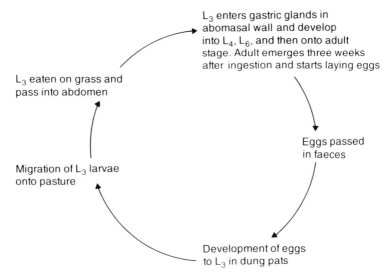

Fig. 2.2 Life cycle of the stomach worm *Ostertagia ostertagi.*

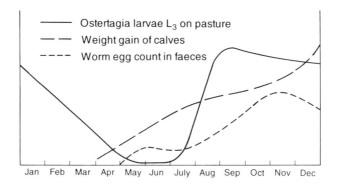

Fig. 2.3 Pattern of summer ostertagia infection, Overwintered L_3 are the primary source of infection, and these are present on pasture until mid June. Disease is caused by the secondary wave of L_3 produced in July (Blowey, 1988).

gen and hydrochloric acid production fall, protein digestion is impaired and this is seen clinically as scouring. Initially the semi-solid dung may simply resemble that of animals on lush grazing. However, as the condition progresses, the scour becomes profuse, watery and bright green and calves lose weight rapidly. Death is uncommon. The main clinical signs are massive weight loss and subsequent retarded growth, precisely what should be avoided for heifers being reared to calve at 2 years old.

Disease is not, therefore, caused by larvae that have overwintered from the previous year, but by the recycling of these larvae by calves turned out in the current grazing season. Towards the end of the grazing season some immunity develops. This has the effect of restricting the life of the adult worm to approximately 1 month and hence only moderate worm burdens are carried. This feature has two important consequences. First, if calves are moved to, and maintained on, pastures free of infection in September, their worm burdens will quite quickly decrease. However, anthelmintic treatment without moving onto a clean pasture will only give temporary relief, as the worms killed by the anthelmintic would have soon died anyway, and because the pasture remains heavily contaminated, new infections are rapidly established from fresh larval intakes. Even if no further worm eggs are passed from July onwards, the pasture grazed early in the spring will remain infected until the end of June the following year, by which time the warm, dry conditions of summer will have killed the larvae.

The incidence and severity of disease caused by ostertagia will therefore depend on a number of factors:

(1) The initial level of pasture larval contamination carried over from the previous year.
(2) The time of turnout. Calves turned out early (e.g. in April) will produce a larger buildup of L_3 on the pasture. By the end of June, if not grazed, larvae will have virtually disappeared and the risk to calves turned out at this time is minimal.
(3) Stocking density. Heavily stocked fields lead to greater larval intakes, more faecal contamination of the pasture and a greater larval rise in July.
(4) Rainfall. Heavy rain physically spreads dung pats and hence spreads larvae over the pasture. In addition, high moisture levels make L_3 more available on grass. It is well known by farmers that worms are much less of a problem in hot, dry summers, even when food is scarce and grazing is tight. Ultraviolet light kills L_3 larvae and lack of rain keeps those that survive in the dung pat.
(5) Concurrent diseases, especially debilitating conditions such as copper and selenium deficiency, reduce the calf's ability to develop an immune response and hence increase the severity of ostertagiasis.

Control: a variety of control measures are available and each farm must choose the system best suited to its requirements. The following are possible options:

(1) Turn calves out onto worm-free pastures. Into this category would fit new leys, especially if planted after an arable crop, or pasture that during the previous year was used only for sheep or conservation. Unfortunately few farmers have sufficient space to graze calves on worm-free pastures for the whole season.

(2) Delay turnout until after the end of June and then turnout onto pasture that has only been used for conservation or sheep earlier in the summer. Overwintered larvae will have died by the end of June.

(3) Worm the calves in early/mid-July, just before the massive larval challenge, and move them onto a worm-free pasture, e.g. an aftermath. The disadvantage of this system is that:

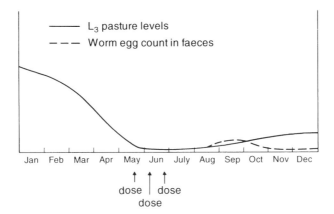

Fig. 2.4 Dosing calves at 3-week intervals (Blowey, 1988).

(a) the pasture that the calves have been grazing will remain heavily infected until June the following year; and
(b) if the 'worm and move' date is delayed, calves will be exposed to a heavy challenge and may suffer clinical signs of disease.

(4) Treat calves with an anthelmintic following turnout, to prevent the mid-July larval buildup. The period between ingestion of L_3 and the appearance of eggs in the faeces is 3 weeks. Therefore if calves are dosed every 3 weeks from turnout, their faecal worm egg excretion remains virtually zero and the July rise of pasture L_3 is eliminated. This scenario is depicted in Fig. 2.4, which should be contrasted with the situation in Fig. 2.3. The 3-weekly dosing can be discontinued by the end of June, since by that stage all overwintered larvae will have died.

There are two additional options to 3-weekly dosing, both of which achieve the same end result. Ivermectin has the unusual property of persisting in the animal to give protection against reinfection for up to 2 weeks after administration. Other avermectins and bambermycin compound have similar or longer duration of activity. In place of 3-weekly worming, therefore, the interval between treatments can be extended by an additional 2 weeks.

For example:

- First dose at turnout and second 8 weeks after turnout where anthelmintic activity persists for about 5 weeks.
- First dose at 3 weeks after turnout gives cover to 5 weeks (invermectin activity persists 2 weeks).
- Second dose at 5 + 3 = 8 weeks after turnout gives cover to 10 weeks.
- Third dose at 10 + 3 = 13 weeks after turnout gives cover to 15 weeks.

Thus, instead of worming at 3-weekly intervals until June, ivermectin can be given at 3, 8 and 13 weeks after turnout and others at 0–8 weeks.

A further option is to use an anthelmintic bolus. One type gives a continuous slow release of morantel for 90 days after administration. An ivermectin bolus

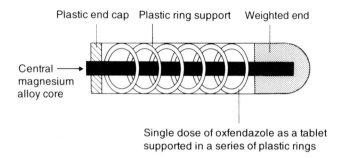

Fig. 2.5   A pulse release wormer bolus.

lasts the whole grazing season as does one for fenbendazole. A more recent version is the pulse release bolus, which automatically delivers a dose of anthelmintic every 3 weeks. Its structure is shown diagrammatically in Fig. 2.5. It consists of five separate doses of 750 mg oxfendazole, each separated by a plastic ring and all enclosed in a PVC case. A magnesium alloy core runs through the centre, attached to a heavy weight at one end. Not only does the weight retain the bolus in the reticulum, but also it reacts with the magnesium core to produce a corrosive galvanic current. The rate of core erosion is constant (11 mm per 3 weeks), allowing one collar to fall off, releasing its dose of anthelmintic every 3 weeks. Calves are given the bolus at turnout and five doses are then dispensed at 3-weekly intervals. Despite its additional expense, the bolus has produced excellent weight gains in treated calves and is very popular with farmers because of its low labour requirement, i.e. removing the need for frequent handling of the calves at a busy time of the year.

The major advantage of regular anthelmintic therapy is that it needs minimal planning, any pasture area can be used, calves can stay on or return to the initial area of grazing throughout the year and that pasture is not heavily contaminated for the following year.

Lungworm (parasitic bronchitis, husk)

Lungworm infestation, husk or parasitic bronchitis is caused by a worm, *Dictyocaulus viviparus*, and is the second most important parasite of young cattle. Adult worms living in the trachea and bronchi of carrier cattle (see Fig. 2.6) lay eggs which rapidly hatch into first-stage larvae (L_1). The development of the infection stage, L_3 is temperature dependent. When mature, L_3 migrate onto blades of grass where they are eaten by the calf and pass into its intestine. Larvae burrow through the intestinal wall and travel via the bloodstream to the lungs. During this larval migration no clinical signs are seen. However, large numbers of larvae penetrating the air sacs (see Fig. 2.6) will produce rapid laboured breathing, weight loss and even death 15–20 days after ingestion of a heavy larval challenge. At this stage coughing will be minimal and no larvae will be detectable in the faeces. This is the prepatent form of husk infestation. As larvae migrate up into the bronchi and trachea, panting continues but coughing, a deep abdominal

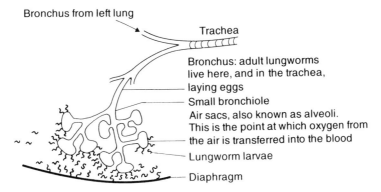

Bronchus from left lung

Trachea

Bronchus: adult lungworms
live here, and in the trachea,
laying eggs

Small bronchiole

Air sacs, also known as alveoli.
This is the point at which oxygen from
the air is transferred into the blood

Lungworm larvae

Diaphragm

Fig. 2.6 Lungworm larvae begin to penetrate air sacs of lungs 10–15 days after being eaten. Signs are first seen at this stage.

cough, becomes much more pronounced. By 30–45 days after exposure to a heavy challenge of L_3, lungworm larvae may be detectable in the faeces of affected calves.

Reservoirs of infection: contaminated pasture, leading to a clincial outbreak of husk, may arise from overwintered L_3 larvae, either deep in the soil or even in earthworms, carrier animals, faecal transmission via boots or tractor wheels, or *Pilobolus* spp. fungus. The latter grows on dung pats and, when ripe, produces a sporangiophore which explodes. Larvae that have migrated onto the exploding *Pilobolus* seed-heads are thus thrown clear of the dung pat and onto surrounding pasture, where they can then be ingested by grazing calves.

Lungworm multiply very rapidly. A single female can produce over 3000 larvae per day, viz. almost 100 000 in 4 weeks. Should pasture conditions suddenly become favourable for their rapid and simultaneous development, a heavy challenge of infection can occur. Disease is usually seen in the autumn, especially if September and October are warm and wet. Unfortunately, the timing of outbreaks of lungworm infestation cannot be predicted with the same accuracy as ostertagia, and strategic anthelmintic medication is not reliable as a control measure.

Control and prevention: both the pulse release bolus and ivermectin administered at 3, 8 and 13 weeks after turnout (see pp. 31–2) will control lungworm during their period of administration, but this gives the calf no protection from September onwards. In addition, there is concern by some that such regimes may be so effective in the early stages that they prevent the calf developing an immunity.

The only reliable way of preventing lungworm is by vaccination. Two doses, each of 1000 irradiated larvae, are given as a drench 6 weeks and 2 weeks prior to turnout. This gives protection for life provided there is exposure to infection to enhance and maintain immunity. Lungworm is probably more common than many farmers realise. A recent serological survey indicated that on farms that had not previously vaccinated against lungworm, two thirds had been exposed to infection but only one farm had reported clinical signs. The effects of subclinical levels of infection on calf growth rates on the remaining farms must be open to speculation.

Liver fluke

The parasite *Fasciola hepatica* or liver fluke can be a serious cause of stunting and poor growth, especially in those parts of the country where the summers are warm and wet. Its life cycle is depicted in Fig. 2.7. Adult liver flukes living in the bile ducts of the liver lay eggs which are passed in the faeces of the host through-out the year, but only when the weather is warm and wet do they hatch. Hatch-ing releases the motile miracidium of the fluke, which swims around in a film of moisture until it penetrates the snail *Lymnaea truncatula*. There is a multiplica-tion phase inside the snail, so that one fluke miracidium entering can lead to the release of over 1000 cercariae from the snail. Cercariae swim onto blades of grass, where they encyst, to become resistant metacercariae, awaiting ingestion by grazing cattle. Once in the intestine, metacercariae hatch into immature flukes, which burrow across the abdomen, into and through the liver and eventually arrive at the bile ducts where they mature to become egg-laying adults, ready to repeat the cycle.

Compared with parasites such as *Dictyocaulus* and *Ostertagia*, the liver fluke has a long life cycle. The various stages are shown in Table 2.7. The period within the snail is highly dependent on favourable conditions existing for the snail habitat, and thus its own growth and multiplication. This is why warm, wet

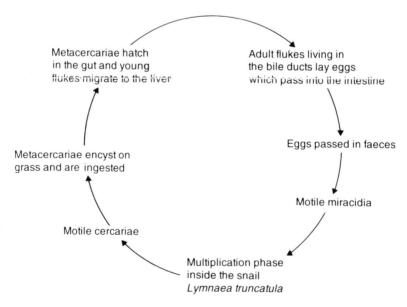

Fig. 2.7   Life cycle of liver fluke, *Fasciola hepatica*.

Table 2.7 Time intervals in the fluke life cycles.

Ingested metacercariae to immature flukes in liver	= 4 weeks	3 months
Immature flukes pass through liver feeding	= 6 weeks	inside the
Flukes mature in bile ducts and produce eggs	= 2 weeks	animal
Egg to miracidium to snail to cercaria to metacercaria	= 2 months *minimum* outside the animal	

summers are so important. Hatching of fluke eggs and snail growth are both stimulated by warmth and humidity, so if June and July are wet, all the fluke eggs which have been passed onto the pasture since December of the previous year may hatch at the same time as the snail population is increasing. This then produces a very heavy infestation of metacercariae on the pasture and a heavy challenge for cattle grazing from September onwards. This is known as 'summer' infection. If September and October are warm and wet, a second wave of snails and fluke miracidia become active. However, by the time the snails are infected, the cold weather arrives and the snails then hibernate for the winter. The resumption of snail activity the following spring/early summer leads to the release of a further wave of infective metacercariae, known as 'winter infection' of snails. However, summer infection is by far the most common.

Immunity to fluke is relatively good once unexposed young stock and adults become infected. This is in contrast to lungworm and ostertagia, which are primarily diseases of young stock in their first or second grazing seasons with immunity following exposure in these seasons. By far the best control of fluke is achieved by pasture improvement, removing or fencing-off the wet, marshy areas which are the classic snail habitats. Known fluke-infested farms should always dose cattle at housing, preferably using one of the newer fluke treatments which has a high degree of efficacy against the immature migrating stages of the parasite. If this is not done, or if cattle are outwintered, a second dose should be given in mid-winter, e.g. January or February.

The clinical sings of chronic liver fluke, casused by the feeding activity of the adults in the bile ducts, are rather non-specific and include weight loss, anaemia and general unthriftiness. Reduced serum protein levels, especially low albumin, lead to oedema, seen clinically as bottle jaw. This is a fairly advanced stage and changes of such severity should not be seen in dairy replacement heifers.

Ticks and tick-borne diseases

The four major conditions in the category of ticks and tick-borne diseases which lead to poor growth and illness primarily in heifers include babesiosis (redwater), tick-borne fever, louping-ill and the direct clinical effects of tick feeding, namely irritation and anaemia due to extensive blood loss.

Ticks prefer coarse, uncultivated pasture, where thick tufts of dense grass provide them with the moisture and protection needed for their complex three-stage life cycle. There are two major species of ticks in Great Britain, *Ixodes ricinus* and *Haemaphysalis punctata*. *Ixodes ricinus* is by far the most common

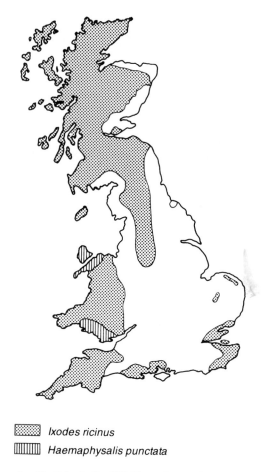

☷ *Ixodes ricinus*
▥ *Haemaphysalis punctata*

Fig. 2.8   Distribution of cattle ticks in the UK (Purnell, 1982).

and is found throughout Scotland, Wales, north and south-west England and in a few coastal areas of Dorset and south-east England (see Fig. 2.8). *Haemaphysalis* is only found in coastal areas of Wales and south England. The complex tick life cycle is spread over 3 years, with only one period of tick feeding each year. Further details are given elsewhere (Blowey, 1988). In addition to their feeding activity, their main effects are in the diseases they transmit.

Redwater (babesiosis)

The disease redwater or babesiosis is caused by a small, single-celled protozoan parasite, *Babesia divergens*, related to malaria in man. The problem occurs in marginal tick areas rather than in the main tick areas or where animals are brought into tick areas and have previously not been exposed to infection. Disease is unlikely to be seen in dairy heifers until towards the end of their first grazing season, because an inherent age resistance exists for the first 6 months. This prevents infection becoming established in animals of less than 9 months old thus indigenous animals are exposed and will then develop premunity rather than infection. In addition, the second annual phase of tick feeding activity does not occur until September or October. Heifers exposed to low levels of infection rapidly establish an immunity and no clinical signs may be seen. However, this immunity is relatively short-lived and as further exposure may not occur for another 12 months, disease can also be seen in heifers during their second grazing season.

Redwater describes the appearance of haemoglobin in the urine caused by haemolysis of red blood cells during one of the multiplication phases of the parasite. In the early stages of disease the heifer will simply be standing apart from the others, having a high temperature, but within 24 hours the urine turns a deep port-wine red colour and froths as it hits the ground. Anaemia may be intense and in some neglected cases even fatal. In the early stages, spasm of the anal sphincter leads to the passage of faeces in a characteristic 'pipestem' propulsive effect. Constipation, associated with severe anaemia, may occur at a later stage. Amicarbalide and quinuronium sulphate are no longer used for treatment; instead treatment is by imidocarb diproprionate. The Divisional Veterinary Manager must be informed before treating. Blood transfusions may be needed in advanced cases. It is best to graze calves under 6 months old. In other countries vaccines are available.

Tick-borne fever

Whereas *Babesia* spp. destroys red blood cells, *Cytoecetes phagocytophila*, another parasite carried by ticks and the cause of tick fever, destroys the white cells. It is a much less severe disease than babesiosis. Affected animals run a high temperature and appear stiff, lethargic and off their feed. Mild cases would probably pass unnoticed, with a spontaneous recovery. Severe attacks can cause abortion in pregnant heifers in their second grazing season. Tetracyclines are effective in treatment.

Louping ill

Louping ill, a flavivirus infection, is primarily a disease of sheep but occasionally occurs in all other species, including man. It is transmitted by the tick *Ixodes ricinus*, and hence occurs only in tick-infested areas. Affected heifers may show a range of clinical signs. Following an initial period of fever, the virus may spread to replicate in the brain, producing nervous signs of trembling, abnormality of gait and staggering, which in severe cases may lead to intense stiffness, recumbency and, very occasionally, death. However, most heifers recover, albeit sometimes retaining mild, permanent central nervous system signs, e.g. twitching. Many infections do not reach the brain, however, and are therefore asymptomatic, but all cases stimulate a good immunity and leave the heifer solidly immune for life. Only sheep and grouse appear to act as a reservoir of infection for ticks. Ticks feeding on infected cattle do not appear to become infected. Vaccination with a formalin-killed oil emulsion vaccine containing louping ill virus can be used. It should not be injected in the last month of pregnancy and an annual booster is advisable.

Fly control

Control of flies in young grazing heifers is important for a number of reasons. Firstly, flies cause irritation and heavily infested heifers will not graze or grow adequately. Certain types of fly even cause panic and groups of heifers may be seen chasing across fields (i.e. 'gadding') in the summer, trying to escape. This can lead to severe physical injuries. Secondly, flies transmit diseases such as New Forest eye and summer mastitis. Summer mastitis is more of a problem in pregnant heifers in their second grazing season and will be discussed in the relevant section (see pp. 43, 220). New Forest eye is most commonly seen in younger heifers.

For young stock the most common form of fly control consists of a large plastic ear tag impregnated with an insecticide, e.g. cypermethrin. As the heifer grooms herself, insecticide from the tag is dissolved by the natural oils of the skin (the sebum) to give an almost complete body covering. The tag gives protection for up to 5 months and is particularly good at reducing fly numbers over the head and back. In heavily infested areas two tags, one in each ear, may be required. Unfortunately the flow of sebum is not particularly good over the teat and this is why additional measures are needed against summer mastitis (see p. 43). Other chemicals may be applied by knapsack spray or simply as pour-on preparations. The latter are increasing in popularity, especially for dairy cows. A small volume (e.g. 20–40 ml) of a synthetic pyrethroid insecticide (permethrin), in a specific chemical carrier, is poured along the animal's back and diffuses over the whole body. One application can provide fly protection for up to 8 weeks. The final measure in fly control is to keep heifers away from areas of high fly density, viz. keep them in open fields where there are no woods, copses or damp areas.

New Forest eye [pink eye, infectious bovine keratoconjunctivitis (IBK)] (see also p. 266)

New Forest eye is caused by the bacterium *Moraxella bovis*, infection spreading from animal to animal by flies, by heifers rubbing against one another, or by indirect contact, for example on feed troughs or posts. Once on the cornea, *Moraxella bovis* multiplies and erodes it to produce an intensely painful ulcer. Affected heifers stand apart from the others, normally with their eyes closed (bright sunlight increases the pain) and watering profusely. If left untreated, the ulcer may erode into the anterior chamber of the eye, rupturing the eyeball. The resultant hole is quickly plugged by tissue from the iris to produce what is known as a staphyloma. Sight has now been permanently lost. Less severe cases, and those that receive prompt treatment, are healed by the eye's own defence mechanisms. In response to bacterial invasion, large quantities of tears are produced containing antibodies and other antibacterial elements in an attempt to wash away and destroy the infection. From the periphery of the eye blood vessels grow across the cornea to carry nutrients and other materials needed to rebuild the area damaged by the ulcer. The red ring of blood vessels progressing across the cornea is known as pannus formation. At this stage the eye will appear almost totally red and sight will be lost. However, this is only temporary, because when rebuilding is complete, the blood vessels regress and sight is regained, with only a small white scar on the centre of the cornea to indicate the original position of the ulcer. Vaccination is used to prevent the disease in some countries (p. 13).

Second winter housing and the service period

Requirements

Autumn-born (e.g. September) calves will need to be served in December if they are to calve at 2 years old. By October, they should have reached 270–300 kg (Table 2.1, Fig. 2.1) and be well-fleshed but not overfat. Depending on the grazing available, supplementary feeding may be necessary during October. Ideally the heifers need to be housed at least 4–6 weeks before service. This allows them to settle into their new housing, establish themselves on their winter rations to reach their target service weight of 330 kg and recover from any routine veterinary treatments before insemination, thus improving conception rates. During their second winter, heifers should (ideally) be housed in the the same type of housing system as the milking herd, thereby adapting them to conditions for the future. For the majority of current UK systems, this involves cubicles. Heifer cubicles can be smaller in both width and length, but it does not seem to matter if full-sized cubicles are provided, or even if (as some do) the heifers lie in them backwards, i.e. facing the dunging passage. It is the acclimatisation that is important. A heifer entering a milking herd has to cope with many new things. Calving itself is a considerable stress, especially if difficult. Having been one of a relatively small group of animals, and possibly well up in the pecking order, after calving she is introduced into a much larger group of animals, all considerably larger than she. Consequently she will be well towards the bottom of the pecking order. She will be fed on food she has probably not been accustomed to and certainly through a feeding system that she has not experienced before. The final insult would therefore be a change in housing. It is for reasons such as these that heifers develop laminitis, sole ulcers and lameness (p. 153) in early to mid lactation. Inadequate access to silage (for example owing to fear and competition) leads to a high concentrate: low fibre diet and acidosis (p. 50). Lack of experience with cubicles, and especially if cubicle passages are narrow or blind ending, or the cubicles themselves are uncomfortable, means that the heifer is reluctant to use them (p. 279). She then spends much longer standing than she ought (60% of time should be spent lying down) and further solar bruising, with resultant sole ulcers, develops.

Routine veterinary treatments at housing

Whatever worm control system was in operation, it is likely that heifers will still have a small worm burden at the end of their first grazing season. In addition, with developing immunity, many of the ostertagia L_3 larvae ingested from September onwards remain dormant as L_4 in the gastric mucosal glands of the abomasal wall. These 'arrested development' hypobiotic forms can lie dormant until February or March of the following year, when their sudden emergence and development into adults can produce an outbreak of profuse watery diarrhoea. This condition, known as winter or type II ostertagiasis, can be fatal if not treated.

Prevention of the condition depends on giving a suitable anthelmintic (avermectins, moxidectin or benzimidazole are widely used) at housing which will kill the arrested development larval forms in addition to the adults living in the abomasal lumen. In unvaccinated heifers, anthelmintic treatment at housing is also a sensible measure to remove lungworm burdens and hence prevent pasture contamination the following year. Similarly, in known fluke areas, treatment should cover liver fluke.

Although now eradicated from British cattle, treatment for warbles was once strongly recommended. If pour-on preparations are used, they should be applied before the end of November. In addition to killing any possible warble larvae, warble dressings also kill lice and mange mites – but not their eggs. If heavy infestations are seen at housing, then a second treatment should be given 2–3 weeks later, to eliminate recently hatched lice and mange (p. 24). No treatment seems to be 100% effective and at least one further dosing during January/February would be beneficial. Avermectin or moxidectin available as a pour-on or injectable preparation must be the treatment of choice at housing, as it is effective against adult ostertagia, inhibited dormant L_4 forms, lungworm, warbles, lice and mange. Where indicated, commercial preparations containing avermectin plus flukicide are available.

If the main herd is known to be infected with leptospirosis, heifers should, ideally, be vaccinated prior to service, thus protecting them from the risk of early fetal death and abortion. If there is to be no contact (either direct or indirect through grazing or streams, etc.) between heifers and cows, then it may be possible to delay vaccination until the heifers are nearer to entering the herd. Two doses are required at an interval of 4 weeks. One trial involving 232 vaccinated and 232 non-vaccinated heifers introduced into known infected dairy herds showed that vaccination conferred a milk yield advantage of 785 litres during the first lactation, despite the fact that no obvious clinical cases of 'milk drop' or 'flabby bag' were reported in the unvaccinated heifers. BVD vaccination may also be necessary.

Preparation for service (see also p. 132)

Choice of sire and service management should be decided well before housing. Natural service, using Hereford or Aberdeen Angus bulls, has traditionally been used for heifers. Not only does this remove the need for heat detection, but also it means that the heifers can be housed some distance away in off-lying buildings, and facilities for artificial insemination are not necessary. More recently, Holstein/Friesian sires have been used. Provided the sire is carefully selected as one that produces an easy calving (this is normally a bull producing calves with

Table 2.8 Heifers from heifers produce higher yields than heifers from cows (from Furniss *et al.*, 1986).

	Dam	
	Heifer	Cow
Weight at first service (kg)	370	360
Weight at calving (kg)	496	503
First lactation 305-day yield (kg)	4977	4742
Per cent rebred	80	80

a short gestation length), problems should not occur. The sire should also be of higher genetic merit than the heifers, otherwise no genetic progress will be made. There are two major advantages in calving heifers to a Friesian bull:

(1) Being born at the start of the year, their calves will be well grown and ready to enter the herd 2 years later, at the start of the calving season. Such a system also produces an even group of heifers for rearing.
(2) Heifers from heifers give higher yields than heifers from cows. Furness *et al.* (1986) recorded the yields from 569 heifers from cows and heifers from heifers (Table 2.8). Despite the probable lower calf weights of heifers from heifers, there was no significant difference in weight at service, weight at calving or the percentage of animals that conceived again. However, the effect on milk yield was quite marked.

Feeding has a dramatic effect on heifer conception rates and supplementary feeding for 6 weeks before until 6 weeks after service is recommended. This boosts fertilisation rates and by continuing the supplementary feeding until well after service (viz. 6 weeks) implantation, which is not normally complete in cattle until 35 days after fertilisation, also benefits. The ration should be formulated to allow the continued growth of around 0.7 kg live weight/day. At housing this normally means supplementing forage with 1–2 kg of a cereal-based ration, depending on forage quality. Drew and Pointer (1977) recorded calving rates on six commercial farms where half of each group of heifers was given a supplementary feed of 20 MJ ME/day for 6 weeks before until 6 weeks after service. The remaining heifers were fed a ration considered by the farmers to be adequate. Their results are shown in Table 2.9. There is clearly a wide variation between farms, but, on average, calving rates increased from 50% to almost 70% in supplemented heifers. Body condition score or, more specifically, the rate of change of condition score at the time of service will also influence conception rates.

Service management (see also pp. 106, 132)

If natural service is to be used, the bull selected should be in good condition but certainly neither fat nor overweight and should have good legs and feet. Ideally

Table 2.9 Effect of supplementary feeding at service on subsequent calving rates of heifers, from Drew and Pointer, 1977.

Farm	Number of heifers	Per cent calved	
		Control	Supplemented
1	62	40	67
2	58	59	75
3	56	32	59
4	37	67	79
5	78	54	69
6	73	53	67
Mean	61	50.0	68.9

20–25 heifers to one bull are enough if good conception rates and a tight calving pattern are to be maintained. Yard surfaces should be kept clean and non-slip to reduce the risk of injury, and if in straw yards, there should be ample space available, e.g. 4.5–5.0 m² per heifer, plus additional loafing/feeding areas.

If Friesian AI is to be used, this is commonly combined with oestrus synchronisation, either using intravaginal progestagens or prostaglandins (p. 132). A combination of the two (viz. prostaglandin administration 24 hours before progestagen removal) probably gives the best synchronisation, although, provided that the heifers are fed and managed properly, there is no reason why conception rates should fall on either system.

It is also common to find combinations of all three systems, viz. synchronisation, heat detection and natural service, in use on the same farm. One such system is to give the heifers two doses of prostaglandin, followed by fixed-time AI, then introduce a bull 24 hours after the second AI. Natural service will then catch those heifers that did not synchronise, plus the repeats. Another option is to give one prostaglandin injection to the heifers, then serve on sight, viz. following heat detection. There will be a surge of oestrous activity 3–4 days after injection. Insemination is continued at observed heat until 10 days after injections, when a second dose of prostaglandin is then given to the remaining unserved heifers, which receive fixed-time AI. Natural service or heat detection plus AI is then used to cover the small proportion of heifers that fail to synchronise and/or return to service.

Whatever system is used, it cannot be stressed too strongly that the heifers should be maintained on a ration that allows a weight gain of approximately 0.7 kg/day and changes in feeding, housing and management should, if at all possible, be avoided until after implantation is complete, i.e. until 6 weeks after service. At this stage it may be possible to reduce growth rates slightly, e.g. down to 0.5 kg/day, especially if the heifers are above target weight. Under practical farm situations, however, they are often all run as a single group and must be fed according to the lower members of that group. If concentrate intakes are reduced or eliminated, some form of mineral or trace element supplementation may be necessary, depending on local farm circumstances. Pregnancy diagnosis 6–8 weeks after fixed-time AI, or even as late as 8 weeks after the bull has been taken out, is a worthwhile procedure. Not only does this identify the non-pregnant heifer (which can then be sold barren if forage availability is limited), but also it gives an early indication of the number of heifers available and therefore the number of cows that can affordably be culled at the same time as maintaining the farm within its milk quota. Following pregnancy diagnosis, heifer management until turnout is minimal, except for ensuring that weight gains are maintained.

Second season at grass and precalving management

Treatments needed at turnout

Pregnant heifers are sometimes the earliest animals to be turned out in the spring. They can be released as soon as there is sufficient grazing available and as soon as the ground is dry enough to carry them. Conversely, a proportion of farms keep heifers housed until May or even June, especially if there is silage from the previous year that needs using up. The heifers can then go out onto an aftermath.

Few routine treatments are required prior to turnout. If blackleg is known to be a problem, then a booster dose would be a suitable precaution. Most consider that second season cattle have sufficient immunity and that no additional worm control is necessary, but this may not always be true. A few still worm and move pregnant heifers in July. This is of dubious cost-effectiveness unless they are very close to calving. With the immunosuppressant stress of imminent parturition, small heifers may show a response to worming prior to entry into the milking herd. Care should be taken to select a product that will not result in milk being discarded. As the heifers will be on grazing alone during their second summer, some form of mineral and trace element supplementation is a suitable precaution. Ensure that the product used contains copper, cobalt, selenium and iodine.

The only other veterinary treatment necessary prior to turnout is a fly repellent to prevent summer mastitis, and precautions against New Forest eye (p. 38) and teat warts (p. 44). Impregnated fly tags are commonly used (see p. 38), but as they give relatively little protection over the teats, additional protection in this area is required. This is discussed in the following section on summer mastitis.

Summer mastitis (see also p. 220)

Summer mastitis is an acute necrotising mastitis which produces a thick, purulent secretion with a characteristic pungent smell. Its importance is that very few affected quarters recover and hence the heifer is damaged for life. It is most commonly seen in mid to late pregnant cows and heifers. Initially the affected heifer will be seen standing apart from the others, often lame, dull, anorexic and with a significantly raised temperature. If left untreated, the pyrexia may be severe enough to cause abortion or, in occasional cases, death. Most sick heifers respond well to antibiotic therapy, although the affected quarter will not recover and may continue to discharge pus for a considerable part of the lactation. In some cases the udder bursts at the rear to release a foul-smelling discharge.

Bacteriological examination of a number of cases has shown that four organisms are commonly involved, namely *Actinomyces pyogenes* (in 78% of cases investigated), *Streptococcus dysgalactiae* (17%), *Peptococcus indolicus* (85%) and a *Micrococcus* (74%). Infection has been shown to be carried by the sheep headfly, *Hydrotoea irritans*, and the annual incidence of disease matches the periods of fly activity. Experimental transmission of disease via infected flies has been disappointing, however (Hillerton *et al.*, 1990), and this has led some to the suggestion that some other factor such as trauma caused by thorns or other plants, or excessive self-inflicted licking is necessary to first reduce the teat end defences. Eggs of *Hydrotoea irritans* overwinter in sandy soils from which they emerge in June or July of the following year. There is only one generation of adults each year and these are found in July, August and September, the months when summer mastitis occurs. High wind speeds (above 20 km/hour) and heavy rain inhibit fly activity. This has two important consequences, namely:

(1)   Summer mastitis is most commonly seen following a period of still, humid weather.
(2)   If the heifers can be kept in high, open fields where there is generally some air movement, and away from sheltered, wooded habitats favoured by *Hydrotoea irritans*, the risk of mastitis will be considerably reduced.

The need for fly protection has already been mentioned, but unfortunately fly tags and pour-on preparations give only limited protection to the teats and udder. Application of a glutinous insecticide (or Stockholm tar) directly onto the teats has been favoured by some. Unfortunately it has to be repeated every 2 weeks, but this is better than losing a quarter. Alternative control measures are to bind tape around the teat ends (this has to be repeated every 3 weeks, but is very effective) or the use of dry cow antibiotic therapy, or either calving or housing heifers in late June, to avoid the period of risk. In heifers the tip of the intramammary tube needs to be apposed against, but not inserted in, the teat canal orifice and the contents infused accordingly. While all these measures help to a certain extent, by far the best control is to keep heifers away from known 'summer mastitis fields' during the danger period, even if this means using the land to conserve forage and feeding it to the same heifers in another field.

Warts

Warts are benign virus-induced tumours of the skin. They are particularly common in 1- to 2-year-old cattle, where they may be seen over the head, brisket, abdomen or teats. In the first three sites they hardly ever cause problems, although unusually large masses may sometimes ulcerate and become infected. Teat warts, however, often persist until after calving, where they interfere with milking, either from the pain of the milking machine pulling on the wart or, by allowing liner slip and entry of air, vacuum fluctuations and teat end impacts are produced, predisposing to mastitis. Even the noise of liner slip can be damaging to an already nervous heifer. It is thought that wart viruses are spread by flies, so fly control is important in prevention. Autogenous vaccines can be used for treatment.

Feeding during pregnancy

It is important that heifers continue to grow during their second grazing season, in order to achieve their target bodyweight (500–520 kg, see Table 2.1) at calving. This necessitates the provision of adequate grazing, plus mineral and trace element supplementation as discussed previously. Heifers that do not achieve adequate bodyweight at calving will have reduced milk yields (see Table 2.2). Conversely, heifers that are overfat will suffer an increased incidence of dystocia. This is likely to be due to excessive fat deposits restricting the size of the pelvic canal. Traditionally it was considered that overfeeding in late pregnancy produced oversized calves, but there is little documentary evidence of this.

In an extensive survey of dystocia in Friesian heifers, Drew (1988) found that the incidence of difficult calvings was greatest at the two extremes of weight gain during pregnancy (see Table 2.10). Calf mortality (i.e. percentage born dead) was therefore greatest for those heifers that grew at less than 0.4 kg/day and those that grew at greater than 0.8 kg/day. In the same study, a detailed comparison between heifers from high- (above 20%) and low- (less than 5%) calf mortality farms failed to show any significant difference in heifer weight or age at service or subsequent calving, nor in the farms' various heights or topographical measurements. There was also little effect of calf weight on dystocia levels. This would suggest that overfeeding in the last 2–3 weeks of pregnancy produces overfat heifers and dystocia due to fat deposition rather than to the size of the calf. Table 2.11 shows that on both high- and low-calf-mortality farms large calves required more assistance than small calves, but it was not the difference in calf size that accounted for the large variation in dystocia between the two groups of farms.

Table 2.10 Effect of weight gain during pregnancy on dystocia rates in Friesian heifers (number of animals in brackets). (From Drew, 1990.)

Weight gain (kg/day)	Calf mortality*	Percentage of calvings		
		Normal	Assisted	Difficult
<0.4 (49)	19	61	35	7
0.41–0.60 (348)	10	74	25	3
0.61–0.80 (854)	11	69	26	5
>8.0 (199)	14	64	28	8

* Percentage born dead.

Table 2.11 Proportion of calves of different sizes at birth on farms with high and low incidence of calf mortality and the effect on calving difficulty. (From Drew, 1990.)

Size of calf	Percentage of calvings	
	Low-mortality farms (<5% calves born dead)	High-mortality farms (>20% calves born dead)
Small	15	14
Medium	66	61
Large	19	25

There must therefore be some aspect(s) of on-farm management at the time of calving which accounts for the difference. These management factors are difficult to quantify. It is this author's opinion that one factor is the length of time that a heifer is allowed to calve unassisted. There is a tendency for some stockmen to provide assistance far too early, before the birth canal and pelvis have fully dilated. This results in the need for protracted assistance and considerably increases the incidence of calves born dead (i.e. calf mortality). Heifers brought in from a field, or simply removed from their group and individually penned in a loose-box become very nervous and stressed. This is likely to lengthen the time taken to calve naturally and may increase the calving problems. Other variables between farms which could have an influence are selenium (pp. 64, 101) and iodine (p. 65) status and vitamin A deficiencies (p. 65), all of which can produce stillbirths.

Preparation for entering the dairy herd

The need to acclimatise heifers to their post-calving housing and the reasons for so doing in the prevention of lameness have been discussed already. If cubicle training was not possible during their second winter, then pregnant heifers can be housed for a few weeks during July and August, when the milking herd is still out. This will have the additional benefit of summer mastitis protection. For the 1–2 weeks prior to calving, heifers should ideally be fed part of their post-calving production ration. This allows the ruminal microflora to adjust to the new diet, thereby reducing the risk of acidosis and subsequent laminitis (pp. 78, 153, 279). Amounts fed (including the forage portion of the ration) should obviously be restricted, otherwise heifers will become overfat. Some herdsmen even walk heifers through the parlour every day, thereby overcoming yet another 'hurdle' in the heifer's life prior to calving.

Competition after calving is clearly an important factor in the way in which a heifer settles into the dairy herd. In a survey of 179 heifers, calving at 2 years old and all sired by the same bull, Drew (1990) showed that heifers that were housed and fed separately performed considerably better than those mixed with the main herd at calving (Table 2.12). The variation in yield according to weight at service was to be expected, but heifers without competition had consistently higher yields

Table 2.12   Effect of weight at service and competition on this milk yield and % survival rates of heifers calving at 2 years. (From Drew, 1990.)

	Weight at service (kg)			
	225–259	260–279	280–299	300–349
	Milk yield (kg); survival rate (%) in brackets			
Competition	2892 (33)	3334 (46)	3639 (18)	3131 (21)
No competition	3852 (37)	4070 (73)	3992 (52)	3857 (32)

than those introduced directly from the main herd. This difference was maintained until the heifers reached their fifth lactation. Survival rates for the two groups also varied. This was at least partly because a greater proportion of heifers in the 'competition' herds were culled on the basis of poor yields.

Vaccinations required prior to entry into the milking herd will, of course, depend on the health status of the adult cows. If rotavirus or K99 *E. coli* are common causes of calf scour, one dose of vaccine should be given between 12 and 4 weeks prior to calving (p. 12). In IBR-infected herds, heifers should receive an intranasal vaccination (p. 13). If leptospirosis is present, either a booster vaccination will be required before the heifer enters the adult herd (where the challenge of infection may be high) or, if not previously vaccinated, the heifer should be given two doses at an interval of 4 weeks, the second being administered at least 2 weeks prior to contact with the milking herd. This 'contact' may simply be grazing over the same fields or drinking from a brook downstream from the cows. Having put so much effort into rearing the heifers to calve at the correct time of the year, at a target weight and at 2 years old, it would be tragic if one aborted in the final months of pregnancy, or suffered a production drop caused by leptospirosis in early lactation, simply because one vaccination was overlooked!

References

Blowey, R. W. (1988) *A Veterinary Book for Dairy Farmers*, 2nd edn., pp. 77–110. Farming Press, Ipswich.

Drew, S. B. (1988) The influence of management factors during rearing on the subsequent performance of Friesian heifers. *British Cattle Breeders Digest* **13**, 41–8.

Drew, S. B. (1990) Heifer rearing 12 weeks to calving. In *Bovine Medicine* (ed. A. H. Andrews, R. W. Blowey, H. Boyd & R. G. Eddy), pp. 45–59. Blackwell Science, Oxford.

Drew, S. B. & Pointer, C. G. (1977) The effect of level of nutrition on fertility in Friesian heifers in autumn and early winter. *European Association of Animal Production 28th Annual Meeting*, Brussels, 22–25 August 1987. Commission on Animal Health and Production Paper 77/8, pp. 1–3.

Furniss, S. J., Stroud, A., Barrington, H., Kirby, S. P. J., Wray, J. P. & Dakin, P. (1986) The effect of dam's parity on first lactation performance of dairy heifers. *Animal Production* **42**, 463.

Harrison, R. D., Reynolds, I. P. & Little, W. (1983) A quantitative analysis of mammary glands of dairy cows reared at different rates of live weight gain. *Journal of Dairy Research* **50**, 405–412.

Hillerton, J. E., Bramley, A. J. & Thomas, G. (1990) The role of *Hydrotoea irritans* in the transmission of summer mastitis. *British Veterinary Journal* **146**, 147–56.

Little, W. & Kay, R. M. (1979) The effects of rapid rearing and early calving on the subsequent performance of dairy heifers. *Animal Production* **29**, 131–42.

Purnell, R. E. (1982) *Tickborne Diseases of British Cattle.* Proceedings of the British Cattle Veterinary Association, Myerscough College, Lancashire, 5–7 April 1982, pp. 103–105.

Stansfield, M. (1983) *The New Herdman's Book*, p. 128. Farming Press, Ipswich.

Tucker, H. A. (1987) Quantitative estimate of mammary growth during various physiological states: a review. *Journal of Dairy Science* **70**, 1958–66.

Chapter 3
Nutrition of the Dairy Cow

Jim Kelly

Introduction

The purpose of this chapter is to give a practical guide to feeding the dairy cow and to emphasise some of the basic principles which are so often forgotten or ignored. Many texts give details of nutrient requirements and the analysis of individual feedstuffs. These can be used effectively only when good husbandry, housing and general welfare are in place. Good nutrition is essential for good health. Health should be regarded as a positive concept embracing complete physical and social wellbeing and not merely the absence of disease or infirmity.

The dairy cow is the most complex farm animal as she can be growing, lactating and pregnant all at the one time. Thus the fate of dietary energy and protein is an interaction between these various physiological demands plus that for maintenance, all of which are themselves changing almost continuously. The main nutrients required are:

- Energy
- Protein
- Fibre
- Major elements
- Trace elements
- Vitamins
- Water

Ruminant digestion

The dairy cow as a ruminant has a highly adapted digestive system to enable it to break down the cellulose and other components of grass and other forages which it has the unique ability to utilise. In order to do this, the ruminant relies on a microbial ecosystem which it has evolved. The microbes feed the ruminant and in turn the ruminant feeds the microbes. Maintaining the correct conditions in the rumen to encourage optimal microbial fermentation is the key to the health and productivity of the high-yielding dairy cow.

The rumen is a specially modified forestomach and is in fact a carefully controlled fermentation chamber which supports a microbial population in an anaerobic environment. The temperature of the rumen is controlled by the cow's homeothermic mechanisms and the pH stabilised by the production of salivary bicarbonate and phosphate. The rumen and reticulum may have a volume of 180–200 litres in an adult cow. It is constantly contracting (every 30–60 seconds), thus ensuring that the contents are thoroughly mixed. Bacteria, which are the main ruminal microbes, secrete a wide variety of enzymes that cleave the linkages of carbohydrates. It is a co-operative effort of a number of organisms acting in synergy as no single organism is capable of digesting the substrate completely by itself.

The organisms that ferment the plant cell wall operate at an optimum pH of around 7. These bacteria are sensitive to acidity and will not function properly at a pH much below 6.2. The principal end product of cellulose fermentation is acetate, an important precursor of milk fat. The organisms that ferment starch and sugar to produce propionic and butyric acids are more tolerant to acid conditions. One species (*Selenomonas ruminantium*) can produce lactic acid and if it predominates can cause depression of rumen pH with resultant rumen stasis and acidosis.

Fungi and protozoa are also found in the rumen. Fungi degrade the bonds between lignin and cellulose. It is thought that protozoa mainly ferment starch and sugar and may digest bacteria, and assist in adaptation of the microflora to new substrates. For the rumen to function most effectively these should be a floating mat of long fibre which serves to trap smaller particles, allowing more complete fermentation.

In summary, the main end products of microbial carbohydrate digestion are acetic, propionic and butyric volatile fatty acids. Acetic acid predominates on high forage diets and propionic on high cereal diets. Butyric acid production is high in animals fed poorly fermented butyric silage. Much of the protein that enters the rumen is degraded to amino acids or ammonia and is then resynthesised into microbial protein. This resynthesis requires fermentable energy, and bacterial growth may be severely limited by lack of energy. It is not appropriate to consider energy and protein requirements in isolation. For optimal microbial growth it is essential to have *diet synchrony* (Fig. 3.1). If the diet is too high in protein relative to energy content excess ammonia is produced and this places further demands on energy to convert it to urea in the liver. A shortage of ammonia in the rumen can likewise result in poor microbial growth.

Factors influencing rumen fermentation

Salivation

The average cow needs to produce 100–150 litres of saliva each day to maintain a preferred rumen pH of 6–7. This saliva will contain in the order of 3.5 kg bicarbonate. The saliva is necessary to buffer the volatile fatty acids produced in the

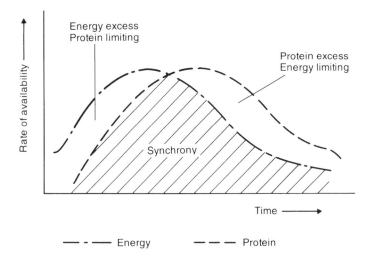

Fig. 3.1   Diet synchrony.

rumen. If the diet is acidic, as frequently will be the case when grass silage is being fed, there is an even greater need for adequate buffering. In order to achieve this level of saliva production the cow will make 30 000–50 000 chewing movements each day. To ensure that sufficient chewing takes place, the cow must ingest 2 kg of long fibre. It is suggested that the average length of fibre in the diet must be at least 2 cm with some at least 4 cm in length. Each kilogram of fibre will stimulate 20–30 minutes' chewing. Ideally the cow will spend 10–11 hours eating and chewing per day. Most of the chewing in adult cows will be done when lying down. At any time, 60% of cows should be chewing their cud when resting.

The formidable saliva production necessary will only be achieved if the cow is 'happy' or content. This means freedom from stress and comfortable lying conditions. Cow comfort and lying time are clearly of paramount importance. Studies have shown that under comfortable conditions a cow will lie for up to 14 hours each day. Under poor conditions such as those found in small, poorly bedded, uncomfortable cubicles the cow may lie for only 6 or 7 hours or less. (Compare the health and productivity of the human after several nights of broken sleep!)

Some cows low in the pecking order or small heifers will be bullied and their productivity will suffer partly due to their inability to compete for food or to digest it properly. Some cows are constantly disturbed throughout the day by cleaning or feeding operations and it is impossible for them to have adequate lying time. Cows perform better if housed in a quiet clean environment and are handled gently and in a consistent manner.

In summary, high forage rations stimulate saliva production and favour a pH over 6. A higher pH favours acetate production and a higher milk fat percentage. Feeding excessive amounts of concentrate stimulates less saliva production and favours propionic acid fermentation, resulting in decreased pH (below 6) and reduced feed intake with impaired microbial production.

Long fibre is necessary

- to stimulate rumination;
- to form floating mat in rumen;
- to stimulate chewing and saliva production.

Insufficient fibre
↓
Poor rumination
↓
Ruminal distension + acidosis

A ration must be balanced, with good sources of long fibre such as straw which are slowly fermented but stimulate saliva production, against quickly fermented feeds such as molasses and ground cereals which stimulate very little salivation.

Nutrient requirements

The high-producing dairy cow does a prodigious amount of metabolic work. The balance between the demands of lactation and pregnancy are closely related and finely balanced. In mammals, nutrients are utilised by tissues involved in maintenance and growth, and for establishing body reserves including energy stores (lipids), glucose reserves (glycogen) and amino acid reserves (labile protein). In the dairy cow two additional tissues utilising a substantial portion of maternal nutrients are the developing fetus and the mammary gland. The nutritional requirements have been published by The Ministry of Agriculture, Fisheries and Food (MAFF) (1980, 1984) the National Research Council (1985) and the Animal Food Research Council (AFRC, 1993).

It has been recognised for a long time that the lactation curve has a characteristic shape. It has been proposed that prediction of the shape of the curve and the amplitude of its peak would theoretically allow matching of energy input with the anticipated energy output in milk. These models are widely used in computer programmes to calculate the daily energy requirements for groups of dairy cows. However, it should be remembered that these predictions are inevitably based on curves modelled on historical data.

During the *first phase*, normally the first 10–12 weeks of lactation, from immediately after calving milk production increases rapidly. Milk fat percentage starts at a high level and inversely follows the lactation curve. These are natural adaptations to the needs of the nursing calf augmented by genetic selection. Dry matter intake rises after calving but lags behind the needs of the rapidly increasing milk production. The cow is able to consume less energy than she is expending. There is inevitably an energy gap and the cow calls on fat reserves to fill the difference between energy intake and energy requirements. Protein intake also has to be high at this time if milk production is not to be compromised. This is a most difficult phase for feeding because the cow has to adjust from eating a high fibre low energy diet during the dry period to a high energy low fibre diet in early lactation. There is also the need to compensate for a dramatic increase in mineral turnover.

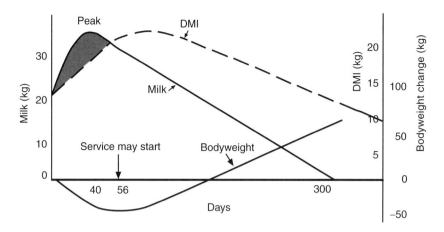

Fig. 3.2 Milk yield, dry matter intake (DMI) and body weight change.

Failure to achieve a smooth transition from the dry to early lactation stage results in poor production and frequently metabolic disease and impaired fertility on many farms.

It is accepted that the cow will lose body weight over this period (Fig. 3.2). The typical Friesian can reasonably lose 35–40 kg or about 0.5 of condition score in the first phase. A Holstein may lose almost twice this body weight. If weight loss is greater than this then metabolic disease may occur or fertility may be compromised.

During *phase two* (weeks 12–24 of lactation) dry matter intake is at its maximum. The use of forage should be exploited to the full and the cow should no longer be in negative energy balance.

Phase three from around week 24 completes the lactation and is the period when yield begins to fall. During this period the cow should be able to restore weight lost in early lactation as well as supporting the increasing demands of the developing fetus.

Phase four is the dry period which ideally should last 6–8 weeks. Rations are predominantly based on forage and should be adequately supplemented with vitamins and minerals. During the latter weeks of the dry period the rumen of the cow should be prepared for the diet it is going to be fed in early lactation. It takes the rumen microflora 10–14 days to adjust to a new substrate.

Dry matter intake (DMI)

When formulating rations for dairy cows by far the most important considera-tion is how much the cow is capable of eating. Small or subtle refinements in diets are of little relevance if the cow is unable to consume it all! Dry matter intake is influenced by numerous factors including body weight, forage quality and digestibility, stage of lactation, milk production levels, exercise, environment, management, cow comfort, social interactions, body condition, balance of ration, palatability and feeding frequency. Dry matter intake is the most important factor in diet formulation and is the most difficult to measure in the on farm situation.

There are many theories regarding the factors that control the cow's appetite, such as concentrations of blood glucose, volatile fatty acids, and various hormones. Recent work has shown the importance of rumen receptors. Whatever the exact mechanisms, probably the main factors are

- the metabolic needs of tissues (hunger);
- the size and digestive capacity of the rumen (rumen fill);
- the effect of palatable food (appetite).

Dry matter intake is the biggest uncertainty in formulating rations for dairy cows. The fact that some cows can get very fat suggests that feed intake is under fairly imprecise control. There is evidence that cattle eat to satisfy their demand for energy for production and maintenance of body weight.

Forage digestibility

Dry matter intake is affected by forage digestibility (D value). Within a plant species, stage of maturity at harvest has a major influence on digestibility and therefore on intake of the forage. On average, intake rises by about 0.15 kg DM/unit increase in D value of the forage.

Forage digestibility governs rate of passage and thus the amount of food consumed. Cell wall is digested less quickly than cell content. Young grass with a large proportion of its carbohydrate in cell content is digested quickly. Slowly digested poor quality forages are retained longer in the rumen, take up space and inhibit further consumption. Digestibility of low quality forage is inhibited if rumen organisms are not there in sufficient numbers because of the lack of energy and rumen-degradable protein for their development. The chemical component of foods that determines their rate of digestion is neutral detergent fibre (NDF), which is in itself a measure of cell wall content; thus there is a negative relationship between the NDF content of feeds and the rate at which they are digested. Some foods that have the same digestibility but differ in NDF (or cell wall content) will promote different intakes, e.g. legumes with less cell wall content will be consumed in about 20% greater quantities than grasses.

Rumen capacity

Rumen capacity governs forage intake. High yielding cows have a large rumen capacity and hence high dry matter intakes. It is policy to encourage rumen development at an early stage by appropriate provision of long fibre. To achieve optimum intakes of forage the amount on offer should exceed actual intake. With concentrates the animal is satisfied long before the capacity of the rumen is reached. Intake is presumably limited by the ability of the animal to metabolise the concentrate. Research findings suggest that somatotrophins enhance metabolism and increase food intake.

Cows will eat more food than is strictly necessary. The taste of food such as sugar beet will increase intake as will factors such as competition and novelty, e.g. a third midday feed. The standard dry matter intake equation for lactating dairy cows is (MAFF, 1984):

$$DMI = 0.0025\,W + 0.1\,Y,$$

where DMI = dry matter intake (kg/day), W = liveweight (kg) and Y = milk yield (kg). In the first 6 weeks of lactation these figures are reduced by 2–3 kg DMI/day.

There is no satisfactory equation for predicting the dry matter intake of dry cows. In pregnant animals two opposing factors can influence feed intake. The need for increased nutrients for the developing fetus causes intake to rise, but by reducing the effective volume of the abdominal cavity limits the room for rumen expansion. This in turn tends to decrease intake, especially if the diet is mainly forage. Fat animals similarly have less capacity for rumen expansion.

During the 2- to 3-week period approaching parturition the cows should be on a rising plane of nutrition to compensate for reduced dry matter intake, to prevent negative energy balance and subsequent mobilisation of body tissue and to meet the requirements of advanced pregnancy. Reasons for a reduction in dry matter intake include:

- Low quality, high fibre diets. Forages with a low digestibility will slow the rate of passage and remain in the rumen longer.
- Chemical feedback from low rumen pH, high levels of blood ketone, non-esterified fatty acid or urea.
- Physical factors such as non-availability of food, restricted feeding space, food that has undergone secondary fermentation.

Cows are like people and they will avoid stale or spoiled food. Maximum dry matter intake will only be achieved when fresh palatable food is freely available.

Energy requirements (Fig. 3.3)

The concept of the requirements for energy and protein of the dairy cow is the subject of ongoing debate. General guidelines on feeding are manifold. A series of AFRC recommendations from the Technical Committee on Responses to Nutrients (TCORN) have been published (AFRC, 1993). The energy systems that have been most improved have been those for the lactating dairy cow. Efficiency of utilisation of metabolisable energy varies less in the cow than in the fattening animal. The energy content of milk is less variable than liveweight gain.

From Fig. 3.3 it would appear that the net energy (NE) system is the most attractive as it directly relates to what is available to the animal. It is the basis of the energy systems adopted in the US and in The Netherlands. The main difficulty

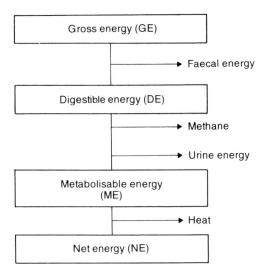

Fig. 3.3 Energy requirements.

in its use is the fact that the animal uses the energy available with differing levels of efficiency:

- Efficiency for milk yield is approximately 60%.
- Efficiency for weight gain is 50%.

This means that three values are quoted for each food according to how they are used by the animal.

The UK uses the metabolisable energy (ME) system (AFRC, 1993). This system relates to the food and means that only one value is given to each feed. In practice, as the systems are further refined, they are moving closer together. The quality of the diet influences the efficiency of the conversion of ME to NE.

- *Maintenance allowances (ME_m), including activity allowance and safety margin*
  $ME_m = 8.3 + 0.091\,W$ (from MAFF, 1975), where W = liveweight (kg).
  $ME_m = 63$–$67\,MJ$ for cows 600–650 kg liveweight.
- *Milk production (ME for milk)*
  ME for milk = 5.3 MJ/kg (4% fat, 3.2% protein).
  Based on ME for milk (MJ/kg)
  $= [(0.376 \times \% \text{ fat} + 0.209 \times \% \text{ protein}) + 0.946] \times 1.694.$
- *Adjustments to allow for weight gain or weight loss*
  Add 34 MJ ME/kg weight gain.
  Deduct 28 MJ ME/kg weight loss.

The first essential is to estimate the energy requirements and then to select foods that can supply these requirements. Energy is always given first consideration because the energy-supplying nutrients in food are present in the greatest quantity. If a diet is constructed to meet other nutrient requirements first and is then found to be low in energy a major revision of its constituents will probably be needed. A further feature of the energy-containing nutrients which distinguishes them from the others is the manner in which liveweight gain or milk production responds to the changes in quantities supplied.

The energy in the diet is derived from several sources. Carbohydrates account for between 50 and 80% of the dry matter in the cow's diet and most are fermented to some degree in the rumen. Microbes break down carbohydrates to volatile fatty acids (VFAs) acetate, propionate and butyrate. The rumen wall can absorb these metabolites. VFAs provide 50–70% of the cow's total energy intake. When large amounts of fibre are fed the predominant volatile fatty acid produced is acetate, accounting for 69–70% of the total VFAs. In addition to providing the energy needs of the cow, acetate is the major precursor of butterfat. When higher proportions of sugars (e.g. molasses) and starches (e.g. barley or maize) are consumed relatively more proprionate is produced.

Fats and oils can also make up an important part of the energy in the cow's diet. Fats have 2.25 times as much energy per unit of dry matter. Caution is required as an excess of fat (over 5% of dry matter of diet available for rumen digestion) may prove toxic to the rumen microbes.

Protein requirements

Traditionally, proteins in foods for ruminants were evaluated in terms of crude protein and digestible crude protein (DCP). This has for some time been regarded as unsatisfactory because it makes no account for the formation of microbial protein in the rumen. The Agricultural and Food Research Council (AFRC, 1993) laid down the principles for meeting the metabolisable protein (MP) demands of the high yielding cow (Fig. 3.4). The metabolisable protein system is now recognised as the official UK system for describing the protein requirements of ruminant livestock and replaces the DCP system. It has also been recognised that energy and protein requirements have very important interactions and that formulating to energy or protein standards in isolation is not sufficient.

Metabolisable protein is defined as the total digestible true protein (amino acids) that is available to the animal for maintenance and production purposes after digestion and absorption of the feed in the animal's digestive tract. Metabolisable protein is made up of two components: an effective rumen-degradable fraction (ERDP) and a digestible undegradable feed protein fraction (DUDP). It is the protein equivalent of the metabolisable energy system.

Microbial protein is synthesised using amino acids and non-protein nitrogen which results from degradation of feed protein in the rumen. This process is energy dependent and emphasises the critical link between supplies of fermentable metabolisable energy (FME) and degradable protein. Fermentable energy represents that portion of the total energy supplied as sugar (e.g. molasses), starch (e.g. cereals) and digestible fibre (e.g. sugar beet pulp). It does

(a) Digestible crude protein

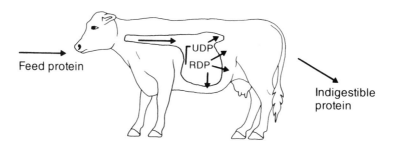

Feed protein

Indigestible protein

(b) Rumen degradable
   (RDP)/undegradable protein (UDP)

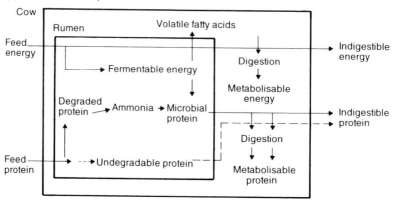

Feed protein

UDP
RDP

Indigestible protein

(c) Metabolisable protein

Cow

Rumen   Volatile fatty acids

Feed energy   Indigestible energy

Fermentable energy   Digestion

                                        Metabolisable energy

Degraded protein → Ammonia → Microbial protein   Indigestible protein

                                        Digestion

Feed protein ----→ Undegradable protein   Metabolisable protein

Fig. 3.4 Protein systems for dairy cows.

not include energy supplied by fat and prefermented products (e.g. silage fermentation acids).

The metabolisable protein requirement is defined by the liveweight of the cow, liveweight change, and the milk yield and protein content. The difference between requirement and microbial protein supply must be met by DUDP. In reality there are two degradable protein fractions: a quickly (QDP) and a slowly (SDP) degraded fraction. Together these make up effective rumen degradable protein (ERDP). By definition the QDP fraction is rapidly available as a source of protein to the microbes. The SDP fraction is more slowly available and the extent of degradation depends in part on duration of time in the rumen. The outflow rate of material from the rumen depends on the level of feeding and, as a consequence, is much faster for a high than a low yielding cow.

The key is not only to provide a balanced supply of fermentable energy and degradable protein in terms of absolute levels, but also to provide the energy and the protein in such a form to ensure synchronous release and thus optimum protein production. Too little fermentable energy results in inadequate bacterial growth with reduced forage intake, lower milk yield and lower milk protein. If fermentable energy is supplied in excess of microbial requirements acidosis may occur with subsequent reduced forage intake and lower milk output.

Fibre

In addition to the fact that fibre contained in forage provides a large portion of energy in the diet, it is necessary for optimal digestibility of the ration, as discussed previously. Fibre levels were expressed as crude fibre, but this has largely been replaced by neutral detergent fibre (NDF), which is essentially lignin, cellulose and hemicellulose. It can be regarded as a measure of the plant cell wall material, and is considered a better measure for predicting total dry matter intake. As plants mature their fibre content shifts from hemicellulose to lignin and cellulose, and their feed value reduces.

Acid detergent fibre (ADF) is essentially cellulose and lignin and excludes hemicellulose, and there is a good relationship between it and the extent to which food is digested. In the UK the ADF method was modified using increased strength of acid and increasing boiling time. Thus the term modified acid-detergent fibre (MADF) evolved.

For the high yielding cow the NDF should be 25–28% of the dry matter of the ration, with at least 22% NDF in dry matter of forages (National Research Council, 1985).

Major elements

Minerals play an essential role in dairy cow nutrition. The total mineral content of the lactating cow's diet is a small percentage of the total dry matter intake. Dairy cows on a good balanced diet with a normal concentrate forage ratio will have a good balance of calcium and phosphorus. Disagreement exists over the nutritional standards with regard to minerals. One of the main difficulties is in the great variability of absorption. Cows do not choose minerals selectively and it is essential to ensure that they are mixed in a ration that they are obliged to consume.

Supplemented minerals are widely available and are frequently fed to excess.

Calcium

Calcium circulates either as calcium ions or protein bound, approximately half in each form. Small amounts are complexed to free fatty acids and phosphate. The calcium ion possesses physiological activity, and is important for function of cell membranes, in muscular contractility, nervous irritability and blood coagulation.

A large part of the body calcium is contained in the mineralised skeleton. Only about 12 g is in the extracellular pool and is freely exchangeable. During the dry period the requirement is low, but at the onset of lactation the requirement is immediately high; 30 kg milk contains 36 g calcium which represents four times the calcium in the blood. The absorption and secretion of calcium are under the very strong homeostatic control of the parathyroid hormone and vitamin D_3 (1,25 dihydroxy cholecalciferol). Calcitonin works in the reverse way to these hormones and is secreted in times of hypercalcaemia.

Calcium content is high in forages, sugar beet pulp, ground limestone and dicalcium phosphate. The recommended level for high yielding dairy cows is 0.66% DMI.

Phosphorus

The phosphorus content of a mature cow is about half that of calcium. It is distributed differently, with the Ca:P ratio 2:1 in bone. Phosphorus is present in higher concentrations in body fluids and soft tissue. Phosphorus has many physiological functions unrelated to calcium. It is a component of nucleoprotein and hence is vital in tissue growth. It is involved in the transport of phospholipids and is a key component of energy-rich compounds such as ATP and creatine phosphate.

In the dairy cow the phosphorus component of the saliva makes an important contribution to metabolism. Most of this phosphate will be recycled via absorption in the lower gut. Phosphate input into the rumen is thought to be essential for healthy microbial growth.

As with calcium, absorption varies greatly. Requirements have been downgraded by one third (TCORN), but there is considerable debate as to whether the lowering of standards was justified. Primary phosphorus deficiency is not common in dairy cows. A phosphorus deficiency is most likely to be secondary to calcium deficiency. An all-grass diet, however, may be deficient in phosphorus.

Phosphorus content is high in cereals, cereal byproducts, and monosodium and dicalcium phosphates. The recommended level is 0.4% DMI.

Magnesium (see also pp. 105–6)

Magnesium is closely associated with calcium and phosphorus. Magnesium is the most common enzyme activator, e.g. in oxidative phosphorylation, in phosphate transferase and in reactions in the tricarboxylic acid cycle. It is therefore essential for the metabolism of carbohydrate and lipids. A deficiency produces irritability in many species. Total magnesium in the cow amounts to about 200 g, around 70% of which is present in the skeleton. Soft tissue accounts for about 29% and only 1% (about 2 g) is circulating in body fluids.

Input of magnesium relies very much on day-to-day dietary supply. The dairy cow giving 25 litres of milk requires 5.5 g per day to remain in balance. As absorption from the diet is very variable a cow requires between 14 g (at 35% availability) and 50 g (at 10% availability). There is little apparent control over input/output regulation and homeostasis is weak, although the kidney appears to play a vital role in preventing hypermagnesaemia.

As with other major minerals, the main difficulty in assessing requirements is the great variability in absorption. Pasture species, fertiliser application, lack of dietary fibre and high rumen ammonia concentrations are all factors that influence magnesium absorption.

Methods of increasing magnesium supply

Cows cannot store magnesium and therefore require an adequate supply every day.

- Inclusion of supplementary magnesium in concentrate is one of the most reliable methods of ensuring regular intake.
- Medicating the water supply with soluble salts, such as magnesium chloride or acetate, can be effective but is relatively expensive. Care must be taken to ensure that no alternative water supplies, such as rivers or streams, are available.
- Pasture dressing with 17 kg finely ground calcined magnesite per ha is used in areas where there is maximum dependence on grass and no supplementary concentrate is fed. It is most effective on controlled systems of grazing such as strip grazing. It may have to be repeated at regular intervals if there is heavy rainfall.
- Mineral supplements. Spreading 60 g calcined magnesite per day per animal on silage or mixing with cereal will prove useful. Magnesium minerals are not very palatable and free access or licks cannot be relied on as the sole source of magnesium.
- High magnesium boluses release magnesium in the reticulum over a period of several weeks. They may not provide sufficient magnesium for high yielding cows and should be regarded as a top-up source of magnesium.
- Magnesium fertiliser may not be effective on all soil types but can provide a longer-term source. Fertilising should be repeated every 3–5 years.

General prevention of hypomagnesaemia

- Sodium and potassium. Ensure plenty of sodium in the diet and control use of fertilisers containing potassium.
- Extra fibre. Provision of fibre in the form of hay straw or big bale silage helps to slow the rate of passage and allows better absorption of magnesium.

- Stress. Protection from cold and wet. Avoid sudden changes in the diet or environment.
- Adequate energy in the diet is important in prevention of hypomagnesaemia. Lack of fermentable energy results in high levels of ammonia in the rumen when excess RDP is available. High levels of ammonia in the rumen reduce magnesium absorption.
- Pasture species. Develop pasture that is slower growing and takes up more magnesium in the spring. Inclusion of clover increases magnesium content of the pasture.

Potassium

Potassium plays an important part, along with sodium, chlorine and bicarbonate ions, in the osmotic regulation of body fluids, and also in nerve and muscle excitability. Potassium content of plants is generally very high. Most normal forage-based diets will have more than adequate amounts. One exception may be diets containing large amounts of distillers' grains ('draff'), which is deficient in many soluble elements including potassium.

Sodium

Most sodium is found in body fluids and soft tissues. Like potassium it is concerned with acid–base balance and osmotic regulation of body fluids. It also plays a part in transmission of nerve impulses and in the absorption of sugars and amino acids from the digestive tract. Most sodium is ingested in the form of common salt. Diets of vegetable origin tend to be low in sodium. Spring grass is often low in salt.

Chlorine

Chlorine is associated with potassium and sodium in acid–base balance. There is evidence that it is sodium rather than chlorine that is the chief limiting factor in salt-deficient diets. The main source of this element is common salt.

Sulphur

Most of the sulphur in the diet is contained in proteins containing the amino acids cystine, cysteine and methionine. The vitamins biotin and thiamine, the hormone insulin and coenzyme A all contain sulphur. Normally it was assumed that as protein was the main source of sulphur, a deficiency of sulphur would indicate a deficiency of protein. In recent years, with increasing amounts of urea in ruminant diets it is recognised that sulphur may limit synthesis of protein in the rumen.

Trace elements

Trace element deficiency should not be a major problem in cattle fed on forage and concentrates, which will in most cases contain ingredients from diverse sources. It is unlikely that all raw materials, cereals, forages and byproducts will be mineral deficient and such mixed diets ensure that trace elements are normally present in sufficient quantities. Cows fed solely on home-grown forage and cereal are most likely to be deficient if the crops are grown on soil known to be deficient in minerals. Most deficiencies will not be primary, as a result of an absolute deficiency of the trace element, but will be secondary, as a result of interaction between elements resulting in impaired absorption.

Copper

Copper is widely distributed in foods and under normal conditions the diet of dairy cows should contain adequate amounts. Copper plays a vital role in many enzyme systems and an important part in oxygen metabolism, in oxidative phosphorylation and is present in certain plasma proteins such as caeruloplasmin.

Most copper deficiencies in cattle are induced. The principal determinants of hypocuprosis in grazing cattle are probably soil molybdenum (Mo), soil sulphur, soil pH (high values encourage Mo intake), sward maturity, rainfall, fertiliser use and soil ingestion (iron depresses copper uptake) rather than copper deficiency of soil or herbage on all but the most impoverished sandy soils.

Certain pastures on calcareous soils in parts of England and Wales have been known for over 100 years to be associated with a condition in cattle described as 'teart', characterised by unthriftiness and scouring. Infertility has long been associated with copper deficiency in cattle, but there is little published evidence that deficiency leads to impaired reproduction unless molybdenum is involved. Molybdenum excess is associated with delays in onset of oestrus, impaired conception and anoestrus.

Supplementation

- Pasture dressing with copper sulphate is possible and inexpensive, but this method does not overcome the inhibition of absorption by molybdenum, sulphur or iron.
- Copper salts can be added to concentrates or forage.
- Copper oxide needles contained in gelatin capsules lodge in the reticulum and are slowly released over a period of months.
- Glass boluses containing copper, cobalt and selenium are another form of oral supplementation, supplying the trace elements over a period of months.
- Copper proteinates appear to give better responses in high molybdenum pastures. They are relatively expensive if used as the only means of copper supplementation.
- Copper injections overcome the difficulties of impaired absorption but are somewhat restricted in use by the danger of toxicity if too large initial doses are given. Slower release injections are often associated with abscesses at the site of injection.

Cobalt

Most foods contain traces of cobalt. Cobalt is required by the micro-organisms in the rumen for the synthesis of vitamin B_{12}. Ruminants have an additional requirement for B_{12} to support glucose synthesis from propionate. Cobalt (and thus vitamin B_{12}) deficiency interferes to a significant extent with intermediary metabolism.

A deficiency of vitamin B_{12} is characterised by pining or wasting, pica and anaemia. There is some evidence to suggest that cobalt-deficient cattle may be more susceptible to parasitic and microbial infection.

Selenium

The principal function of selenium in animals relates to its intracellular presence in the antioxidant enzyme glutathione peroxidase (GSHPx) which uses various potentially dangerous peroxides as substrates. Vitamin E shares the role of antioxidant defence with selenium. Selenium is believed to enhance immune function, antibody production and neutrophil bacteriocidal activity. Selenium deficiency is usually attributed to shortage of element in the diet due to low selenium content in the soil.

At parturition, cows of low selenium status are more likely to retain their placentas than selenium-supplemented cows and they may be more susceptible to metritis, mastitis and cystic ovaries. Supplementation can be carried out via the feed, but there is a danger of toxic overdose as the safety margin is not high. Glass boluses are reliable. For growing heifers, see p. 25.

Iodine

Iodine is widely spread throughout body tissue, but its only known role is in the formation of the hormones triiodothyronine and tetraiodothyronine (thyroxin). The thyroid hormones accelerate reactions in most organs and tissues in the body, thus increasing basal metabolic rate, accelerating growth and increasing oxygen consumption. A diet deficient in iodine decreases the production of thyroxine, stimulating a compensatory hypertrophy of the thyroid gland (goitre).

Reproductive abnormalities are one of the consequences of reduced thyroid function; calves may be born weak or stillborn. Usually they will have evidence of goitre. Occasionally there will be some areas of alopecia. Iodine deficiency can be caused by a primary lack of iodine in the diet or by a secondary deficiency resulting from a high intake of brassicas, high calcium intake, heavy bacterial contamination of water or food or the intake of linseed meal or other sources of cyanogenetic glycosides.

Iodine occurs in traces in most foods, but foods of marine origin, e.g. fish meal, are rich sources. Iodised salt can be used in diets when a deficiency is suspected.

Vitamins

The fat-soluble vitamins, A, D and E are all essential for cattle.

Vitamin A

Vitamin A occurs in plant materials in the form of carotenoids – its precursors. The most important precursor is B carotene. The following disorders have been attributed to B carotene deficiency: silent or poorly detectable oestrus, delayed ovulation, poor insemination rate, lowered progesterone synthesis, increased occurrence of ovarian cysts, death of fetus in first trimester and higher disease rate of calves.

The effect of B carotene is still under discussion. Overall, the numerous scientific and field studies carried out in many countries show that B carotene supplementation is only successful in improving fertility in cows that were previously shown to be deficient, as shown by plasma analyses.

Fresh grass is an excellent source of B carotene, but a large proportion of the B carotene content may be destroyed in silage making. Vitamin A is stored in the liver and a cow that has been at grass for 6 months may store enough to meet her needs during the winter. Compound rations for dairy cows may be supplemented with vitamin A.

Vitamin D

Dairy cattle synthesise vitamin D_3 through the action of sunlight. Green plants are also a rich source. Vitamin D regulates the absorption of calcium through the gut wall and its concentration in extracellular fluid. The direct use of vitamin metabolites to prevent milk fever has been investigated by numerous workers. For growing heifers, see p. 26.

Vitamin E

The main function of vitamin E in the body is as an anti-oxidant, protecting cells from oxidative destruction. The role vitamin E plays in fertility is disputed. The fact that the endocrine glands have comparatively high levels of vitamin E would support the hypothesis that it has an effect on reproduction. Vitamin E is thought to promote release of FSH, ACTH and LH. Retained placenta is often associated with deficiencies of vitamin E and selenium. Vitamin E is thought to be important in udder health. Supplementation of deficient cows with selenium and vitamin E reduced infection rates at calving and throughout the lactation.

In normal circumstances the typical diet of a dairy cow containing grass or silage should supply sufficient vitamin E. For growing heifers, see p. 26.

Vitamin B complex

The water-soluble vitamin B complex including vitamins such as thiamine, riboflavin and biotin is synthesised in adequate amounts by the rumen microbes.

Water

Water is an essential nutrient, although it is commonly overlooked. A 600-kg cow eating maize silage and producing 45 kg milk may drink 113 litres at an environmental temperature of <16 °C and 140 litres of water at >20 °C.

Lactating cows require 2–2.5 kg drinking water for each kilogram of milk produced. Cows will drink about 14 times a day. Length of drink is short (about 1–3 min). They also like to drink immediately after being milked. Grazing cattle drink 2–5 times a day if they have free access. If access is limited, milk production falls. There should be at least one watering space per 20 head of cattle.

Feeds for dairy cows (see also Chapter 2)

In most high yielding herds in the UK cows are fed forage and some form of concentrate feed. Concentrate feed by definition contains a high concentration of nutrients (mainly energy) per kilogram of fresh weight. When the price of milk is greater than the price of purchased concentrate it is economical to feed purchased concentrates to dairy cows. If the price of concentrate rises or the value of milk falls then it may no longer be a viable proposition to feed large amounts of concentrate. In order to meet the energy requirements of high yielding cows some receive up to 70% of their rations as concentrate with the other 30% made up of forage. At this level the rumen microflora are finely balanced and rumen pH may drop, resulting in acidosis (p. 78) and other digestive upsets. Such high levels of concentrate feeding demand good access to high quality forage.

In general, where they have facilities, more farmers are attempting to maximise the utilisation of home-produced forage to meet the nutrient requirements of their dairy cows.

Forages

Grazing

The research carried out on grazing systems has shown that using the best techniques, it is possible to obtain a very high milk production per hectare grazed. The level of intake is, however, very variable, from 8 to more than 17 kg dry matter by 600-kg cows. It is inversely related to the filling effect which depends on the crude fibre content. Therefore cows have to be fed young highly digestible material if the intake is to be optimal. Spring grass about 10 cm in height has a D value of about 75% and an energy density of around 12 MJ/kg DM (referred to as the metabolisable energy ME or M/D of the food). It can in theory support a milk yield of around 30 litres. After midsummer D value may fall to around 60%, with an ME value of 9.5–10 MJ/kg DM.

Forage intake is also influenced by the amount of material available. Maximum intake is ensured when around 140% of intake is offered. Lower intakes in late summer and autumn seem to be linked to an increased area contaminated by defaecation.

Concentrates given during grazing reduced forage intake. The higher the quantity of concentrate the greater the reduction in forage consumption per kilogram of extra concentrate.

The main factors that have an effect on milk production per hectare would appear to be the stocking rate, the fertilisation level and supplementation with concentrates.

Grazing strategies

- Strip grazing whereby each day cows are given a fresh strip of grass is effective for utilising the growth of high quality grass. Little is wasted and cows defaecate on areas already grazed.
- Rotational grazing involves moving cows from pasture to pasture, allowing periods for recovery. Pastures may be rested for 4–8 weeks for regrowth.
- Set stocking means having a sufficient stocking density so that the rate at which grass is eaten matches growth.

It has been suggested that the effects of different systems are small compared with those due to stocking rate. There has been a trend in recent years for farmers to return to simple grazing systems, but the development of more complex systems with the increased use of nitrogenous fertiliser has highlighted the potential productivity of grassland.

Silage

Silage is the material produced by the controlled fermentation of a crop of high moisture content. Almost any crop can be preserved as silage, although the most common crops used are grasses, legumes and whole cereals, especially maize.

The first essential objective is the achievement of anaerobic conditions. In practice this is done by chopping the crop during harvesting, by rapid filling of the silo and by adequate consolidation and sealing. The second main objective is to discourage the activities of undesirable micro-organisms such as clostridia and bacteria which produce objectionable fermentation products. These bacteria can be discouraged by reducing the pH of the silage by encouraging the growth of lactic acid bacteria or by using chemical additives. The lactic acid bacteria ferment the naturally occurring sugars to a mixture of acids, mainly lactic. This increases the hydrogen ion concentration to a level at which undesirable bacteria are inhibited. The pH at which this occurs varies mainly with the dry matter content and buffering capacity of the crop. With grass crops with a dry matter content of 20% the achievement of a pH of around 4 will normally preserve the crop satisfactorily.

The type of silo is variable, ranging from plastic bags to large purpose-built structures of concrete, steel or wood. Probably the most common type is the clamp or bunker, which consists of three solid walls some 2–3 m in height, often built beneath a Dutch barn to protect it from the elements. When full it is covered with plastic sheeting and weighted with straw bales or rubber tyres. In recent years there has been a dramatic increase in the amount of silage conserved in big plastic bales weighing 0.5–1 tonne. Provided the plastic is not punctured this is a satisfactory method, allowing flexibility of usage.

Analysis of the ideal silage

Dry matter (DM) is the residue left after oven drying. For most grass silages it is corrected to recognise the presence of volatile components (18–50%).

Metabolisable energy (ME) is the energy value of the food (9.6–11.2 MJ/kg DM).

Crude protein (CP) is calculated from the nitrogen content of the feed.

Digestible crude protein (DCP) is predicted from the crude protein content of the feed (80–120 g/kg DM).

Digestibility (D value) is a measure of the digestible organic matter (60–70%).

Ash is a measure of the mineral content (less than 90 g/kg DM).

Ammonia N increases as protein is degraded during the ensilage/fermentation process (less than 100 g/kg TN).

pH is a measure of the acidity of silage and is a good indicator of fermentation quality (3.8–4.2).

Acid detergent fibre (ADF) indicates the level of cellulose and lignin present. A high level indicates a more mature forage of lower digestibility (150–400 g/kg DM).

Neutral detergent fibre (NDF) indicates the level of total fibre fraction present that is cellulose, lignin and hemi-cellulose (400–600 g/kg DM).

Fermentable energy (FME) reflects the proportion of metabolisable energy potentially available to the rumen microbes (8–9.5 MJ/kg DM).

Rumen acetate + butyrate/propionate ratio is an estimate of the likely pattern of fermentation when grass silage is on offer as the sole feed. Higher levels tend to be more supportive of milk fat production (2–5).

Quickly degraded protein (QDP) is a measure of the soluble protein as a proportion of total protein (0.5–0.7).

Slowly degraded protein (SDP) is a measure of the insoluble protein as a proportion of the total protein (0.25–0.35).

SDP rate reflects the potential rate of digestion of the slowly degraded protein (0.05–0.15).

Amino acid N is a measure of how much soluble nitrogen has been broken down. The larger the percentage, the less the breakdown, the better the silage (60–80% total soluble N).

VFA represents the less desirable fermentation acids (acetic and butyric) in silage. The lower the percentage the better the fermentation (20–40% total acids).

Lactic acid is the more desirable fermentation acid in silage. Higher values reflect the dominance of a lactobacillus fermentation (5–30 g/kg fresh weight).

Residual sugar is a measure of the sugar remaining after fermentation. Higher values are associated with higher intakes (0–15 g/kg fresh weight).

Neutralising value index is a measure of the amount of saliva needed to neutralise the acids in silage and raise the pH to rumen optimum levels. Values range from 0 to 5, with higher values associated with silages of lower intake potential.

Intake potential is a statement of the likely intake of a silage. It reflects the nutritional status of the silage in terms of overall digestibility and the consequences of the fermentation process, e.g. the extent of protein breakdown as described by the amino acid N status.

Starch in maize silage is a measure of maturity of the crop at the time of harvest. Higher starch figures are associated with a more mature crop and one that is likely to have higher intake characteristics (150–300 g/kg DM).

Intake of silage is also affected by time of access. There is an increase in silage intake of up to 30% when access time is increased from 5 to 24 hours. Chop length may have an effect on silage intake; 1–2 cm particle size increased intake.

Badly preserved silages are frequently produced from crops that are ensiled at too high a moisture content and that contain low levels of soluble carbohydrates. Silages of this type have pH values in the range 5.0–7.0. The main fermentation acid present is either acetic or butyric. The ammonia levels are above 200 g/kg. The productive performance of cows consuming this type of silage is poor as a result of depressed voluntary food intake and poor utilisation of silage nitrogen.

Additive-treated silages

Silage additives can be classed as fermentation stimulants, such as sugar-rich materials, inoculants and enzymes, which encourage the growth of lactic acid bacteria, and fermentation inhibitors, such as acids and formalin, which partially or completely inhibit microbial growth.

The use of acids has decreased due to the dangers of handling the material. The use of inoculants has increased, but the success depends on the inoculation rate and the presence of rapidly fermentable carbohydrate.

Ensiled whole crop cereals

Maize silage if cut at the correct stage is an excellent feed for dairy cows. Maize should be harvested when the ears are fully mature and the tops of the kernels have begun to dent. At this stage the corn is 30–35% DM. Silages harvested earlier tend to lose nutrients through seepage once ensiled. If it is too dry there may be problems with secondary fermentation. Trial work has shown that intakes of maize silage increase with dry matter content. In typical UK conditions maize silage has a dry matter content averaging above 30%, with an average dairy cow able to consume around 12 kg per day. It is an excellent source of energy but is low in ERDP. (Grass silage normally has an excess of ERDP.) In the UK it is now grown extensively on farms in the southern half of England and in Wales. Cows have been shown to perform well on a forage with a 50–50 mixture of grass and maize silage.

Whole crop wheat or barley has created interest in the past few years. The crop is cut before maturity and treated with urea which hydrolyses to ammonia and preserves the crop at around a pH of 5. It is becoming more popular in areas where it is not possible to grow maize.

Hay

Hay has a poorer nutritive value than silage because it is cut when the grass is more mature and fibrous. Typical M/D value is 8.5 which limits its use as an energy provider for the high yielding cow. A little hay (1–2 kg) is, however, an excellent source of digestible fibre, encourages rumination and is valuable when balancing the lack of fibre in young spring grass.

Straw

Straw has a low feed value but can play a part in increasing the dry matter of very wet silage and in buffering the lowering of butterfat produced by spring grass. Straw can be nutritionally improved by treating with sodium hydroxide or ammonium hydroxide. This can have the effect of increasing the M/D to around 8.5, which is similar to hay.

Other green food

Cows are fed brassicas such as kale, rape, cabbage and the tops of turnips and sugar beet. Kale and rape are good sources of energy and protein. However, they may contain toxic substances which can interfere with iodine utilisation. They are best cut and fed, as feeding kale in the field in autumn or winter can expend as much energy as is derived from the crop and leads to dirty udders and foot problems. Not more than one third of total DM intake should be of kale or rape.

Root crops

Root crops include turnips, mangolds and fodder beet. They vary in dry matter content (10% for turnips and 18% for fodder beet). They have the advantage of being highly palatable and are a good source of fermentable sugar. They are low in degradable protein and may provide a good balance with some grass silages. Fodder beet can be very dirty and this depresses intake.

Cereals

The major cereals fed are barley, maize, wheat and oats. These provide a good source of energy provided they form part of a balanced diet. The starch in cereals is fermented to volatile fatty acids in the rumen with a relatively higher proportion of propionate than acetate. The starchy cereals are of great importance in feeding dairy cows as they provide a source of energy of a higher density than can be obtained from forage and help to meet the energy requirements within the constraints of dry matter intake; 4–5 kg of a cereal at any one feed is considered to be the upper limit, otherwise rapid fermentation will cause a drop in pH and metabolic acidosis. The protein content of cereals is relatively low and around 80% is degraded in the rumen, making it a good source of microbial protein.

Oil seeds

The major oil seeds are grown in the tropics or semi-tropics. They include soya bean, ground nut, cottonseed and linseed. In recent years rape seed has been grown very successfully in the cooler temperate zones. The oil seed cakes and meals are residues after extraction of the oil. They are rich in protein, mostly rumen degradable and are also good sources of energy. They are excellent to complement cereals in a diet.

Soya is the most popular protein-rich vegetable-based product in animal feeding. It is rich in protein of a high biological value, having an excellent balance of amino acids. It is high in RDP and has to be treated in order to 'protect' the protein from rumen degradation if a substantial contribution of undegradable protein (DUDP) is required.

Groundnut meal is rich in crude protein and is a good source of ERDP. The balance of amino acids is not as good as that of soya bean. Reliable suppliers and correct storage are essential to avoid aflatoxin contamination.

Linseed is highly palatable and rich in oil. The oil is digested in the duodenum and provides a useful energy contribution. It is said to put a good 'bloom' on the animal's coat.

Rapeseed has a protein content comparable to soya bean meal. There was some evidence of toxic substances in some strains, e.g. erucic acid and glucosinolates, which affected palatability and in some cases fertility. The use of 'double zero' varieties which contain minimal levels of toxins are now mandatory in Europe. Compound manufacturers restrict its inclusion to within defined limits (<10%). There can be batch to batch variation.

Animal protein concentrates

The Bovine Spongiform Encephalopathy (No 2) Order 1988 forbids the sale for feeding to bovine animals of any feedingstuff in which protein of bovine origin has been incorporated. Subsequent orders have prohibited the use of animal or poultry protein in the diet.

Fish meal is an excellent source of DUPD. The meal is produced by cooking fish (mainly oily species) and, according to the amount of heating, the digestibility of the protein can vary from 0.95 to as low as 0.6. Recent trials have indicated that fish meal may have additional synergistic effects on silage digestibility. It also has a high mineral content.

Feeding animal protein to cows has received adverse publicity following the BSE outbreak and many farmers and some feed manufacturers no longer use it. There is also concern about the world's dwindling fish resources.

Feather meal is produced by hydrolysing, drying and grinding poultry feathers. Feather meal has a high energy and protein content but poor palatability. There is also the danger of salmonella contamination.

By-products

Brewer's grains are commonly delivered as a wet slurry from the brewery, although dried grains are available. They are a good source of ERDP and are reasonable in energy content. They are extremely palatable and useful for extending forage supplies. As they are 80% water the amount that can be incorporated into a diet is a maximum of 15–20 kg per cow per day.

Beet pulp is a product of the sugar beet industry. It is a palatable food and is a good source of digestible fibre.

Maize gluten is a by-product of starch extraction from maize. It is a good source of energy, most of which is in the form of digestible fibre. It can be a good source of protein (problems have arisen due to overestimation of protein contribution). Different batches of the product can have variable analysis, especially of protein. Regular analysis is essential if this by-product is making up a significant part of a diet.

Wheatings (also known as wheatfeed, pollards or thirds) is one of several by-products from flour milling. It is a useful source of energy from digestible energy and starch and has moderate protein content. It is a common ingredient in commercial diets.

Citrus pulp is similar in energy and digestible energy value to beet pulp. It generally has a low protein content. Palatability may be variable if there is a large proportion of lemon present.

Molasses is a by-product of the manufacture of sugar. It appears to stimulate ruminal fermentation and is high in energy, with little or no protein or fibre content. It is often used to improve palatability and increase food intake.

Purchased compound feeds utilise cereals and by-products of industrial processes to produce a balanced feed formulated to meet the requirements of the dairy cow. They are formulated to have an energy, protein and fibre content that will complement the forage and other feeds available on the farm. The type of concentrate required will also depend on the yield and hence energy and protein requirements of an individual herd.

Feeding strategies

Feeding strategies are adopted for reasons that may not be strictly nutritional. They are governed by the facilities available on a farm, the type of forage that can be grown successfully and the machinery and labour available to handle it.

'Steaming up'

Very few farmers now practise feeding large amounts of concentrate before calving in order that the cow can store resources to be drawn on in early lactation (known as 'steaming up'). Cows tended to calve down with large swollen udders. They frequently had to be premilked and were very prone to metabolic disease and mastitis. There are, however, great benefits to be gained from introducing up to 2 kg of concentrate 14 days prior to calving in order to condition rumen flora to post-calving diet and to stimulate the restoration of the rumen villae which in turn increases post-calving absorption from the rumen.

Feeding to yield

Feeding to yield involves attempting to meet the calculated requirements of the cow using standard allowances for maintenance and production. Most cows will be fed some concentrate and forage, usually grass in summer and silage in winter supplemented by concentrate.

One of the constraints to the achievement of high yields was the limitation of feeding concentrate in the parlour at milking time. With ever increasing yields cows had difficulty in consuming sufficient concentrate in the parlour. There was the problem of rumen acidosis (p. 78) and slowing down of fibre digestion. The limit is 4–5 kg/day for single concentrate feeds. To increase concentrate intake, a third feed usually at mid-day of cereal, compound or by-products such as sugar beet pulp is commonly given.

With the advent of computerised cow identification, out-of-parlour feeders provide the facility to feed a cow little and often. It is possible to divide the daily concentrate ration into up to 12 feeds per day. They have the added advantage of being able to record the amount of concentrate actually consumed. Feeding to yield depends on the accuracy of the estimations of the nutritive value of the diet and as always the uncertainty of dry matter intake. It also depends on accurate and current information on milk yield. If historical information is used yields may be chased 'downhill'. Further inaccuracies can occur due to errors in calibration of the feeders both in and out of parlour.

Lead feeding

Lead feeding was a strategy to encourage cows to reach their full potential, i.e. they were fed extra concentrate in addition to their calculated requirements. In early lactation the substitution rate of concentrates for forage is high. However, this practice has largely been discontinued partly because of quotas and partly because of the increased awareness of metabolic problems associated with overfeeding concentrate.

Flat-rate feeding (see also pp. 96–7)

The principle of flat-rate feeding is that all cows receive the same amount of concentrate, irrespective of their actual or potential milk production, together with silage ad libitum. The system works best when there is a compact calving pattern, with most cows at the same stage of lactation, and when input of concentrates is relatively low. Its success does depend on the cows having free access to good quality silage, so large quantities of good quality silage are required.

A variation of this system is the less extreme *stepped-rate* system where cows are fed a higher rate of concentrates, say 8 kg for the first 16 weeks, then 4 kg for the remainder of the lactation.

Complete diets (total mixed ration)

The main principle of the complete diet system [total mixed ration (TMR)] is that the animal receives slow and rapidly fermentable feeds in an intimate mix, thus balancing the inflow into the rumen of feeds of widely differing rates of fermentation, and thereby maintaining stable conditions in the rumen. When a portion of grass silage is replaced by an alternative forage, feed intake generally increases. The system has generally meant fewer metabolic problems and better butter fat. It is most useful for a farmer buying and feeding by-products and it affords the opportunity to buy the most competitively priced ingredients and incorporate them in a balanced diet. This does, however, require a degree of skill and nutritional knowledge.

When first introduced, some cows tended to over-eat and overfat cows with fatty liver syndrome resulted. The system is expensive to set up as a relatively costly mixer wagon and facilities to group cows are required. Unless there is a very tight calving pattern, two or three different rations may be required to accommodate the requirements of cows at differing stages of lactation.

Many farmers now adopt a partial complete diet system, feeding a large portion of the ration through a mixer wagon, topping up with concentrate in the parlour.

Buffer feeding

Buffer feeding was developed as a way of reducing losses of output from grazed pasture. It is now commonly used when cows are calving at grass during the summer. Typically, silage, maize silage, hay or straw is used. It is often fed after each milking before cows return to grazing. Best results will be obtained by holding cows in a paddock or yard before milking and making buffer feed available. It may be more satisfactory to make buffer feed available 24 hours a day. However, there is a danger than buffer feed may merely substitute for grass.

Dry cow feeding (see also pp. 96–7)

The dry cow period should be seen as the beginning of the next lactation. As nutrient requirements are much less than for the lactating cow, dry cows are often fed poorly balanced rations of inferior foodstuffs. Many postpartum diseases including hypocalcaemia, 'downer cow', ketosis, delayed conception, retained placentas, uterine infection and displaced abomasa find their beginnings in the dry period.

More than 60% of the total weight of the conceptus is gained during the last 2 months of the dry period. During the last 1–3 weeks of the dry period the cow must make the transition from body and fetal tissue deposition to tissue mobilisation to support lactation. There are really two stages of the dry period: the early stage up to 30 days precalving and the last 2–3 weeks precalving. The nutrient requirements of the two stages are rather different and the best method of management is to treat them separately.

The dry cow can have much of her requirements met with forage. It is essential that dry cows do not get too fat. The high forage diet helps to restore the health and function of the rumen. Excessive amounts of grass close to calving raise the calcium intake and may predispose to parturient paresis. Magnesium is an important cofactor in the absorption and mobilisation of calcium postcalving and adequate magnesium intake in the run-up to calving is also required to prevent hypocalcaemia.

Some concentrate should be fed in the second stage of the dry period in order to condition rumen flora to the post-calving diet and as a vehicle for mineral and vitamin supplementation. At this stage, dry matter intake will have dropped very significantly and it is important to increase the energy density of the ration in order to reduce the risk of fat mobilisation.

Trough space

In order to allow cows optimal opportunity to maximise dry matter intake they must be given sufficient trough space. The commonly recommended width is 24 cm in the UK when 24-hour access is allowed. When width is reduced to below 20 cm, intake is reduced. The recommended level for access to a clamp is 30 cm. Intake from a clamp may be 20% lower than for similar cows eating from a trough.

In a study of the behaviour of Friesian cows it was found that many high ranking animals demonstrated a strong preference to feed at a particular section of a feed barrier. Lower ranking animals will feed less if the trough space is not long enough to allow all cows to feed simultaneously.

Assessment of nutritional status

Diet formulation for dairy cows is not an exact science. There are many unknown factors that can influence dry matter intake, etc. There is frequently too much reliance on computer-based formulations and so it is essential that the veterinary practitioner is in a position to be able to check how the cows are dealing with a given feeding regime.

Feed quality

Analysis of both forage and concentrate may be available. This can be regarded as a useful starting point, but the value of the analytical results depends very much on how representative the sample was of the batch of food being currently fed.

Dry matter intake

Dry matter intake is possible to estimate more often on a group rather than an individual basis. Mixer wagons often have weigh cells enabling group intakes to be measured accurately. Unless the cows in the group are all at the same stage of lactation and of the same yield potential then individual intakes may be very variable. This will certainly be the case if cows more than 100 days calved, on full dry matter intake, are grouped with early lactation animals.

- Observe cows when undisturbed. This gives a good indication of cow comfort. At least 60% should be lying ruminating.
- Observe feeding behaviour.
- Check access to trough. Make sure trough height is not too great; 45 cm or higher will discourage less dominant cows. If many cows are observed with feed on their backs, troughs are probably too high.
- Physical condition of the trough may affect intake. Rough pitted surfaces may result in food spoilage.
- Food must be fresh and not piled on top of stale food.
- Make sure water supply is clean and accessible to all cows. Dominant cows may control availability. There should not be too many cows around the water trough at any one time.

Faecal consistency

- The gross appearance of fresh faeces can provide valuable guidelines as to the nutritional status of the cow. The consistency of the faeces depends on its water and fibre content. This in turn depends on the type of food and subsequent rate of passage.
- Normal faeces should have a medium porridge-like consistency. Ideally, the pats should have a concave surface and should be able to support a rose stem in the centre!
- A liquid or runny faeces with no real form suggests a diet low in fibre with too much degradable starch or protein in the diet, e.g. spring grass. Excessive mineral supplementation, e.g. magnesium, may also be the cause.
- Stiff or thick faeces are typical of diets high in fibre and low in energy, e.g. dry cow diets. Some diets low in ERDP will produce stiff faeces.
- Slow rate of passage may result in a mucoid covering of the faeces, e.g. acetonaemia.
- The presence of whole or partially digested grain may indicate incomplete digestion or accelerated rate of passage.

Milk production

Peak and persistency of yield should be monitored on a regular basis:

Peak $\times$ 200 = lactation yield (to achieve a lactation yield of 6000 litres a cow must peak at least at 30 litres).

After 100 days, yield declines by 2.5% each week or approx. 10% each month. If milk drop is more precipitous then cows are probably being underfed.

Milk quality

Details of the composition of milk are now available to farmers on a regular basis and provide valuable information on nutritional status. Milk quality is influenced by the genotype of the parents and many farmers have significantly altered the milk quality of their herds by strategic breeding policy.

Butterfat levels are influenced by fibre levels in the diet, i.e. an acetic fermentation in the rumen. When concentrate to forage ratio exceeds 60:40 butterfat percentage may fall. Butterfat traditionally falls in the UK when cows are eating lush spring grass, which, because of its low fibre content, is fermented in the rumen like a concentrate. Low butterfat levels respond quickly to the addition of long fibre to the diet in the form of hay, big bale silage or straw.

Milk protein is largely dependent on the supply of microbial protein which requires a balance of fermentable energy (FME) and rumen degradable protein (RDP) for its development. Generally, milk protein falls after a period of inadequate energy intake. Falling milk protein often occurs in parallel with a drop in body condition (milk protein below 3%, condition score below 2.) Initially the cow will respond by mobilisation of her own body resources. When these have been depleted, milk protein falls. On many UK farms milk protein falls in January and February as a result of underfeeding in late autumn and early winter. Low milk protein and low body condition scores are frequently accompanied by poor fertility.

Milk protein levels are notoriously difficult to raise in the short term. Given more food the cow will first restore body reserves before increasing milk protein production. Some undegradable proteins or 'protected', amino acids will undoubtedly increase milk protein. They may, however, not be cost effective. It is much more sensible to optimise rumen function and achieve high levels of microbial protein production.

When investigating an apparent fall in milk quality it is important to take account of the calving pattern. If there are many recently calved, high yielding cows fall in milk quality may simply be a dilution factor. Milk quantity broadly follows an inverse relationship with milk quality.

Body condition score

It is important for the individual farmer or herdsman to establish a consistent technique for body condition scoring. The five point scoring scheme is based on an assessment of two areas, namely the lumbar and sacral areas. Condition score ranges between 5 (obese) and 1 (very thin). The sacral area is useful when assessing fatter animals >3. The lumbar, on the other hand, is more useful at the other end of the scale (<3). The ideal score at calving is 3, falling to 2.5 in early lactation. Cows should enter the dry period at score 2.5–3.

This is a very valuable technique especially when used to compare groups of cows on individual farms. Scoring groups of dry and early lactation cows will clearly demonstrate the magnitude of condition score loss in the first critical weeks of early lactation. Cows should be regularly scored on all advisory or fertility visits. A condition score loss of > 0.75 points has been associated with reduced fertility. A condition score point approximately equates to a loss of 30–50 kg body weight depending on breed type.

Presence of disease

Monitoring the incidence of metabolic disease is a very useful tool for the practitioner in the assessment of a feeding regime.

Rumen acidosis

Subclinical or clinical acidosis can be a common problem in postpartum dairy cows. Cud dropping may be one of the observed signs. Rumen pH declines below 6 with a resultant drop in dry matter intake and milk yield. Acidosis often results from inadequate preparation of the rumen papilla and flora during the run-up to parturition. A smooth transition from dry period to early lactation is essential and sudden changes in feeding must be avoided. Invariably the early lactation diet will have a concentrate to forage ratio of > 60:40 on a dry matter basis. (See also p. 39.)

Prevention

- Improve the transitional diet from 10 to 14 days before calving. Include the forage to be fed post-calving. Introduce some post-calving concentrate (maximum 2 kg) to condition rumen flora and allow rumen papilla to be restored more quickly to optimum size.
- Limit daily increase of concentrate post-calving to 0.5 kg/day.
- Increase long fibre in the diet.
- Add buffer such as sodium bicarbonate (250 g/day is required). However, it is much cheaper to improve the supply of long fibre and cow comfort. Cows will produce 3.5 kg bicarbonate/day in saliva under optimum conditions.

Fatty liver syndrome

Fatty liver syndrome is a metabolic disorder which has been associated with decreased hepatic gluconeogenesis (Fig. 3.5). Evidence suggests that it may precede clinical ketosis. Fatty liver has been associated with reduced production,

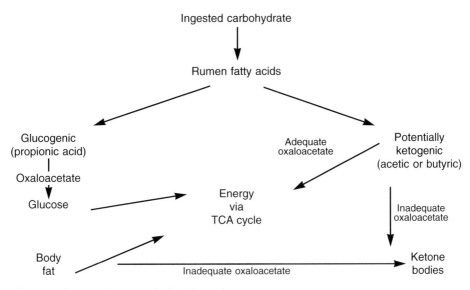

Fig. 3.5 Carbohydrate metabolism in ruminants.

reproductive performance and immune competence. During periods of excessive fatty acid mobilisation from adipose tissue ruminants are prone to the development of fatty liver. Hepatic uptake of fatty acids (NEFAs) is positively related to plasma concentration. When fatty acids are taken up by hepatocytes they are either oxidised to CO_2, partially oxidised to acetyl-coenzyme A and released as ketone bodies, or esterified mainly to triglycerides. Storage of triglycerides is increased as NEFA levels increase. Some triglycerides can be exported as lipoproteins, but the capacity of the bovine to do this is low. Fatty liver is commonly thought to develop postpartum, but it is likely that fat is often deposited from around day 17 prepartum to day 1 postpartum.

Liver fat levels can de determined using liver biopsy. An alternative method is to measure prepartum plasma NEFA, β-hydroxy butyrate (BHB) and glucose levels. These parameters are strongly correlated with liver triglyceride levels at day 1 (Fig. 3.6).

Animals with over 35% hepatic lipid concentrations will be clinically ill and have a poor prognosis. At 25–35% levels there will often be clinical signs. At 15–25% there may be no clinical signs but animals will be more susceptible to disease such as toxic mastitis.

Acetonaemia (ketosis) (see also p. 92)

Acetonaemia or ketosis is a metabolic disorder of the periparturient period and is interrelated with fatty liver. Clinical signs include diminished appetite, starting with concentrates, decreased milk production, loss of weight, hypoglycaemia, hyperketonaemia and sometimes nervous signs.

Primary acetonaemia occurs when not enough food is consumed to meet requirements and body reserves are utilised, resulting in ketonaemia. Secondary

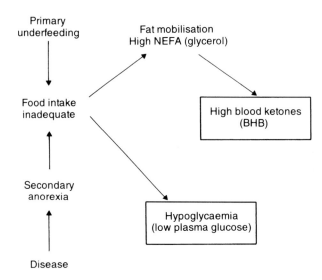

Fig. 3.6   Energy parameters.

acetonaemia occurs when other diseases, e.g. mastitis or metritis, cause a reduction in food intake and nutrient demands are not met. Acetonaemia may also occur if large amounts of ketogenic precursors are fed in the diet, e.g. butyric silage. An imbalance of nutrients in the diet, e.g. a high concentrate to forage ratio, can also result in ketosis.

The diagnosis of one case of primary acetonaemia will usually indicate that the whole of the early lactation group of cows are unhappy with their current diet.

Both fatty liver and acetonaemia are a result of fat infiltration into the liver and negative energy balance. When the dietary supply of glucose and that produced by glycogenesis are insufficient to meet requirements, fat is mobilised. A decrease in the availability and concentration of oxaloacetate is a major causal factor in acetonaemia. Fat mobilisation may result in excessive fatty acid uptake by the liver and production of ketone bodies. Both conditions are characterised by elevated plasma NEFA and ketone levels. Excessive fat accumulation reduces glycogenesis. Liver output of glucose is reduced, resulting in lowered insulin output with the vicious circle of further increase in fat mobilisation.

Prevention of acetonaemia and fatty liver

- Ensure dry cow management is given a high priority. Tender loving care is indicated.
- Environmental and group changes all cause stress.
- Make sure that cows do not get too fat in the dry period. Condition score 3 at calving is ideal.
- Cows should be introduced to an early lactation diet during the last 14 days of the dry period. This enables rumen flora to become adapted to the diet

they will receive in the lactation period and will ensure that the transition from the dry to early lactation stage is as smooth as possible.

- Dry matter intakes tend to drop sharply as parturition approaches. It is essential that cows at this stage are comfortable and have fresh food and water available.
- The best forage available should be given to cows immediately before calving and in early lactation. Frequently, dry or newly calved cows for convenience are fed poorer quality second or third cut silage.
- Any changes in diet should be made gradually.
- Ensure that supply of protein and energy in the diet is well balanced.

Displaced abomasum

Displaced abomasum usually occurs 1–3 weeks post-calving. In 90% of cases it is a left-sided displacement (LDA). A right-sided displacement (RDA) involves a twist or torsion on the right side. The aetiology is unclear, but risk factors include:

- Lack of dietary long fibre.
- Too high a concentrate to forage ratio in the diet.
- Too fat at calving.
- Sudden feed changes with rapid increase in concentrates.
- Lack of sufficient exercise.
- Poor quality forage before calving.

Milk fever or parturient paresis (see also p. 105)

As the milk yield of dairy cows in the UK has increased over the past 30 years, so has the overall incidence of milk fever, from around 3% to over 7%. Milk fever is a metabolic disease usually occurring between 12 hours before and 72 hours after parturition. It is most commonly seen in cows from their third calving onwards. The reason for hypocalcaemia is that some cows are unable to match their rapidly increasing requirements for calcium for milk secretion by absorbing sufficient calcium from their gut or by mobilising calcium from their own skeleton. Preventive strategies are aimed at ensuring that the strong homeostatic mechanisms that control blood calcium levels are well prepared. Stimulation of the release of parathyroid hormone (PTH) and the formation of 1,25-dihydroxy vitamin D_3 with the resultant increased absorption of calcium from the bone takes at least 24 hours (Fig. 3.7). The timing of preventive procedures is therefore important.

Prevention

- Avoid high concentrations of calcium in the diet during the dry period. This can be difficult in practice as most forages, including grass, have a relatively high calcium content. Clover, lucerne, beet pulp and kale all also have a high calcium content. It may be necessary to restrict grazing and feed low calcium

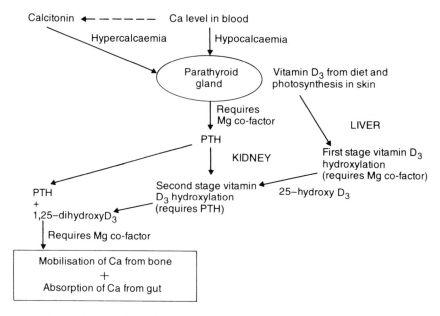

Fig. 3.7 Regulation of calcium homeostasis in the cow.

forage such as maize. Cereals are low in calcium, but milking cow concentrate will have a relatively high calcium content.
- Supplementation of the diet with monosodium phosphate may be indicated if hypophosphataemia has been identified as a concurrent problem. Ca:P ratio does not seem to be so important in the ruminant if vitamin D status is kept high.
- Avoid cows being too fat at calving.
- Avoid 'steaming up'. Milking cow concentrate is high in calcium.
- Magnesium supplementation may be required especially if dry cows are being fed on wet autumn grass. Magnesium is an important co-factor in the absorption and mobilisation of calcium.
- Drenching with a solution of calcium chloride for 3 days immediately post-calving can be successful especially if used following a low calcium diet in the dry period.
- Provision of long fibre in the form of hay, straw or big bale silage is considered to be effective in milk fever prevention. Long fibre will slow the rate of passage of ingesta and increase absorption of magnesium.
- Alteration of the ionic balance by increasing the acidity of the diet may facilitate the absorption of calcium. In the dry period cows are fed mainly forages with high K+ cation content. This results in a mild alkalosis (this can be checked using urine pH). There is some evidence to show that bone and kidney may be refractory to the effects of PTH in an alkaline metabolic state and the stimulatory effects are enhanced during metabolic acidosis. This has led to the use of mineral acids or acid salts in dry cow diets. Magnesium chloride, ammonium sulphate, calcium chloride and aluminium sulphate have all

been used with varying degrees of success. The feeding of silage which is relatively acid with or without additional salts has also proved to be effective. There is the possibility that prophylactic measures involving induction of acidosis only work when alkalosis is the predisposing factor.

- Large doses of vitamin D have been used successfully to prevent milk fever. The response is rather slow and to be effective injections must be given between 8 and 3 days precalving. The difficulty in predicting accurate calving dates may limit use.
- Vitamin D analogue (hydroxycholecalciferol) bypasses one of the hydroxylations in the kidney. This analogue therefore acts more quickly than vitamin D_3, and can be used at a lower dose rate closer to calving.
- Induction of calving and injection of vitamin D analogue has been used successfully when calving date is uncertain and the cow is judged to be a high risk animal.
- Reduce the amount of calcium required by not milking the cow out fully in the first few days. Milk production is limited by back pressure and demand for calcium is reduced.
- Calcium solution is frequently given as a prophylactic measure to cows that are about to calve. Injudicious use of calcium at this time, i.e. large depots of calcium solution injected subcutaneously, may be contraindicated because of the suppression of normal hormonal control mechanisms.
- Housing has been shown to reduce the incidence of milk fever in autumn calving herds when other preventive measures have proved ineffective.

Many of these preventive measures will not be effective in isolation. Once again, it is essential to have good dry cow management in place.

Infertility and lameness (see also Chapters 5 and 6)

Infertility and lameness are two of the most important production problems of dairy cattle and both are responsible for major economic loss. There are undoubtedly important connections between nutrition and both these conditions, but the links are by no means well established and some of the scientific evidence is equivocal. The aetiology of lameness and infertility is multifactorial and it is not always clear how much faulty nutrition is a contributing factor. It is, however, important, whenever possible, to make sure that nutrition is not playing any part in what might appear to be a complex equation.

Lameness has been highlighted as a major welfare problem for the UK dairy industry. The Dairy Herd Health and Productivity Service (DHHPS) suggests that the average dairy unit will have on average 30 cases of lameness per 100 cows. Some farms will experience two to three times that level. Factors involving husbandry, management, infectious agents and genetics may well be involved as well as nutrition.

Mineral imbalance resulting in rickets, copper deficiency causing developmental problems involving tendons and joints, and selenium deficiency associated with muscular dystrophy are all clearcut examples of cases where faulty nutrition undoubtedly results in lameness. Such examples are, however, comparatively rare in the modern dairy herd.

Laminitis, which is considered by many to be the forerunner of two of the most common manifestations of lameness, namely solar ulcer and white line disease, is most likely to have its starting point in the digestive tract. Difficulty in closing the energy gap in early lactation when the cow may only be attaining 75% dry matter intake frequently results in proportional overload of concentrate, with the concentrate : forage ratio being too high. It has been postulated that the rumen pH may drop below 5.5 with excessive production of lactic acid, histamine release and bacterial endotoxin production. These toxins may result in micro lesions in the laminae.

The causes of laminitis can be manifold. Experimental work with calves has produced foot lesions when toxins were injected, but this work does not appear to have been repeated in dairy cows. Other toxic conditions such as metritis and mastitis have produced laminitis. Diets too high in protein have been implicated in causing laminitis, but again experiments and trials have produced equivocal results. Grazing cows often have protein intakes far in excess of requirements without any deleterious effects. If protein does play a part it is unlikely to be the protein intake per se but rather the ratio of fermentable energy (FME) to rumen degradable protein (ERDP) in the diet. Low pH silage has also been associated with laminitis. This is another example where the explanation will not be as straightforward as low pH silage on its own but more importantly how well the total ration is balanced to counteract a high intake of acid material.

Nutrition and fertility (see also Chapter 5)

Energy

Energy is the first limiting dietary component to optimal dairy cow performance in early lactation. The modern dairy cow with high genetic potential will make milk production her first priority. This means that when energy output exceeds intake the cow will mobilise her own body resources. This is perhaps inevitable, but it is the magnitude of the deficit that may influence subsequent fertility. The extent and duration of negative energy status of the cow is one of the most important factors influencing when she will return to normal ovarian function after calving. The degree of energy deficit in the first 20 days post-calving can have a very significant effect on the time of first ovulation.

Experimental work has shown that it does not appear to be the volume of milk produced, but rather the dry matter intake that governs energy deficit. Intake of feed of anoestrous cows continually lagged behind that of cycling cows. Not only did anoestrous cows consume less at week 1 postpartum but also the difference in dry matter intake increased with the elapse of time. Anoestrous cows may eat 2.5–4 kg per day less than their fellow group members who are cycling normally. *It must be emphasised that the energy status during the first 2 weeks is of paramount importance.*

The movement back towards positive energy status appears to be important in the initiation of oestrus. It has been calculated that ovulation occurred approximately 10 days after the most negative stage was reached.

Linoleic and other fatty acids have been shown to be effective in increasing prostaglandin concentrations and the growth of ovarian follicles. Excessive linoleic acid has, on the other hand, been shown to inhibit the synthesis of prostaglandin. It may be possible to formulate diets that will specifically enhance fertility, but such development is still at the theoretical stage.

Crude protein

The effect of high *crude protein* intakes on reproduction of the dairy cow is controversial. The results of experimental work have been equivocal and research is ongoing. If more rumen degradable protein is fed than the cow can utilise then urea levels in body tissues can rise. Raised blood urea levels have been related to delay of first ovulation, to lowered conception rates, increased embryonic death and general reproductive inefficiency.

The manner by which high protein intake may negatively affect reproductive performance is a matter for speculation. Possible effects on gametes, hypophyseal–pituitary–ovarian axis, embryo viability or its implantation have all been suggested as the cause of infertility. Perhaps the most likely explanation is not so much excess protein in the diet but an excess of protein in relation to the amount of energy available. The excess ammonia produced as a result of excess dietary rumen degradable protein needs to be detoxified and this places an extra energy cost on the animal which is probably already in negative energy balance. It could be argued that the effects attributed to excess protein in the diet are in actual fact ultimately due to energy deficiency.

Copper, iodine, manganese and vitamin A deficiencies have all been implicated in affecting fertility. They may be important on individual farms. Other symptoms of deficiency are also likely to be present.

To ensure that nutrition is not adversely affecting fertility or causing lameness, the transition from dry to early lactation stage must be as smooth as possible in order to optimise dry matter intake in early lactation. Feeding and management of the dry cow is once again of paramount importance. Avoid abrupt changes in diet or environment.

Metabolic profiles

Metabolic profiles (see also Chapter 4) do not replace all the basic techniques which have been discussed but rather serve to provide additional *current* information about the nutritional balance of key groups of cows in the herd. Metabolic profiles are of most use when used as an integral part of a planned preventive medicine programme. The technique can identify potential problem areas before they are reflected in lost production, health or fertility problems or disappointing profitability.

Blood sampling

The first cows in the group to experience new dietary or management conditions should be sampled in order that any necessary changes can be implemented before the majority of cows enter the group, e.g. in early lactation.

When to sample

- May or June when grass is generally of optimum quality and availability. This test provides a valuable base line for comparison with results obtained later in the season under less favourable conditions.
- July or August can be a valuable time to test summer calving herds. Grass growth and quality are often unpredictable and variable at this time of year. It can often be difficult to assess whether the nutritional requirements of high yielding cows are being satisfied.
- Autumn grazing period blood analysis frequently identifies potential problems resulting from an overestimation of the contribution from grass, especially for high yielding cows.
- Winter feeding period. A test 2–3 weeks after the cows have been exposed to the winter feeding regime gives a good balance of the total diet. This allows adjustments to be made before expensive health and production problems manifest themselves.
- After major management or feeding change, for example change of silage pit or introduction of maize silage.

Correct timing of the test

Because of biological variations associated with feeding it is essential to allow 2–3 hours to elapse after the animal has had a major concentrate feed. This delay is less important when small feeds are provided regularly or when a total mixed ration is being fed. It is also essential to wait until 2 weeks have elapsed after a major dietary change. The rumen microflora takes time (10–14 days) to adjust to a new substrate.

Cow selection

Addressing the correct questions to the correct animals is essential if the test is going to be of any value.

Early lactation group (10–20 days post-calving): this group is likely to yield most information. High yielding cows will almost certainly be in energy deficit at this time. The greatest energy gap will generally be around 2 weeks post-calving. It is the extent of the energy deficiency that will indicate whether failure to attain peak productivity, development of metabolic disease, or, in the longer term, adverse effect on milk quality or reproduction are probabilities. On the other hand, if cows are sampled too long after calving they may respond to underfeeding by dropping milk yield and quality and have normal biochemical results. Normally five to seven animals should be sampled from this group.

Mid-lactation group: normally these cows should be around 100-days calved. They will be achieving full dry matter intake and should be pregnant again. This particular group is invaluable as a control group for comparison with the early lactation cows. It is particularly important to monitor body condition at this time. It is often possible to assess the potential contribution of the forage at this stage and then to adjust concentrate levels accordingly. Five cows are normally included in this group.

Dry cows: dry cows were for so long the neglected animals in the herd. It is now well recognised that the management and nutrition of the dry cow are vital for the optimum health and productivity of the cow in early lactation. Cow condition and biochemical status 2 weeks prior to calving give valuable clues to potential problem areas (too fat, high plasma NEFA levels, low magnesium status, deficiency in dietary RDP, etc.). Sampling two groups of dry cows for comparison (one group at 60–30 days precalving and one at 5–14 days precalving) can reinforce the need for management change and permit some remedial action to be taken.

Common errors in cow selection

- Cows that have calved more than 3 weeks should not be included in the early lactation group. If cows have been underfed over a period of time they may well have adjusted yield accordingly and all biochemical parameters will be within the normal range. This is the main reason that metabolic profiles used as a troubleshooting exercise as a last resort have fallen into disrepute.
- Inclusion of too many cows that are not representative of the herd. Given a free choice the herdsman will often include 'problem' or 'odd' cows, which can lead to a misleading interpretation of the results.
- Cows with long-standing health or reproductive problems.
- Sampling immediately before or after a major management or dietary change is a waste of resources.

Background information

At time of sampling it is essential to record cow identification, calving date, condition score, body weight (by body band is an accurate and easy method), milk yield and quality, lactation number and full dietary details.

Attempting to interpret biochemical data in isolation is futile and can be extremely misleading. However, used properly as an integral part of a health programme, this technique will enable the veterinary surgeon to become involved in all aspects of dairy management and diet evaluation. Metabolic profiles should not be regarded as a 'quick fix'.

References

AFRC (1993) *Energy and Protein Requirements of Ruminants.* An advisory manual prepared by the AFRC Technical Committee on Responses to Nutrients. CAB International, Wallingford.

MAFF (1975) *Energy Allowances and Feeding Systems for Ruminants.* Technical Bulletin 33. HMSO, London.

MAFF (1980) *Nutrient Allowances and Composition of Feeding Stuff for Ruminants.* Booklet 2087. MAFF Publications, Alnwick, Northumberland.

MAFF (1984) *Energy Allowances and Feeding Systems for Ruminants.* Technical Bulletin 433. HMSO, London.

National Research Council (1985) *Nutrient Requirements of Domestic Animals.* No. 3 Dairy Cattle. National Academy of Sciences, Washington.

Chapter 4
Use and Interpretation of Metabolic Profiles

David A. Whitaker

Introduction

The metabolic profile approach to dairy herds should be used as a means of 'asking the cows what they think of their diet'. Rations are planned using *in vitro* feed analysis and rationing programmes, but these cannot take fully into account variation in cow size, performance and stage of lactation within herds. Nor can they guarantee that the right amount of food is put out and that all the cows get the opportunity to eat what is programmed. Assessment of how the planned ration is actually working is therefore important. This can be done by observation of daily milk yields, peak yields, lactation curves, body condition changes, fat and protein content of milk, strength of oestrous signs and conception rates. Unless the original ration was severely unbalanced, it can be months before it is clear that some of these parameters are not satisfactory. Even then it may be far from clear which aspect of nutrition is or was the problem. Metabolic profiles properly planned and organised will tell that something is wrong or about to go wrong, what it is and what is the best/most economic solution.

Proper planning means an understanding of the importance of three vital factors: the timing of the blood test, the selection of the cows and the collection and assessment of relevant information about the cows and the farm. Anyone can collect blood samples. Anyone can do laboratory analysis. Whether the valuable information obtainable is delivered depends greatly on these three factors.

Timing of blood tests

In relation to feeding

As there can be short-term biochemical changes associated with feeding itself, cows should not be blood sampled soon after a larger concentrate feed. It is best to wait 1 hour after feeding anyway, but 2 hours if cows are receiving more than 2 kg of concentrates at milking time.

In relation to feed changes

Due to the manner in which the rumen functions, cows should not be sampled within 2 weeks after a major diet change – particularly a change in forage type. This is to allow the rumen environment to become fully adapted to the new ration and so to utilise its potential. Changes in the quantities of existing components of a ration do not require the same wait.

In relation to calving pattern and feeding season

As the earliest indication of the cows' opinion of the diet is the aim, blood sampling should therefore be done as soon as possible after any major diet change. So 2 weeks after cows are housed fully for the winter is an important time, rather than in the middle of winter. Then any constraints can be identified and put right quickly for the benefit of the bulk of the season. Other times might be after maize silage or second cut grass silage are introduced or after turnout to grass in the spring. If the diet is changed in response to a blood test, a test 2 weeks later to assess the effect should be done too. As cows in early lactation and late pregnancy are the most important, tests should also be planned near the start of each period of increased calving activity – again to allow constraints to be identified in time for correction to benefit the majority.

Selection of cows

Failure to select the right cows for testing can result in optimum biochemical values from thin, infertile cows which are underperforming. This is because of the animal's ability, when faced with an inadequate diet – energy in particular – to adapt its performance downwards to the level that could be met by that diet. Then its biochemistry is also adapted to optimum. Cows must be blood sampled before they have had the opportunity to do this.

Individual variations are such that the biochemical results from single cows are not helpful and may even mislead. Groups of five cows at least in each of the described categories should be sampled. Those that are as typical as possible in the herd of that stage should be selected – not the lowest or the highest yielders and not at random. Cows with apparent problems should be excluded as the type of testing in metabolic profiles is not likely to identify causes and the results may undermine the group picture. Cows that are failing to conceive hardly ever show abnormal results and so should be excluded too unless they fall into the mid lactation category or are included separately in addition to the other groups.

Early lactation group

The most important cows to test are those in early lactation, i.e. 10–20 days calved. If tested closer to calving, their yields may still be quite low and their biochemistry may still be affected by calving and the introduction to the herd rather than their nutritional status. If tested later in lactation, adaptation to an inadequate ration may be under way and a significant constraint missed.

Mid lactation group

Some cows well in to lactation – 100 days calved approximately – should always be sampled as well. They provide a very useful within-herd comparison with the early lactation cows and allow confirmation that abnormal results are not due to prandial effects.

Dry cow group

The dry period is very important for the success of the following lactation. Problems are usually at their greatest at the end of pregnancy. So cows in the last week or 10 days before calving should be sampled. It can be informative to test for comparison another group with a month to go.

Other groups

Maiden, heavily pregnant or first lactation heifer groups might be considered for special reasons, but they should be included with mature cow groups to ensure that within-herd comparisons are available.

Background information

Knowledge of the feeding and housing systems, calving pattern, herd size, aspirations and problems is essential to being able to put results into a useful and practical context. In addition, if full value from the metabolic profile approach is to be obtained, the following data should accompany blood samples to the laboratory: cow identification, calving/expected calving date, body weight preferably by heart girth measurement, body condition score, current daily milk yield, lactation number, daily supplementary feed intake, daily estimated forage intake, analytical description of feeds, herd milk quality.

On-farm interpretation

However skilled laboratory-based interpretation may be, there are always going to be common circumstances where, although the diagnosis is correct, the resolution of the problem can only be worked out by discussion at the farm. Farm advisory meetings should therefore always take place as soon as the results are available. These should include the farmer, his staff, the local veterinary surgeon and any other advisers involved with nutrition on the farm. The benefit from a team working together is far greater than from the individuals working separately.

Written reports

All advice given should be supported in writing and copies circulated to partici-
pants in the team. The advice is then clear to all and it can be charged for with
confidence.

Metabolites regularly measured

A wide range of metabolites can be measured in blood, but their number as part
of a nutritional advice programme needs to be kept to a usable minimum on
grounds of cost and to avoid overcomplication of results and interpretation.
When selecting those to be measured it is important to bear in mind that aspects
of dietary energy and protein are most likely to influence productivity and so
should be looked at primarily. Practically the metabolite needs to be stable in an
unseparated sample after collection for 2–3 days while in transit to a laboratory.
The method of analysis needs to be rapid, accurate and not expensive. It is
necessary for those interpreting the results to be able to identify with confidence
what variations from optimum levels actually imply on the farm.

It is an obvious prerequisite that laboratory results are accurate. To ensure that
this is so, each laboratory analysing metabolite levels should belong to an
independent quality assessment scheme.

'Normal' or perhaps more appropriately 'optimum' metabolite values quoted
here were derived originally from looking at the population mean plus or minus
two standard deviations in the thousands of samples submitted every year to the
Dairy Herd Health and Productivity Service (DHHPS) laboratory since 1978.
However, as some values have a skewed distribution, this approach has been
modified using a lognormal transformation. There is a large body of anecdotal
evidence from farms using the DHHPS – where samples are accompanied by
background information about the cows and followed up and reported on by the
farm's veterinary surgeon – that the optimum values used are realistic as such.
In addition, trials where there has been close monitoring of performance, weight
and condition change and feeding together with regular blood sampling have
allowed more scientific confirmation of this. Nevertheless, *optimum values and
ranges are guides only and should not be used too precisely*. In looking at metabolite levels in blood samples, group means from a minimum of five cows should
be considered. So should variations within the group with both the number of
'abnormal' values and the extent to which they vary from the optimum examined. Individual values should be considered against individual performance,
weight, body condition, feeding and stage of lactation.

Energy balance (see also pp. 79–81)

β-hydroxybutyrate (BHB)

The optimum level of β-hydroxybutyrate (BHB) for milkers is below 1.0 mmol/-
litre and for dry cows at the end of pregnancy below 0.6. BHB is a ketone body

present in the blood of all animals. The concentration increases as the animal is under increasing energy stress. BHB is stable in blood after collection and in transit. Butyric acid from grass silage in the rumen can, on rare occasions, be absorbed into the blood as BHB. In interpretation this situation can be detected by within-herd comparisons of BHB level against performance and stage of lactation.

Non-esterified fatty acid (NEFA or free fatty acid)

The optimum level of non-esterified fatty acid (NEFA) for milkers is below 0.7 mmol/litre and for dry cows at the end of pregnancy below 0.4. NEFA is a more direct measure of fat mobilisation than BHB. It is of especial value in dry cows. However, it is not as stable in transit. From 48 hours after collection it may start to rise. Cows severely upset at testing may show rises not relating to nutrition. Practically neither of these potential causes of confusion should be a problem provided there is background information accompanying the cow's sample, allowing within-herd comparisons against yield and stage of lactation.

Glucose

The optimum level of glucose in plasma is over 3.0 mmol/litre. This is different from values in whole blood or serum, neither of which are as accurate. Glucose is not as sensitive to changes in energy balance as BHB or NEFA because of homeostatic control. However, within the optimum range there is some evidence that plasma glucose can reflect weight change. Deterioration can occur in the sample in transit with loss of glucose, especially if the anticoagulant is inadequately mixed or the expiry date of the sampling tubes has passed. Cows severely stressed at sampling may have very high values.

Interpretation: cows in milk

When cows in milk have high BHB and/or high NEFA, with normal or low glucose, this indicates a dietary energy *problem* but not necessarily a dietary *deficiency*. Uncorrected, this situation constrains milk and milk protein yield and fertility, with the effect on protein and fertility frequently not obvious at the time but rather delayed weeks or months. Resistance to disease may be reduced. More supplementary feed may be required, but the same biochemical situation can be brought about by too much, inducing an excessively high non-forage to forage ratio and not enough fibre in the rumen. Then the total energy intake may be adequate or even in excess, but it is being underutilised and partly wasted. The resolution can therefore be to supply less supplementary feeds or to alter the manner in which they are supplied. Without background information on stage of lactation, milk yield, body weight and feeding the correct judgement is difficult if not nearly impossible.

Table 4.1 shows the range of factors that should be considered on the farm. The extent and character of these factors indicate why it is so important that

Table 4.1 Factors to consider where energy problems have been diagnosed in cows in early lactation.

- Not enough concentrates fed in total – expected forage ME unreasonably high.
- Too much concentrates being fed overall – concentrate to forage ratio at or over 3:1 on a dry matter (DM) basis. Silage, hay, straw and grazing count as forages, everything else as concentrates, although sometimes referred to as roughages such as brewer's grains.
- Too much concentrates fed at each milking – 4 kg is the target maximum. Above this, rumen acidity may be increased inefficiently.
- Too much concentrates fed at a single feed in a trough unmixed with silage other than at milking time – 2 kg per cow per feed is the maximum. More than this and greedy cows get too much and the new-calved – those most at risk – get too little.
- Not enough silage offered – rationing information available will include an estimated daily DM intake of the ration per cow. This should be the same as or greater than the theoretical DM intake calculated from body weight, milk yield and content and stage of lactation. Modern high yielding cows are capable of achieving average DM intakes of 25 kg per day with good feed management. To take advantage of the ability to eat forage, 5–10% more than the group will eat should be offered so that there is always food available. The excess should be removed every day. It is common to find that food runs out overnight or that the amount offered is restricted so that the cows clean up the trough; many troughs are designed so that it is very difficult for people or machines to do this.
- Silage/silage mix stale – if troughs are not cleared out daily. Secondary fermentation in silage/concentrate mixes can also occur under some circumstances in feed in front of the cows. It will feel hot in the middle and steam may rise off it on cold mornings. Loss of nutrients by starlings removing grain from mixed rations appears to be significant on some farms.
- Unpalatable conserved forage – modern forage analytical techniques allow quite precise assessment of intake potential of silages, but some still confound science. Observation of the cows is always advisable. In general, very wet or very dry grass silage in the UK is not eaten as well although there are exceptions. Sometimes unpalatable forage from the top or sides of a clamp is mixed with good material in a wagon, inhibiting overall intakes. Low pH grass silage can lead to the rejection of cuds.
- Access to conserved forage restricted – trough space inadequate, trough space adequate but length not all filled routinely, cows eat all they can reach quickly and rest not pushed up, trough unprotected from elements, route to trough/self-feed area unprotected; self-feed face too narrow, barrier not moved far enough/often enough, electrified barrier too savage, silage too tightly packed in clamp; not enough ring feeders. Observation of what happens can reveal constraints; particularly note where and when heifers and new calved cows are feeding.
- Deteriorating silage – poor management of the clamp, particularly of the face letting in air and water, can allow secondary fermentation with loss of nutrients and lower intake because of reduced DM content.
- Unmixed forages – lower total forage intakes always result when conserved forages such as grass, maize or whole crop cereal silages are fed separately rather than mixed in a wagon. The full potential advantages of feeding maize and whole crop with grass silage are rarely fully gained unless they are mixed before feeding.
- Conserved forage of low energy content – if the forage is palatable, rationing can compensate provided its low energy content is recognised and provided access to it is not restricted.
- Grass silage very low in fibre – a rare event but can occur in silage of very high quality in other respects made very early in spring. Incorporating 0.5–1.0 kg chopped straw per cow in the forage mix is usually enough. Alternative free access to long fibre sources does not usually work satisfactorily due to lower and variable intakes.
- Restricted grazing – not enough grass available, set stocking systems which allow uneven and fibrous growth, overrestricted strip grazing, changing paddocks too infrequently. Zealous desire to utilise grazing to the last leaf is not suitable for high yielding early lactation cows.
- Buffer feeding to grazing not working – forage in it of poor quality/palatability, timing of access inappropriate for new calved cows, length of time of free access inadequate, site of access not suitable.
- Excess digestible rumen undegradable protein (DUP) – in relation to dietary energy.
- Salt deficiency.
- Water deprivation – trough size, siting, filling rate and/or cleanliness.
- Changes in diet at calving, particularly the introduction of concentrates or new forages can have a large effect on energy balance in the very important first 2–3 weeks of lactation.
- Lack of reasonable cow comfort.

final diagnoses and decisions should be taken in discussion with the farmer and his nutritional adviser at the farm rather than in the surgery or over the telephone.

Cows in milk can have high BHB, high NEFA and low glucose where there is no dietary energy problem, i.e. where milk yields are good and condition is not being lost. The reason may be because blood testing was carried out too close to feeding or to major diet changes. Silage type can very rarely be involved, but then NEFAs remain 'normal'.

To identify this situation, it is necessary to look at the individual variations of yield level and stage of lactation between cows within the metabolic profile test – one of the reasons for including groups at different stages of lactation. For example, if a mid lactation cow giving 20 litres of milk has the same high BHBs, etc. as a cow calved 14 days giving 35 litres, then dietary energy deficiency is unlikely to be the cause.

More precisely the individual cow's energy expectation from the forage component of the diet can be looked at:

Required ME – Fed concentrate ME = expected forage ME.

The required metabolisable energy (ME) in megajoules (MJ) required is calcu-lated from the body weight, milk yield and milk quality. From this is subtracted the ME that is being supplied by the non-forage component of the diet. The amount of concentrates being supplied per cow is usually fairly accurately available from the farm compared to the amount of forage consumed. Actual ME or book values for non-forages are used. This difference is the amount of energy the cows are being expected to get from the forage component of their diet as a consequence of the quantity of concentrates provided – the expected forage ME. If these figures are widely different between cows but the BHBs, etc. are raised to the same degree, then a dietary energy problem is unlikely to be the main cause.

If milking cows have BHB, NEFA and glucose values within optimum ranges, this means cows are having their energy requirements met. However, are those requirements for 5 litres of milk only or for 40? Are they in early lactation cows or in mid lactation animals. The answers to questions like these can provide much useful information on how well a diet is working and whether adjustments to the use of the various foods can be safely and economically made. For example, in cows at grass receiving only concentrates at milking time the expected forage ME represents what they are being expected to get from grazing. If their metabolite results are good, it represents what they are actually getting from grazing. In Table 4.2 cows 1, 2 and 3 are having their energy needs met as shown by their metabolite results. So they are achieving their expected forage ME figures from grazing. All cows in the herd more than 50 days calved should be able to get 170 MJ from the grass available – especially those in mid and late lactation. So, cows 4, 5 and 6 are receiving more concentrates than their performance requires and reductions can be made. Similar within-herd assessments of concentrate use can be made on winter rations, but where there is a forage/concentrate out-of-parlour

Table 4.2   Individual cow result examples for interpretation of energy contribution of forage.

Cow	NEFA (mmol/l)	BHB (mmol/l)	Days calved	Expected forage ME (MJ)
1	0.5	0.7	45	181
2	0.4	0.4	63	175
3	0.3	0.8	32	173
4	0.4	0.5	78	154
5	0.3	0.4	180	115
6	0.4	0.3	212	97

mix it is less accurate individually. On winter rations concentrate reductions in mid and late pregnancy on the grounds of modifying energy input can cause the ration to become deficient in protein and thus loss of milk yield. So more caution is needed than in grazing cattle which are usually receiving an excess of protein anyway.

It should be remembered that optimum metabolite values may be found in cows that have previously experienced an energy problem and have failed to yield to their potential already because of it. They may at the time of sampling be in energy balance, but only because their requirements are lower than they should be. They may have lost body condition before but no longer be doing so when blood sampled. This is a trap into which it is quite easy to fall when early lactation cows on modern feeding systems are sampled later than 3–4 weeks calved.

Interpretation: dry cows (see also pp. 74–5)

In cows within the last 1–2 weeks of pregnancy, BHB and/or NEFA above the optimum is a sign of negative energy balance which can have important implications for production and fertility in the following lactation. Recent surveys have shown loss of condition during the dry period and low body condition score at calving to be associated with poor performance, including lower fertility. NEFA is a particularly sensitive measure of this. It may occur in any dry cows, including those overfat or thin. Individuals carrying twins tend to have abnormal results when close to calving.

In cows in the early part of the dry period, BHB, plasma glucose and NEFA results tend to be normal, but this often changes as appetite drops because of the increasing volume of the pregnant uterus. If results are abnormal in the early dry period, it may mean condition is being lost. Only if cows are too fat at this stage – body condition score >3.5 – will it not matter. However, then steps must be taken to arrest that situation by the time they get to 3–4 weeks before calving. Controlling fatness is best done in late pregnancy, but this is not always successful. So, confining overfat cows on straw and a suitable effective rumen degradable protein (ERDP) source may be advisable for a week or two at drying off.

Table 4.3 illustrates the ideal approach to dry cow management and thus areas of likely problems. Only blood sampling in the last week or two of pregnancy is likely to show up variations from the reference values, but the origin of difficulties may be earlier on. Sampling five cows close to calving and five with 4–5 weeks

Table 4.3 Dry cow management.

- Manage cows so that they go dry at body condition score 2.5–3.0 and maintain this until calving.
- Confine those overfat on straw and ERDP for 1–3 weeks. Do not restrict the quantity of forage offered.
- Feed generously cows very thin at drying off – below condition score 2.
- Provide free access minerals in the early part of the dry period.
- Treat the last 4 weeks of pregnancy as a unique opportunity to maintain and restore resources.
- During the last 4 weeks before calving provide cows with the best nutrition and environment.
- Provide 24-hour access to quality forage of the type(s) cows will receive in pregnancy. Some chopped straw can be mixed in. Feeding quality forage for 12–18 hours and expecting cows to fill up on straw usually means that total food intake is lower than it could be and frequently means that total energy intake is inadequate as well. Failure to provide full-time access to quality forage is the most common cause of energy problems and fat mobilisation prior to calving.
- Feed 2–3 kg of high quality concentrates per day. This increases the energy density of the diet, compensating for the dropping appetite of the heavily pregnant, acclimatises the rumen flora to concentrates and allows the development of an increase in the area of rumen lining available. The last two processes require a minimum of 2 weeks to be completed and are necessary if the vital first 2–3 weeks of lactation are to work properly.
- Ensure that these concentrates contain the type of DUP that will enhance milk protein production, where desired.
- Ensure that the forages – grass silage or grazing – on offer provide adequate ERDP. Specialist dry cow concentrates are usually formulated making this assumption. Overenthusiastic use of straw, maize or whole crop silage commonly results in a dry cow diet deficient in ERDP unless specifically supplemented.
- Ensure that these concentrates or the silage mixture contain adequate and appropriate dry cow minerals and vitamins for the restoration and maintenance of reserves and for the control of hypocalcaemia.
- Provide fresh concentrates, forage and water in calving boxes.
- Include pregnant heifers in this close-to-calving group.
- Overfatness comes from overfeeding in late lactation or the eighth month of pregnancy.
- Outsize calves come from overfeeding in the seventh to eighth month of pregnancy, the genetic makeup of the dam (underdeveloped heifer with the potential to grow much more) or extended gestation (a function of the genetic makeup of the sire). The rate of growth of the calf in the last month of pregnancy is at its greatest, but it cannot be increased or decreased by feeding during that time.

to go can provide a useful within-herd comparison and also the opportunity to see what is being practised earlier on. Energy problems with fat mobilisation before calving most commonly come from failing to supply enough quality forage and/or enough concentrates.

Protein

Urea-nitrogen (ureaN)

The optimum level of urea-nitrogen (ureaN) is over 1.7 mmol/litre. Urea is often analysed for, but interpretation is no different provided the correct range is used.

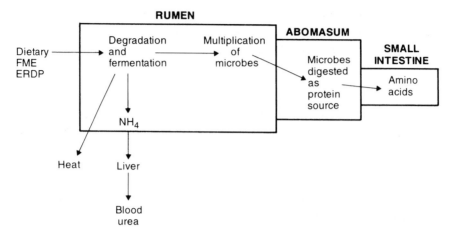

Fig. 4.1   Schematic of the degradation and digestion of ERDP and FME by ruminants.

Urea is 2.14 times ureaN. So the optimum range for urea is over 3.6 mmol/litre. Blood ureaN reflects very well the intake of effective rumen degradable protein (ERDP) and its balance with fermentable metabolisable energy (FME). Figure 4.1 illustrates the relationship.

If cows at any stage have low ureaN values in their blood, this shows inadequate ERDP in the rumen and represents a situation inhibiting productivity, but it does not distinguish between a low dietary content and a low intake of a diet containing an adequate proportion of ERDP. A cow that does not eat properly during the previous 12–24 hours will have a low urea the next day, for example, but will recover the level if it starts eating again. General constraints on feeding can therefore cause low urea results in addition to low ERDP content of the total food intake, although in the former instance biochemical parameters for energy may be abnormal too. Within a group of cattle some may have lower urea results than others simply for potential appetite reasons, e.g. newly calved cows, first lactation heifers. Cows fed maize silage over night and grass silage during the day will have low urea results if tested in the morning. While their total diet may not be short of ERDP, the method of feeding means that the rumen will not be utilising the ration to its potential.

Where a diet is deficient in ERDP, cows will usually respond to supplementation with more milk within 24–36 hours. However, they will need to be able to eat more silage for the change to work fully and so management must expect and allow for this in planning. Current rationing programmes and forage analysis are relatively weak in assessing ERDP adequacy. Mistakes are quite common, with nutritional advisers reluctant to acknowledge them because the solution is usually to feed something cheaper than included in the original plan. This can appear commercially embarrassing.

Low ureaN results in dry cows are common for the reasons outlined in Table 4.3 and require correction for the system to work and for cows to achieve their potential.

Where cows have high blood ureaN there is an excess of ERDP in relation to FME in the diet. This is a common situation in grazing cows in temperate climates and at worst usually reflects just a waste of nitrogen. In housed cows high urea results may be associated with an excess of dietary protein leading to an energy inadequacy. Where possible, dietary balances should be adjusted to achieve better utilisation and productivity. So, increasing the proportion of dietary FME is the best option theoretically but practically may be difficult to bring about. Reducing ERDP should be approached with caution because it is difficult to achieve in isolation from digestible undegradable protein (DUP) and may result in loss of milk yield. It is usually not possible to make sufficient feeding adjustments in cows at grass to reduce blood urea levels significantly without removing access to grazing and so the attempt may be better not made. So far the reported association between high blood/milk urea and poor fertility has not been demonstrated to be a direct link, with the question remaining controversial. Many cows retain good fertility in spite of high urea levels.

Albumin

The optimum level of albumin is over 30 g/litre. Albumin is a protein that is synthesised by the liver. When levels are low this reflects liver health or a poor amino-acid supply from the diet. This effect is usually long term. Severe prolonged underfeeding or significant disease are usually required before there are noticeable changes in albumin level. Clotted blood samples produce lower albumin results than those collected into anticoagulants.

There is no way of directly assessing through blood metabolites the adequacy of digestible undegradable protein (DUP) or metabolisable protein (MP) in a diet. Practically, however, if milk/milk protein performance is below expectation and if there is definitely no negative energy balance (normal BHB, NEFA and glucose in early lactation and body condition gain) and no shortage of ERDP (normal ureaN results), then additional DUP is worth trying. However, as with additional ERDP, more forage must be made available at the time, with allowance made for more to be consumed during the rest of the winter.

Globulin

The optimum level of globulin is below 50 g/litre. Globulin level is not measured itself but rather total protein is and albumin subtracted from it to give globulin. Therefore total protein results have no relevance themselves to nutritional balance and probably should not be quoted on final reports. Globulins are antibodies of the type formed in response to chronic inflammation. The level does not relate either to the severity of the condition or to how recently it took place. The most common causes are things like mastitis, metritis or lameness. Infections such as *Fasciola hepatica* may be involved. Where clinical explanations are not apparent and more than one or two cows are involved, herd investigations should be carried out to check on such possibilities. The inclusion of globulin in a metabolic profile test can provide unexpected opportunities for constructive discussion of disease control and preventive measures.

Minerals and trace elements

Magnesium

The optimum level of magnesium is between 0.8 and 1.3 mmol/litre. Plasma levels reflect current daily intake rather than reserves which are not quickly available. In milking cows hypomagnesaemia can occur at any time of the year in temperate climates. Low blood values are an early warning of the possibility of clinical problems. Subclinical deficiency can affect appetite and so milk yield. Because of the complex nature of the factors that interfere with magnesium absorption, changes in the supplementation approach should be followed by a check test 7–10 days later.

In dry cows, low plasma magnesium may be associated with a depressing effect on the calcium mobilisation system and consequently hypocalcaemia around calving. When this is happening blood magnesium levels may not drop until a day or two before calving. Clinical hypomagnesaemia is rare but possible in dry cows.

Inorganic phosphate

The optimum level of inorganic phosphate is between 1.4 and 2.5 mmol/litre. Plasma values reflect current dietary intake principally. Cows can tolerate low levels for some weeks while remaining productive and fertile. As follow-up tests, especially on grazing cows after rain, often reveal normal results, it is advisable to check test before embarking on expensive supplementation.

Calcium

Variations in blood calcium are small except in the immediate periparturient period and have no relationship with dietary intake due to the strong homeostatic control mechanism. Estimation is therefore of little value in routine metabolite testing and should only be done as part of individual cow clinical investigations.

Sodium and potassium

Homeostasis renders measurement of blood level of both sodium and potassium meaningless as a means of assessing dietary intake or content.

Thyroxine (T₄)

Thyroxine (T_4) is a measure of iodine status, particularly useful in dry cows. Optimum level is above 20 nmol/litre. Low T_4 in plasma reflects poor iodine status as opposed to inorganic iodine measurements which reflect current daily intake.

Low values in milkers may be associated with poor production, but the main interest is low values in dry cows or pregnant heifers associated with abortions or the birth of dead calves. Weighing the thyroid gland of such calves does not provide adequate information but histopathology may in the absence of access to T_4 analysis. There are several other causes of abortion and stillbirth which should be investigated as well.

Copper

The optimum level of copper is over 9.4 µmol/litre for plasma and 7.5 µmol/litre for serum. Blood copper values are not an accurate guide to body and liver status, where most of it is found. If levels are low, productivity and health may be affected as copper is such an important part of many biochemical processes. However, normal values may be found in animals with clinical problems. Diagnosis then depends on liver analysis and/or response to supplementation. A copper-responsive fertility problem is only likely to be found where the forage contains 5 mg molybdenum kg DM or more.

Glutathione peroxidase (GSHPx)

The optimum level of glutathione peroxidase (GSHPx) is over 50 units/haemoglobin or over 15 units/ml of cells. GSHPx is a selenium-containing enzyme. Estimation of it allows a judgement to be made of selenium intake over the previous month or two. Direct measurement of selenium in blood can be done but is too expensive as a routine.

It is important to appreciate that GSHPx levels can be dropping while dietary selenium intake is rising and vice versa. So, because values reflect selenium intake over a long period, low results may disguise an already improving situation. Equally, normal results may disguise a deficiency situation which has taken place and caused problems. Clinical judgements are therefore important. Poor fertility in growing heifers, retained fetal membranes, stillbirths and muscular dystrophy are conditions that may be related. Because of relationships in the body, analysis for vitamin E in cows on conserved forage may be advisable as well. (See also pp. 25, 64.)

Vitamin B₁₂

The optimum level of vitamin B_{12} is supposed to be over 90 ng/litre. Interpretation is difficult, however, with lower values than this sometimes being found in apparently normal, healthy and fertile cattle. There is some doubt as to whether the chemical analysed is biologically active. Low values should therefore be approached with some caution. Injection with vitamin B_{12} and observation for a response is a sensible initial step.

Measuring metabolites in milk

If the same rigour – selection of cows, timing of tests, assessment of background information in conjunction with biochemical results – already described in this chapter was applied to measuring metabolites in milk and if the relationships between milk metabolites were established, then milk testing could have considerable value. At the time of writing, however, the approach is in danger of falling into some of the same traps metabolic profiles did 30 years ago – assumptions that milk levels reflect dietary intake accurately and/or that daily dietary intake rather than nutritional status is what matters. Furthermore, dry cow nutrition cannot be assessed from milk.

The best available measurement in milk about which there is enough known is urea. It mirrors accurately the blood level and so in individual cows can be used to assess in part the protein/energy dietary situation in cows. However, as this is not simply a question of too much or too little protein (Fig. 4.1), reliable interpretation without a measurement of energy status alongside and without within-herd groups for comparison to assess the effect of variation in intake is not possible and could be wrong. At the moment there is no measurement of energy status through milk which is practically available and sensitive enough. β-hydroxybutyrate has been suggested, but it does not correspond to blood levels because it is involved in milk fat synthesis in the udder.

Bulk milk urea testing is of little use because the results represent the average for the milking herd. It takes no account of the range of values which are always present from variations in intake because of stage of lactation, lactation number, etc. Very low bulk milk urea values would indicate a shortage of ERDP in the diet and would be worth responding to. 'Normal' or 'high' values reflect so many different situations, many of which are quite 'normal', that they can be hazardously misleading and should either be ignored or responded to by a metabolic profile blood test carried out with the rigour described earlier in this chapter.

Measuring minerals and trace elements in milk has major pitfalls as well. This is partly because many nutrients such as calcium are concentrated in milk to supply the suckling calf's needs. Others may just reflect current intake rather than nutritional status and so can give entirely the wrong impression. Doubts about the practical value of some blood analyses such as vitamin B_{12} exist even after many years. Too little research has been done and there is no body of anecdotal information available for milk analyses to be a reliable way to approach perceived trace element problems which are often difficult enough to sort out with any certainty anyway without controlled trials.

Problems likely to be encountered

Failure to achieve expected peak yields; rapid decline from peak; cases of ketosis; loss of condition

A metabolic profile including end-of-pregnancy dry cows, a group calved 10–20 days and a group of mid lactationers should confirm the presence of energy problems. The full range of potential influences in Table 4.1 should be discussed.

Disappointing milk protein

The first step is to convert weekly protein percentage figures into protein yields to confirm that protein production is dropping. Where dilution is taking place because there are many cows at peak yield, butterfat percentage will have dropped too. The most common cause of poor milk protein is a long-term energy problem. So a metabolic profile should be carried out to determine whether there is a current energy constraint. However, as, for example, low protein in the New Year is usually because cows had energy problems in the autumn, a metabolic profile may miss this. It may be too late because the cows that were on the troublesome ration have got themselves back into energy balance but have inadequate reserves for full protein production. Furthermore those currently in early lactation are on different, better rations. So a look at body condition of the milkers which are passed peak and comparison with any dry cows available may confirm the cause. Farmers should be questioned whether there was noticeable condition loss in the newly calved in the autumn. They may be reluctant to accept the diagnosis. Thus a plan to do a metabolic profile test next autumn is important – early enough in the calving pattern for a change in nutrition for the benefit of most of the cows at risk to be carried out.

Providing better energy status in cows that are thin and past peak yield should halt the decline in protein production but is unlikely to restore it fully within less than a month or two. Some specialised compound concentrates may have a more rapid effect but not if the cows have become very thin.

If loss of condition is not obvious, a metabolic profile test should confirm the absence of an ERDP shortage – something more likely to inhibit total milk yield than protein production – and it is necessary to confirm the absence of a current energy constraint. Cows experiencing a shortage of dietary DUP, which can affect milk protein, will look fit and in good condition. Supplying additional DUP will then usually result in a response in milk and protein yield but not usually in protein percentage for some weeks at least. Additional DUP will make matters worse and may even precipitate cases of ketosis if there is an energy constraint in the diet. It may not produce the desired response either if cows are not enabled to eat more forage.

Low butterfat percentage

Under modern milk marketing circumstances a low butterfat percentage is only likely to be a problem for the farmer if the percentage is so low that the milk purchaser is starting to complain. A metabolic profile test is unlikely to be helpful directly but may be desirable to confirm the absence of some nutritional constraints and to ensure veterinary involvement in the investigation. The most likely cause of very low butterfat is a concentrate to forage ratio on a DM basis of over 3:1. If this calculation is not possible because of the uncertainty about the amount of forage being eaten, then an expected forage ME calculation (see 'Interpretation cows in milk') may come out below 50 MJ where butterfat is poor. It is sometimes even negative. If the ration cannot readily be changed, feeding sodium bicarbonate may work. It needs to be incorporated in a silage/concentrate mix. Intakes will not be adequate if sodium bicarbonate is offered *ad libitum*, 300–400 g per cow per day is needed to produce the required effect. This amount cannot be incorporated successfully in compound concentrates.

High butterfat percentage

Cows in significant negative energy balance tend to produce milk with a high butterfat content. So if this is the complaint, a metabolic profile test should be carried out to check. There are specialised commercial concentrate rations on the market designed to enhance milk protein and suppress milk fat. It is advisable for veterinary surgeons not to get involved in predicting responses to these. Diets high in conserved forage and/or digestible fibre will tend to produce milk higher in fat content.

Failure to yield to expectation, no loss of condition

A metabolic profile test is essential to define which constraints are present and those which are not. The latter is just as important. Groups of cows included should be in the last week of pregnancy, pre-peak (10–20 days calved) and in mid lactation. The most common causes of this type of complaint arise from dry cow management, a short sharp energy problem in early lactation, ERDP dietary shortage and/or DUP dietary shortage. Very rarely herd subclinical hypomagnesaemia will do this. Then it is usual to find herd excitability, but a metabolic profile test is necessary to confirm it.

Poor fertility

Poor fertility of course is a very common complaint, with farmers expecting blood tests of subfertile cows to provide the answers. They hardly ever do, but they provide opportunities for misdiagnosing endless trace element red herrings. As the main nutritional causes of poor fertility occur in late pregnancy and early lactation, i.e. well before the symptoms of poor fertility are apparent, a standard metabolic profile of a group in the last week of pregnancy, a group 10–20 days calved and some mid lactation cows, which can be those failing to conceive thus keeping the farmer happy, will frequently allow accurate diagnosis. There is a problem if the early lactation and dry cows available are on a different regime from those with poor fertility when they were at the same stage. Then all metabolite values may be within the reference ranges. Analysis of fertility records may allow a particular season to be identified and plans to be made to blood test earlier next time. Analysis may also show that fertility in groups of cows calved on the regimes currently experienced by dry and early lactation animals is reasonable by comparison. Where historical nutrition is the cause of cows failing to conceive now, milk protein may be low and a contrast in condition scores between the dry period and peak yield may have been noticed by the farmer or the vet at routine visits. In addition, analysis of records may show second service conception rate greater than first, higher conception rates in first lactation heifers than in cows and an increase in conception rate with days calved after 7–8 weeks calved. It is always worth remembering that most cows conceive eventually anyway. So, interventions including expensive mineral supplements are often perceived to have worked when in fact they have had no influence.

A run of stillborn calves

A metabolic profile of a group of dry cows/pregnant heifers at the end of pregnancy and some 10–20 days calved including some that gave birth to dead calves should be carried out. Severe precalving energy problems/acute fatty liver syndrome and magnesium, iodine, copper, selenium and, in winter, vitamin E deficiencies should all be investigated. For interpretation of the results, refer to earlier sections of the chapter. Investigations for the possibility that infectious disease, such as *Leptospira hardjo* or bovine viral diarrhoea (BVD), are involved should also be carried out.

A run of retained fetal membranes (RFM)

Mini-epidemics of retained fetal membranes (RFM) are common. Frequently, by the time investigation has produced no clear reason, the epidemic has stopped anyway. Severe precalving energy problems can be involved. Thus, a metabolic profile of some cows in the last week of pregnancy is advisable and it will be perceived by the farmer as action. Selenium deficiency is supposed to be a possibility, but current experience raises some doubts. Because of the delayed relationship between selenium intake and glutathione peroxidase (GSHPx) blood level, dry cows that are experiencing a dietary selenium deficiency may have GSHPx blood levels within the reference range but low values in lactation even after they have started a satisfactorily supplemented diet. Firm diagnosis therefore may depend on injecting one of a number of paired dry cows and seeing what happens. *Brucella* infection and other abortifacient agents cause a high incidence of RFM. It is possible that the mini-epidemics of RFM are caused by some relatively trivial systemic infection which has passed through the group unnoticed at an earlier stage of pregnancy.

Hypomagnesaemia/staggers (see also pp. 60–62)

One unexpected dead cow may be the first sign of hypomagnesaemia or staggers, but post mortem findings are never conclusive. Circumstantial evidence may be quite strong, but cases can occur in milking cows in temperate climates in any month of the year. So a metabolic profile should be done because if there is one cow dead from hypomagnesaemia, others will have low blood levels and be at risk. The blood test will allow an assessment also of the possible involvement of low energy and high ammonia in the rumen in the inhibition of the absorption of dietary magnesium. British dairy farmers are well aware of the risks of hypomagnesaemia and act accordingly. However, dropping milk price and the consequence of depending more on forages increases the risks. Routine blood testing at times such as spring and early summer may therefore be a wise precaution. Only between 10 and 35% of dietary magnesium is absorbed; 30g of magnesium per day (equivalent to 60g of calcined magnesite) in the diet is the average target for a milking cow. The need is a daily one as the cow cannot effectively draw on reserves. An inclusion of magnesium in concentrates is the most sure way to deliver this, but even then the variations in the inhibition of absorption make prevention not possible to guarantee. Other methods of magnesium supplementation have all failed on occasion because a level daily intake is so difficult to achieve. On lush grazing, the enforced feeding of conserved long fibre may help. The timing of the application of nitrogen and potash fertilisers may be worth discussing for next season. However, without doubt the most successful control and prevention measure is to ensure a daily dietary intake of enough magnesium.

Hypocalcaemia/milk fever (see also p. 81)

Mini-epidemics of hypocalcaemia or milk fever are common, with 90% of cows calving over a short period sometimes affected. Metabolic profile testing is of limited use. It should be done nevertheless in cows close to calving to make sure that a dietary magnesium deficiency is not involved. Blood samples taken from clinical cases immediately prior to treatment are only of use for diagnosis. Levels of calcium, magnesium and phosphate then reflect the metabolic disturbance of the condition and they do not provide indications of potential predisposing causes. As four fifths of the diet of heavily pregnant cows consists of forage, the first preventive action should always be to change the forage source in the ration – another field, introduce silage, off grass and onto silage, another silage clamp, big bale silage instead of clamp, bales of silage from another field. The effect can be dramatic. Otherwise, maintain as low a calcium intake as possible until calving is imminent. Then increase it. Maintain a high magnesium level in the late dry cow ration. Maintain a high input of anions – chlorides particularly. Sulphates and phosphates exert the same effect, but supplementing with either has some theoretical hazards. Magnesium chloride is the supplement of choice. It can be most effectively supplied by maintaining some coarse crystals/flakes all the time in a permeable container in the ball tap compartment of all water supplies to which the cows have access. Failures with this approach occur when the container is allowed to remain empty for periods or unmedicated water sources are also available.

Low conception rate in maiden heifers (see also pp. 41–3)

ERDP and trace element deficiencies are quite common in heifers brought to service on straw or low quality silage-based diets. Insufficient supplementation with ERDP frequently occurs. As these are growing animals, trace element needs are different to those of adults and shortcomings particularly with selenium may be present. A metabolic profile test should therefore be carried out, but the possibility of a problem with DIY AI technique or semen storage or with a bull being used needs to be considered.

Summary

In the early days of the use of metabolic profiles – the late 1960s and early 1970s – there was a tendency to assume that all blood biochemical values were a precise indication of the nutritional situation of a group of animals. The ability and, for some metabolites, the absolute life-maintaining need for homeostatic mechanisms to control blood levels has meant that some measurements are valueless as a reflection of nutritional status and others only of value if the timing of sampling is carefully thought about in advance. In addition, as there are a number of different reasons and so solutions to each biochemical pattern, the value of metabolic profiles depends on a thorough understanding of what is happening on each farm at the time when blood samples are taken. With increasing emphasis on prevention, the full use and interpretation of metabolic profiles provides a major opportunity for the modern veterinary surgeon to exercise both the art and science of veterinary medicine to the positive benefit of productivity. Using the notion that the technique 'asks the cows' – the end-users – what they think of their nutrition, planning of the timing of tests can allow checks on each nutritional situation soon after it is in place. So constraints can be identified and rectified before loss of productivity or fertility is apparent. Metabolic profiles are widely used in the UK in this way, but the technique is also widely used as part of the resolution of problems already in existence.

Further reading

AFRC (1995) *Energy and Protein Requirements of Ruminants.* An Advisory Manual prepared by the Agricultural and Food Research Council Technical Committee on Responses to Nutrients. CAB International, Wallingford.

Brand, A., Noordhuizen, J. P. T. M. & Schukken, Y. H. (1996) *Herd Health and Production Management in Dairy Practice.* Wageningen Pers, Wageningen, The Netherlands.

McDonald, P., Edwards, R. A., Greenhalgh, J. F. D. & Morgan, C. A. (1995) *Animal Nutrition*, 5th edn. Longman Scientific & Technical, Harlow.

Webster, J. (1993) *Understanding the Dairy Cow.* Blackwell Scientific Publications, Oxford.

Chapter 5
Fertility and Infertility

David Noakes

Normal structure and function of the genital system

A knowledge of the normal, gross anatomical structure of the genital system is an important requirement for good clinical examination of the cow and the bull.

The cow

The external genitalia comprise the vulval labia which are covered with soft, thin skin and a minimum of hair. At the ventral commissure the length of the hair at the mucocutaneous junction is greater, giving a characteristic tuft. In the freemartin heifer it may be more obvious. The vulva, particularly the constrictor muscle, provides an effective physical barrier to the entry of opportunist bacteria from the environment. Trauma, which impairs its function, can be followed by temporary or permanent aspiration of air (pneumovagina) with consequential bacterial contamination.

The vestibule is approximately 8–10 cm in length. At the vestibular/vaginal junction the urethra and sub-urethral diverticulum open ventrally (Figs. 5.1–5.3); the latter is a blind pouch about 3.5 cm in length. In some cows the canals of Gartner, remnants of the Woolfian ducts, can be identified as thickened quill-like or cystic structures in the floor of the anterior vagina. The vagina is about 30 cm in length although it can appear to be very variable because of the mobility of the cervix. It is lined by a smooth, pink mucosa. It is only a potential cavity because other than at coitus, at parturition or immediately post partum the walls are closely apposed. If the vulval seal is broken, air is aspirated and dilates the vagina.

Ventrally in the anterior vagina a number of mucosal folds arise which often become more distinct and merge with the cervix (Fig. 5.4). The cervix is an important physical barrier which is only breached at calving and during artificial insemination (not at natural service since the bull serves into the anterior vagina). It protrudes into the anterior vagina and is surrounded by a well-developed fornix which is deeper dorsally than ventrally. The cervical canal opens at the external os and is surrounded by a number of folds to give it a 'rosette-like' appearance (Fig. 5.5). Location of the external os can be difficult in some individuals because

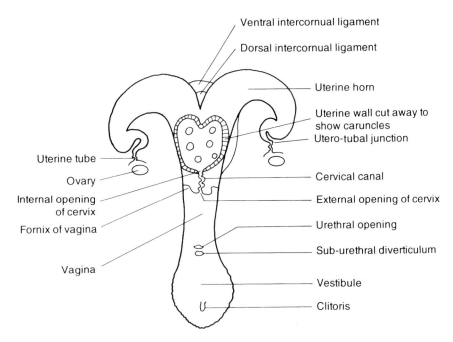

Fig. 5.1   The cow's genital system viewed from the dorsal surface; note that uterine body wall, cervical and vaginal/vestibular walls have been removed.

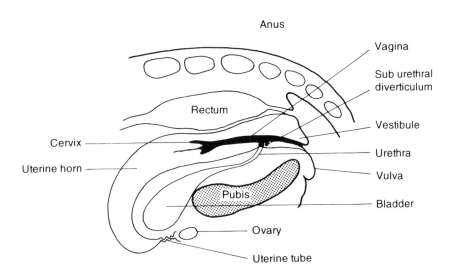

Fig. 5.2   Sagittal section of pelvic area of the cow, showing the genital organs.

of these folds and indentations. The cervix is 5–12 cm in length and 2–8 cm in width, being smallest in prepubertal and nulligravid individuals, larger in pluri-para and largest during pregnancy.

The cervical canal is irregular, with transverse folds which can interfere with the passage of cervical intra-uterine catheters. The uterine body is 3–4 cm in

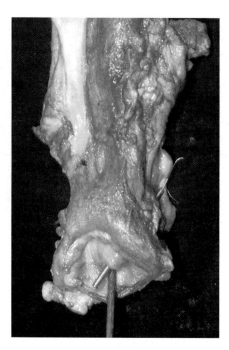

Fig. 5.3 Vestibular/vaginal junction. Note metal probe is inserted into the urethra (and can be seen protruding from the severed end); wooden probe is inserted into the sub-urethral diverticulum.

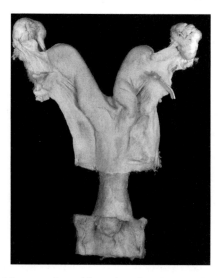

Fig. 5.4 Genital tract of the cow viewed from dorsal surface, with cranial dorsal vaginal wall incised (to show cervix protruding into anterior vagina) and cervical folds extending onto ventral surface of vagina.

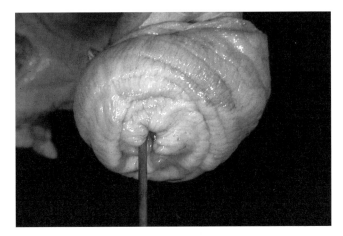

Fig. 5.5 Cervix protruding into anterior vagina with characteristic 'rosette-like' appearance surrounding external opening of cervical canal into which a probe has been inserted.

length and quickly divides to form two uterine horns which are about 30–45 cm in length in post-pubertal, non-gravid genital tracts. The horns curve outwards (laterally) caudally and ventrally and at the same time taper to about 2–3 mm in diameter, almost merging imperceptibly with the uterine tube at the utero-tubal junction (Fig. 5.6). The uterine tubes comprise three parts: immediately after the utero-tubal junction there is a narrow, convoluted portion – the isthmus – which then widens to form the ampulla where fertilisation occurs, before opening into the abdominal cavity via the ostium or infundibulum which is surrounded by the funnel-shaped fimbrae. The uterine tubes are 20–30 cm in length, the isthmus is 2–3 cm long and the ampulla 5–6 mm in diameter (Fig. 5.7). The uterine horns are suspended in the pelvis and caudal abdomen by the broad ligament which is attached to the lesser curvature of each horn; it contains smooth muscle and fat, and the blood and nerve supply to the uterus and uterine tubes.

Ovaries

The ovaries are essentially ovoid although extremely variable both in outline and in size. This is because during the oestrous cycle they undergo constant change associated with the growth, regression and ovulation of follicles, and the formation and regression of the corpus luteum (CL). The ovaries are attached to the cranial border of the broad ligament, there is a well developed utero-ovarian ligament which is attached to the medial surface of the ovary and is supported dorsally and laterally by a portion of the broad ligament – the mesovarium. In the post-pubertal animal, normal ovaries range in size from as small as $1 \times 1 \times 0.5$ cm to up to $5 \times 4 \times 2$ cm. Pathological conditions (see below) can result in much larger structures.

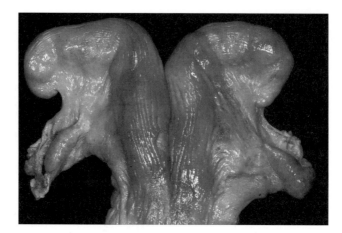

Fig. 5.6   Uterine horns showing curvature and tapering towards utero-tubal junction.

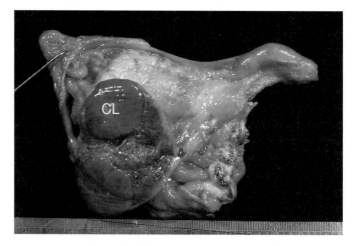

Fig. 5.7   Tip of uterine horn, utero-tubal junction and uterine tube with adjacent ovary, which has been sectioned to show the corpus luteum (CL).

Ovarian structures

Mature follicles just before ovulation reach a maximum size of about 2 cm in diameter, although it must be stressed that on palpation they do not feel as large as this. Ovulation occurs at any point of the surface of the ovary following rupture of the *tunica albuginea* which covers the surface of the ovary. After ovulation there is slight haemorrhage into the space occupied by the previous mature follicle; at this stage it is sometimes possible to palpate rectally a softened depression on the surface of the ovary and sometimes slight crepitus can be identified. The granulosa cells of the follicle hypertrophy and become luteinised to form the CL. This results in enlargement of the ovary and, in some cases, but not always, a distinct ovulation papilla can be identified. The CL generally has a 'rubber-like' texture on palpation as it develops, reaching a maximum size at about 7 days after ovulation when it is about 2–2.5 cm long. The CL remains this size until about 17–18 days when it becomes smaller in size and harder in consistency. Throughout the time that the CL is present in the ovary (dioestrus or the luteal phase) the ovaries are continually changing in size and shape because of waves of follicular growth and regression. In some individual cows there are two and in others three follicular waves (and in a very small number four waves). Thus, the presence of follicles palpable on rectal palpation in association with a CL is quite a common occurrence.

The ability to identify accurately a CL on rectal palpation is dependent upon its size, shape, degree of protrusion from the surface of the ovary and the prominence of the ovulation papilla. Figure 5.8 shows the different types of CLs. In up to 25% of CLs there is a central, fluid-filled cavity or vacuole. These are sometimes incorrectly designated 'cystic corpora lutea' (Fig. 5.9) since they are not pathological, do not cause aberrant cyclical activity and result from a normal ovulation. They should not be confused with a luteal cyst (see 'Oestrus not observed') and in order to prevent confusion are better referred to as vacuolated CLs.

In some instances, luteinisation of anovulatory follicles occurs particularly in the immediate post partum period before the establishment of normal hypo-thalamic/pituitary/ovarian function. Their lifespan is not greater than that of a CL and, although they do not normally cause aberrant cyclical activity, they can be associated with a short luteal phase. More ovulations occur from the right than the left ovary.

The bull

The external genitalia comprise the testes and epididymides enclosed within the scrotum, and the penis enclosed within the prepuce except when erect (Fig. 5.10). The testes descend in the foetal bull calf mid-way through gestation. Puberty occurs at about 9–10 months of age at which time obvious changes occur. Firstly, the testes increase in size and, secondly, there is physical separation of the attachment of the penile mucosa to the prepuce.

The testes of the adult bull are about $13 \times 7 \times 7$ cm, weigh about 350 g and are very similar in size. The tail of the epididymis can be readily palpated at the ventral (most dependent) pole of the testis as a soft swelling; palpation of the head and body of the epididymis is difficult.

The *ductus deferens*, which originates from the tail of the epididymis, passes in the spermatic cord via the inguinal canal into the abdomen. Before the ductus deferens enters the pelvic urethra it dilates to form the ampulla. Each ampulla is about 10–15 cm in length and about 12–15 mm in diameter. The penis originates from the ischial arch of the pelvis as a tough, tubular structure which extends cranially and ventrally, forming the sigmoid flexure just caudal to the scrotum. As a result of erection the sigmoid flexure is straightened. The penis tapers slightly to form the *glans penis* which is about 8 cm in length and which becomes flattened and twisted near its tip, with the urethra opening at the

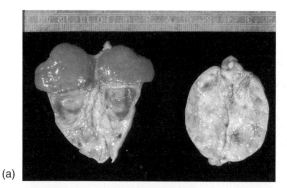

(a)

Fig. 5.8a Both ovaries sectioned along the sagittal plane showing presence of mature CL in the left ovary, together with a 1-cm follicle. The right ovary is smaller and there are no structures of note.

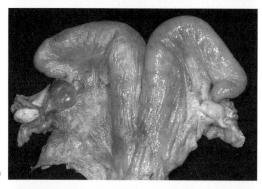

(b)

Fig. 5.8b The left ovary is large with a mature CL and a mid-dioestral follicle. The right ovary is smaller and there are no structures of note.

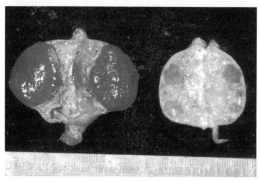

(c)

Fig. 5.8c Both ovaries sectioned along the sagittal plane showing mature CL in the left ovary and remnants of regressed CLs in the right ovary.

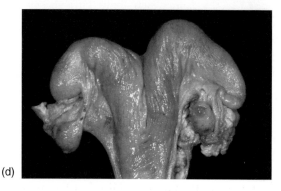

(d)

Fig. 5.8d The left ovary is large and contains a mature CL (with ovulation papilla) and surface antral follicle. The right ovary is smaller and there are two antral follicles apparent on the surface.

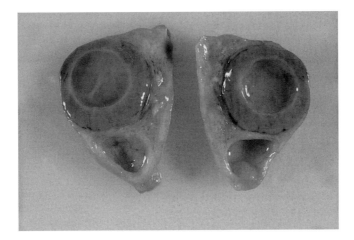

Fig. 5.9 Sagittal section of an ovary of a cow, showing vacuolated CL with thick layer of luteal tissue, together with a follicle.

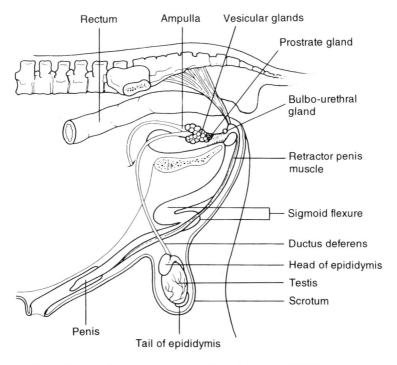

Fig. 5.10 The bull's genital system. (Redrawn from Ashdown, 1986.)

end of a groove formed by the twist. The overall length of the penis in the adult bull is about 90 cm.

The prostate gland comprises two parts. One part is stretched across the dorsal surface of the neck of the bladder at the origin of the urethra, whilst the other part surrounds the pelvic urethra. The paired vesicular glands are compact, soft,

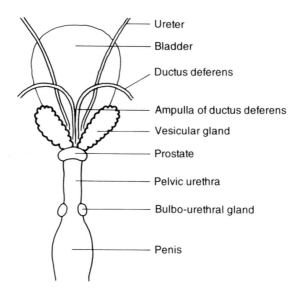

Ureter

Bladder

Ductus deferens

Ampulla of ductus deferens

Vesicular gland

Prostate

Pelvic urethra

Bulbo-urethral gland

Penis

Fig. 5.11   The bull's intra-pelvic genital organs viewed from the dorsal surface.

lobulated structures about 10–12 cm in length and 5 cm wide, lying lateral to the ampullae of the ductus deferentia (Fig. 5.11). They frequently differ slightly in size.

Clinical examination

The cow

Clinical examination of the genital tract is performed as a method of diagnosing pregnancy when there is evidence of reproductive disease shown by an abnormal discharge, after abortion, at parturition if dystocia is suspected, as part of a routine prebreeding examination in cows that are at risk (see pp. 145–6) before sale, and when there is evidence of infertility (see pp. 140–45).

Traditionally, clinical examination has been restricted to either visual inspection or palpation, the latter being vaginal or rectal palpation. Whilst these are still of major importance, the use of other techniques is emerging, notably ultrasound imaging, and, indirectly, changes in progesterone concentrations in the peripheral plasma or milk. Whilst more specialist techniques such as the PSP dye test to determine uterine tubal patency can be useful, routine microbiological culture and endometrial biopsies have a more limited application.

Visual inspection

Visual inspection of the vulva and vestibular mucosa, together with the appearance and volume of any discharge, is readily performed. The vulva should be sym-

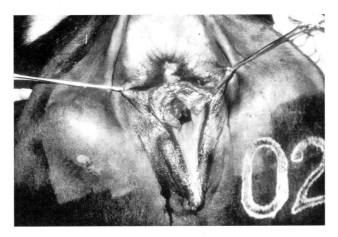

Fig. 5.12 Cow with third-degree perineal laceration. Note the breakdown of tissue between rectum and vestibule/vagina creates a cloaca. (From Noakes, 1997.)

metrical with no evidence of recent or previous trauma; Fig. 5.12 illustrates a cow that suffered a third-degree perineal laceration at the time of calving. The labia can be parted to examine the vestibular mucosa and the appearance of any discharge; the mucosa is normally pink and moist. Generalised or localised inflammation or the presence of any lesions such as papules, pustules or ulcers should be noted.

The presence and appearance of any vulval discharge should also be noted; this may be attached to the ventral commissure of the vulva, or it may be attached to the tail just below its point of contact with the vulva. Normal discharges are: (1) clear elastic mucus around oestrus, (2) bright-red blood-stained mucus in metoestrus, and (3) reddish-brown puerperal discharge 7–14 days post partum. Abnormal discharges will be associated with placental retention (see 'Abnormal vulval discharge') and with infection of the genital tract comprising inflammatory exudates or mucopurulent fluid originating from the vestibule, vagina or uterus.

The vagina and cervix and their mucous membrane can be examined visually using a speculum. This is a useful procedure where there is an abnormal discharge, particularly in order to confirm the presence of a vaginitis due to some specific infectious agents such as bovine herpes virus (infectious pustular vulvo-vaginitis), granular vulvovaginitis or the presence of vaginal urine pooling or a vaginal tumour. For each examination a sterile speculum or guard is necessary to prevent the spread of venereally transmitted infectious agents, and also to reduce general contamination.

Vaginal palpation

Vaginal palpation is performed to investigate the parturient animal or where there is an abnormal discharge. At parturition, the degree of cervical dilation can be assessed or the disposition of the calf determined. When there is an abnormal discharge the quantity and appearance of the discharge can be assessed by scooping material from the anterior vagina just caudal to the cervix. The presence of major lesions or the presence of urine pooling can be detected.

Vaginal palpation in the normal animal, especially around oestrus just before insemination or natural service, should be discouraged. Vaginal palpation should be performed as cleanly as possible.

Rectal palpation

Rectal palpation is an important technique used in both normal and abnormal animals, requiring regular routine to prevent omissions; a repeat examination at a later date may be necessary for confirmation of the reproductive status of the animal. Unless a pneumovagina is created it will be difficult to identify this organ, so that the first structure to identify by palpation is the cervix. This is an important landmark in the clinical examination of the genital system, especially for beginners. The cervix will be within the pelvis in nullipara, on the brim of the pelvis in most non-pregnant, parous individuals, and on or over the brim in pregnant and immediately post parturient individuals. The cervix is slightly conical in shape, being wider caudally than cranially. It increases in size during pregnancy, and increases incrementally with each succeeding parity. It becomes less mobile as pregnancy advances. Note its position, size and mobility.

The bifurcation is just cranial to the cervix and can usually be identified as a cleft with the horns eventually diverging (Figs. 5.4 and 5.6). The ease of identification of the uterine horns will depend upon the stage of the oestrous cycle; thus at oestrus there is increased tone and the horns become tubular and more coiled but during dioestrus there is flaccidity. During early pregnancy the tone increases, but the horns are of different sizes, the walls of the uterus become thin and the contents fluctuant. Uterine infection results in oedema of the uterine wall, hence they feel doughy on palpation. The presence or absence of adhesions can sometimes be determined. The uterine tubes are difficult to identify by palpation if normal; enlargement or induration makes identification simpler.

The ovaries in the non-pregnant animal are usually within 5 cm of the cornual bifurcation and close to the pelvic brim (Figs. 5.1, 5.2, 5.4 and 5.6). They cannot be palpated rectally beyond 5 months of gestation in most cows. At oestrus, because of increased uterine tone and the tendency for the horns to become coiled, they are generally more cranial in relation to the uterine horns.

The ovaries should be examined for size and the nature of any palpable structures. Normally, the ovaries are largest when they contain a fully formed, functional CL. In a pluriparous cow such an ovary will be at least $4 \times 3 \times 2$ cm, with the fully formed CL being about 2.5 cm at its largest dimension (Figs. 5.8a, 5.8c and 5.13). Less marked changes will be associated with follicular growth and regression. Although the mature follicle is about 2–2.5 cm in diameter at the time of ovulation, follicles as large as 1.5 cm are frequently palpable during dioestrus; these subsequently regress and become atretic. Waves of follicular growth occur throughout the oestrous cycle (Fig. 5.13), (see, pp. 124–5). The important structure to identify is the CL; if it is palpable it indicates

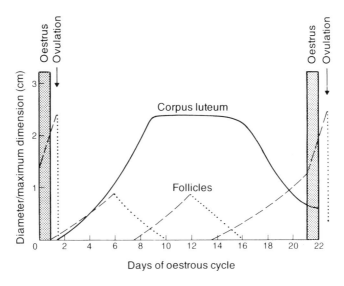

Fig. 5.13 Growth and regression of follicles and CL during the oestrous cycle (this is an example of a cow with three waves of follicular growth).

that the cow has ovulated and thus may be in dioestrus, pregnant, or it may be persistent due to infection (see pp. 142–3). The accuracy of identifying ovarian structures by palpation is probably not greater than 70% even by experienced clinicians. Estimation of the size of ovaries can be made using the comparison with finger thickness.

Ovaries that contain no palpable structures and are small are probably, but not definitely, associated with acyclicity. However, this cannot be determined accurately following a single examination and requires sequential palpation for confirmation. Ovaries that are larger than normal, i.e. >4 × 3 × 2 cm, probably contain cysts (see Fig. 5.14). A cyst is defined as a fluid-filled structure present within the ovary and >2.5 cm in diameter, i.e. larger than a normal mature follicle. Cysts may or may not be responsible for cystic ovarian disease (see p. 142). An enlarged ovary can also be due to the presence of a granulosa cell tumour, but these are rare. An ovary with twin CLs due to twin ovulations can be much larger.

Other fluid-filled structures which develop are luteinised follicles and cavitated or vacuolated CLs (see pp. 140–41).

Ultrasound

The development of B mode real-time ultrasonography has enabled the genital system to be imaged using the transrectal approach. Whilst it has been shown to be very accurate in the identification of pregnant cows from as early as 14–15 days (Pierson and Ginther, 1984) using a 7.5-mHZ transducer probe, and from 25–26 days using a 5-mHZ probe, the accuracy of identifying all ovarian structures has been somewhat disappointing. Whereas it is very accurate in

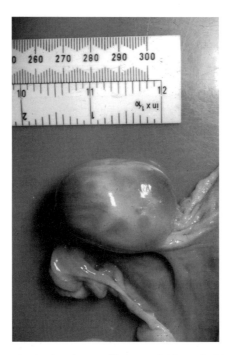

Fig. 5.14 Ovary of nymphomaniacal cow with several thin-walled follicular cysts.

identifying follicles and detecting CLs, the ability to determine the age of CLs, particularly early or regressing, has been shown to be little better than rectal palpation (Pieterse *et al.*, 1990). Figures 5.15a and 5.15b show examples of echograms of ovaries.

Hormone assays

Reproductive function can be monitored using progesterone assays in the peripheral circulation and in milk. The measurement of other hormones, with the exception of oestrone sulphate in plasma or milk to diagnose pregnancy after 100 days, is of no practical value. The measurement of progesterone in plasma or milk, except after 100 days of gestation when the placenta commences the synthesis, enables assessment of luteal function, since the rise and fall of progesterone is directly correlated with the functional state of the CL.

With the availability of simple qualitative ELISA assay kits it is possible for routine progesterone assays to be done on the farm and in veterinary practice.

The bull

Before sale or purchase and when infertility is suspected it may be necessary to examine the reproductive system. However, the only absolute proof of fertility is the bull's ability to sire offspring. Initially, it will be necessary to determine the

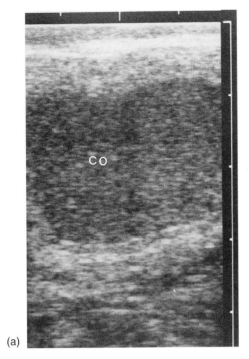

(a)

Fig. 5.15a Ovary showing CL (CO) which has a distinctive 'speckled' echotexture and defined border from the rest of the ovarian stroma. (Scale: 6 mm.)

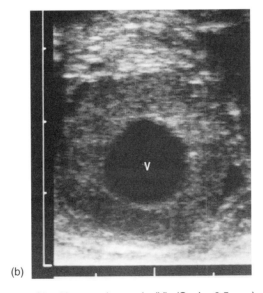

(b)

Fig. 5.15b Ovary with CL with central vacuole (V). (Scale: 6.5 mm.)

bull's libido. This is best done by presenting a cow or heifer in oestrus (usually induced to occur at a specific time using prostaglandin F2α) to the bull in its normal environment in which it serves. Methods of quantification can be used, e.g. measurement of the reaction time (the time from access to the female and first mounting), time to first service and the number of repeated services. In some cases a quantitative measurement is made and is referred to as the libido score (Chenowith, 1986).

It is then necessary to determine: (1) if the bull is capable of mounting a cow in oestrus and performing service normally; (2) if the penis is protruded normally; (3) if normal intromission is achieved with thrusting, and, as a consequence, ejaculation. During the preliminary teasing phase the penis can be visually inspected, for although there are methods of causing relaxation of the penis using cranial epidural or pudendal nerve blocks (Hall and Clarke, 1995) these are either fraught with some danger or are difficult to perform.

The next component of the clinical examination involves the assessment of the external genitalia. This should be performed systematically: firstly, palpation and visual inspection of the scrotum, vestigial mammary glands, testes, epididymides and spermatic cords (see Fig. 5.10). Consistency and size of the testes are important, as is the consistency and size of the epididymides, especially the *cauda epididymis*. The testes should be of the correct size for the age and breed of bull. This is usually assessed by measuring the scrotal circumference at its greatest point; in yearling bulls normally it should be greater than 30 cm, whilst in mature bulls it should be approaching 40 cm. Testes size has been shown to be correlated with a number of fertility parameters in the bull, such as sperm output and sperm quality. The testes should be of approximately equal size, obvious disparity should be viewed with concern, and be painless on palpation and freely mobile in the scrotum. They should be soft, but not flaccid, when compressed between thumb and finger with the surface capable of being depressed very slightly. The tail of the epididymis should be soft and full. The head and body of the epididymis is difficult to identify.

The prepuce should be soft and pliable, the preputial opening capable of accommodating 3–4 fingers; the preputial mucosa should not protrude. The penis can be palpated within the prepuce and should be of equal diameter along its length (except for the tip) and freely mobile in the prepuce. It is usually just possible to palpate the sigmoid flexure cranial to the scrotum (see Fig. 5.10). There should be no evidence of blood or dried discharge on the hairs surrounding the preputial opening.

The internal genitalia can be palpated per rectum. The vesicular glands, a site of infection in young bulls, are paired, soft, lobulated structures (Figs. 5.10 and 5.11). If infected and inflamed they are usually painful, enlarged and, because they are harder, they can be palpated more easily. The prostate gland feels like a collar at the cranial end of the urethra. The ampullae of the vas deferens can be identified as paired 'pencil-like' tubular structures about 1.5 cm in diameter and 12 cm in length. They can be rolled under the fingers against the brim and floor of the pelvis (Figs. 5.10 and 5.11).

Visual inspection of the penis is best done at the time of teasing when the degree of protrusion, the absence of curvature or deviations and the appearance of the integument can be assessed.

Semen evaluation is an important part of evaluation of the bull, especially if the bull is unproven or has evidence of abnormality or suspect fertility. This should be done routinely at the time of purchase, hire or, for a home-bred yearling, *before* he is required for service. Considerable expense can be incurred and time lost if a sub-fertile bull is used. Whilst it is possible to aspirate semen from the anterior vagina after natural service, and to examine it for the presence of spermatozoa which may or may not be motile, because it will be diluted with mucus and is only an aliquot of the total ejaculate, quantitative tests are not possible. The most reliable method is collection using an artificial vagina (AV) (Figs. 5.16 and 5.17). For this, a teaser cow or heifer in oestrus is required. The bull

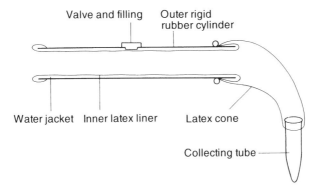

Fig. 5.16 An artificial vagina.

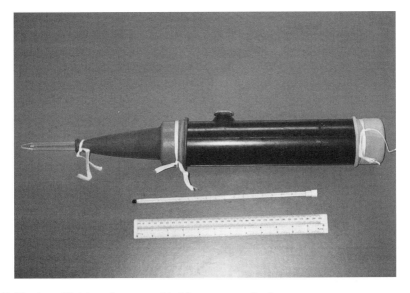

Fig. 5.17 An artificial vagina assembled for semen collection.

should be rested for a week before collection. Some bulls, especially if their libido is suspect or they are nervous or resent the restraint necessary for safe handling, are reluctant to serve into an AV. Patience will usually be rewarded. It is important to check regularly the temperature of the water in the AV liner frequently whilst waiting, so that it is about 44 °C when used. Ejaculation can be assumed to have occurred when the bull thrusts vigorously.

The following are normal semen parameters:

- Volume: 4–5 ml
- Colour: white to creamy with marbling
- Mass motility: vigorous swirling movement when examined under low power
- Individual motility: after dilution with physiological saline or minimal essential medium (MEM) vigorous progressive movement of individual spermatozoa.

Following eosin-nigrosin staining there should not be more than 30% dead and 30% abnormal sperm in the ejaculate, depending on the duration of the rest period before collection.

Some abnormalities are induced by faulty technique. Assessment of a single ejaculate should not normally be used to evaluate a bull. Some degree of compensation can be made between good and bad facets of the ejaculate, particularly in relation to the number of sperm in each ejaculate and the number of normal, live, vigorously motile spermatozoa.

Endocrine control of reproduction

Female

Puberty in the heifer is heralded by the onset of cyclical ovarian activity; thus she will come into oestrus, accept natural service, and be capable of becoming pregnant. The time of onset of puberty is dependent upon breed, body weight and age; it generally ranges from 7 to 18 months, with dairy breeds being more precocious.

After the onset of puberty the heifer or cow undergoes continuous cyclical ovarian activity; the only time that cyclical activity ceases is during pregnancy and for a few weeks post partum. Cyclical ovarian activity is controlled by the interaction of hormones produced by the hypothalamus, anterior pituitary, ovary and uterus. The CL occupies a pivotal role in the control of cyclical activity.

The hypothalamic neurones secrete a decapeptide hormone, gonadotrophin (GnRH). This substance is transferred, via the hypothalamic/hypophyseal portal system, to the anterior pituitary, and stimulates the release of both follicular stimulating hormone (FSH) and luteinising hormone (LH). These are glycoproteins of molecular weight 25 000 and 40 000, respectively. Basal or tonic FSH secretion stimulates follicular growth and, in combination with basal or tonic LH secretion, stimulates the larger Graafian follicles to secrete oestrogen. The rise in oestrogen exerts a stimulatory effect (positive feedback) on the hypothalamus, which, via the secretion of GnRH, stimulates an episodic surge of LH secretion causing ovulation. LH is also luteotrophic, stimulating the formation of the CL.

Follicular growth and regression is a feature of the oestrous cycle of the cow. Some cows have two and others three waves of follicular growth; those with the latter pattern tend to have a longer cycle length (Fig. 5.13). As well as the role of gonadotrophins in stimulating follicular growth, ovulation and CL formation, there are also intra-ovarian hormones, notably inhibin, which have an important role. Inhibin, which is secreted by the granulosa cells of the developing antral follicle, is a peptide which, in combination with oestradiol, exerts a negative feedback on FSH secretion and possibly prevents FSH binding to the granulosa cells. Other intra-ovarian peptide hormones, namely activin and follistatin, are also believed to play a role in controlling folliculogenesis, particularly in association with inhibin in ensuring that normally only one dominant follicle develops to the preovulatory stage.

Once the CL develops there is a rise in peripheral progesterone concentrations since the luteal cells of the CL secrete progesterone. Progesterone suppresses the release of episodic gonadotrophin and hence prevents oestrus and ovulation. The lifespan of the CL is terminated by the episodic release of prostaglandin F2α (PGF2α) from the endometrium, induced by the secretion of oxytocin by the CL, which mediates its effect via oxytocin receptors in the endometrium. These increase during the luteal phase of the oestrous cycle due to stimulation by both progesterone and oestradiol, particularly the latter which is associated with the wave of follicular growth that occurs. Once the CL regresses then the negative feedback effect on the hypothalamus and anterior pituitary is removed, allowing gonadotrophins to be secreted and resulting in follicular maturation, oestrus and ovulation.

A schematic representation of the main hormone changes in the peripheral circulation is shown in Fig. 5.18.

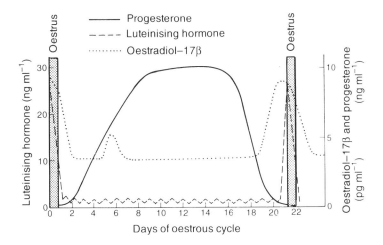

Fig. 5.18 Hormone changes in peripheral blood during the oestrous cycle.

The oestrous cycle

The interval between the onset of successive behavioural oestral periods is generally assumed to be 21 days; however, there are considerable variations, with 60–70% of cows having a cycle length of 17–25 days (Hafez, 1993; Peters and Ball, 1995). Opinions vary on the duration of oestrus in the cow with figures ranging from 2 to 30 hours. The duration of oestrus is influenced by factors such as breed of cow, presence of bull, presence of other cows in oestrus, time of day, ability to express signs. An average figure is probably about 15 hours. Ovulation, which is spontaneous, occurs about 30 hours after the onset of oestrus.

Signs of oestrus

The signs of oestrus are many and varied and can be listed as follows:

- Increased restlessness
- Grouping of cows in or around oestrus
- Bellowing, if isolated
- Reduced milk yield
- Slight increase in body temperature
- Abrasions of tail head
- Scuff marks around flanks
- Clear, elastic, vulval mucous discharge
- Standing to be mounted or rarely head to head mounting

Cows will frequently mount other cows when they are approaching the onset of oestrus, or at other times, hence this is not a sign of true oestrus. A fresh blood-stained vulval mucous discharge is indicative that the cow has been in oestrus a few days before (metoestral bleeding).

Traditionally, the oestrous cycle is divided into four stages. Proestrus is the period just before behavioural oestrus when the CL with be regressing and the cow may show more mounting behaviour. Metoestrus is the period after ovulation when the CL is developing. Dioestrus (luteal phase) is the period when the CL is fully formed and when progesterone concentrations are elevated. Oestrus is the only readily discernible phase of the oestrous cycle. However, the use of the terms 'luteal phase' for that part dominated by the CL and 'non-luteal' or 'follicular phase' for the remainder of the cycle is more appropriate.

Male

Reproductive function in the bull shows no signs of seasonality. Thus, once a bull has reached puberty, libido and spermatogenesis remain fairly constant. As in the female, the hypothalamic-pituitary-gonadal axis plays the major role in regulating reproduction. The testis has two functions: (1) it is responsible for gamete production and (2) it is an endocrine organ. Early stages of spermatogenesis are primarily under the control of FSH, although testosterone produced by the

Leydig or interstitial cells also has a role, particularly in the latter stages and in sperm maturation. Testosterone secretion is regulated via LH secretion, with testosterone exerting a negative feedback on the anterior pituitary and hypothalamus. FSH secretion is modulated by inhibin, a polypeptide hormone produced by the Sertoli cells.

Spermatogenesis is the process of spermatozoa production. It takes about 60 days from the first cell division on the seminiferous tubule to the formation of a mature spermatozoon. In addition, 8–14 days are required for maturation and transport through the epididymis. This time interval is important in relation to the frequency of examination of bulls suspected of being infertile (see pp. 146–7).

At natural service, about 6×10^9 spermatozoa are deposited in the anterior vagina and over the surface of the cervix. At artificial insemination, much lower doses of about 20×10^6 are deposited just cranial to the internal os uteri in the uterine body, although a substantial number of these will not have survived freezing. Following natural service the sperm have to negotiate the cervical mucus before reaching and residing in the cervical crypts, whereas following AI, this phase of sperm transport is largely bypassed. The sperm need to traverse the uterine horns and utero-tubal junction before reaching the ampulla of the uterine tube. Sperm transport is, to a limited extent, dependent upon the direct motility of the spermatozoa themselves; however, the contractions of the uterine horns and the uterine tubes and also the movement of the cilia in the uterine tubes provide the main propulsive effort.

During their passage through the female tubular genital tract, capacitation and the acrosome reaction occur, so that penetration of the oocyte by spermatozoa can occur when they reach the ampulla of the uterine tube. Spermatozoa can probably remain fertile for 30–48 hours (Hafez, 1993). After ovulation, the oocyte, surrounded by the *cumulus oophorus*, is harvested by the fimbria of the uterine tube, and transported to the ampulla so that fertilisation can occur. The oocyte remains fertile for 20–24 hours after ovulation (Hafez, 1993). After fertilisation the zygote spends about 72–84 hours in the uterine tube before traversing the utero-tubal junction to the uterine horns as an 8- to 16-cell morula.

Embryology, initial placentation and maternal recognition of pregnancy

The blastocyst hatches from its *zona pellicida* at 9–10 days and then undergoes rapid elongation from a 3-mm sphere at day 13, to a 25-cm filamentous structure at day 17. By 18 days it has usually extended into the contralateral horn. The earliest evidence of a loose placental attachment has been identified at 22 days.

As described above, the continuation of normal cyclical activity is dependent upon the CL regressing under the influence of PGF2α. Pregnancy results in the persistence of the CL. There is good evidence that the bovine conceptus produces a signal which results in prolongation of the lifespan of the CL – this was first described by Short (1969) as the 'maternal recognition of pregnancy' and occurs from about 14 days after insemination. The signal produced by the bovine conceptus is a trophoblast-derived protein, a type-1 interferon (IFNγ) which inhibits the formation of oxytocin receptors in the endometrium, thereby preventing luteal-derived oxytocin from stimulating PGF2α secretion; luteal oxytocin is finite and after depletion cannot be replenished during pregnancy. The practical significance of the maternal recognition of pregnancy is that, if the embryo dies before days 14–15 (early embryonic death), then the cow will return to oestrus at a normal interval, whereas if it occurs after this date (late embryonic or early fetal death) then the interval to the next oestrus will be extended.

Detection of pregnancy

Although much emphasis is placed upon the detection of pregnancy, it is really the early detection of the absence of pregnancy which is important in the reproductive management of dairy cows. Ideally, it should be before 18 days after insemination, so that a return to oestrus could be predicted, oestrus identified and the animal re-inseminated.

Detailed descriptions of the various methods available are described elsewhere (see Arthur *et al.*, 1996). The methods and the earliest and optimum times that they can be used are summarised below:

- Transrectal ultrasonography. Earliest at 13 days but optimum time for routine use from about 28 days.
- Milk or plasma progesterone assay. Sequential sampling from day 16 or 17 after insemination can be used to predict the likelihood of non-pregnancy if values decline. A single sample at 24 days after insemination, especially if combined with a sample on the day of insemination to confirm oestrus, is reliable.
- Observed return to oestrus at 18–24 days.
- Pregnancy-specific protein B (BSPB), also referred to as bovine pregnancy-associated glycoprotein (bPAG), produced by the binucleate cells of the trophoblast ectoderm, can be detected as early as 24 days.
- Identification of allantochorionic membrane by transrectal palpation. Can be used as early as 33 days, more reliable at 42 days, possible danger of inducing late embryonic death.
- Identification of gravid horn. Changes in the texture of the gravid horn, namely thinning of the uterine wall, disparity in size of the horn, soft, fluctuant texture. From 35 days.
- Palpation of placentomes. From 80 days.
- Unilateral enlargement of middle uterine artery with subsequent fremitus. From 85 days.
- Oestrone sulphate in plasma or milk. Earliest from 105 days but more reliable from 120 days.

Normal breeding practice

Sire and dam selection

Before breeding a cow or heifer there is an obvious need to select the correct sire. In the case of natural service where a sweeper bull is used to serve those animals that are not pregnant to AI, the most likely determining factor in sire selection will be the availability of the bull, the main requirement being that he should be fertile and disease-free. In the case of heifers, an important requirement is that the bull will sire calves that will not result in dystocia due to feto-maternal disproportion.

If AI is used, then semen from a reputable organisation will generally be from a bull of superior genotype. In the case of dairy cattle, the main objectives will be the improvement of milk yield, milk quality, body conformation (particularly teats, udder and locomotor system), and if beef from dairy cows is the objective, such factors as liveweight gain and carcass quality will be important (provided it is not at the expense of an increase in dystocia). It is interesting to note the wide variation in the heritability of certain traits; with milk yield it is 25–35%, whereas for percentage solids-not-fat it is 55–65%. Traditionally, sires at AI studs have been evaluated by progeny testing by assessing the first lactations of their daughters in comparison with first calving contemporaries sired by other bulls. This technique is both time consuming and expensive. However, with the advent of multiple ovulation and embryo transfer (MOET) technology, sibling testing can be performed. Dairy sires used for AI are now assessed on their predicted transmitting ability (PTA) for particular production characteristics such as milk yield, weight and percentage of milk fat and protein; this predicts the genetic merit of the particular sire to his offspring. In addition, individual PTA values can be used to derive an index that measures the overall profitability of using a particular sire. This is referred to as a PIN value and is a measure, in monetary terms, of the bull's genetic potential for milk yield, milk fat and protein production, taking into account production costs. Methods of assessing beef sires are not so well developed; however, indices are available, such as the Beef Index and Beef Value which, importantly, take into consideration the ease of calving.

Selection of dams is usually done on simple subjective measurements, although PTA and PIN values can be calculated for cows.

Natural service

In many cases natural service is not controlled, the bull being allowed to run with a group of cows or heifers and serving at will. There are problems associated with such a system and the following need to be considered:

- The bull must be known to be free from venereally transmitted disease (see p. 148).
- The bull must be observed to mount and serve cows or heifers normally; ideally his fertility should be evaluated beforehand.

- In the case of young bulls, there is a need to ensure that he is not subject to overuse or bullying.
- Harems are not formed within the herd.
- The bull should not be used too soon after transportation.
- The number of cows or heifers should not exceed 20 for a young bull in his first season, or 50 for a mature bull at pasture.
- Where possible, ensure that the bull does not suffer injury.

When controlled mating is used, the following should be considered:

- A suitable, preferably consistent, environment, with a good floor surface to prevent slipping and possible injury.
- Not more than 3–4 services per week for a young bull and 8–10 for a mature bull.

Artificial insemination

If artificial insemination is used, then provided that the semen originates from a reputable organisation, it can be assumed to be free of venereally transmitted disease. If AI is used it can either be provided by inseminator service from an AI organisation or performed by farm staff (DIY AI). Whichever method is used, it is imperative that:

- Cows and heifers have been identified in oestrus.
- They are inseminated at the correct time, unless oestrous synchronisation is used with fixed time AI (see pp. 132–4).
- They are inseminated using the correct technique.

Because of the time taken for sperm transport, capacitation and their longevity, together with the time of ovulation in the cow, it has been shown that best fertility is obtained when cows are inseminated towards the end of behavioural oestrus, i.e. about 15 hours before ovulation (Trimberger and Davis, 1943). Traditionally, a cow seen in oestrus for the first time in the morning should be inseminated in the afternoon, whilst those showing signs in the afternoon should be inseminated the following morning. However, if there is doubt about the precise time of onset of oestrus, it is preferable to inseminate earlier than the ideal time, rather than later. This is because of the time required for sperm transport and capacitation, and because spermatozoa have a greater longevity than the oocyte. Surprisingly good results have been obtained when cows have been inseminated in relation to a decline in milk progesterone, i.e. on the second day of a low milk progesterone (Foulkes *et al.*, 1982). Many cows are inseminated during dioestrus when there is obviously no possibility of conception.

AI technique

Extended bull semen is stored in liquid nitrogen at a temperature of $-196°C$, usually in 0.25-ml, *or* 0.5-ml polyvinyl tubes or straws. Provided that the straws are retained at the correct temperature, by ensuring that the correct levels of liquid nitrogen are maintained, and the straws are handled properly when the baskets are withdrawn, frozen semen will survive for years.

The insemination technique is as follows:

(1) The correctly identified cow should be adequately restrained.
(2) The straw should be removed from the holding basket after carefully ensuring that it is the one required. The straws are usually colour-coded for breed with the bull's identity on the side. Once a straw has been removed and allowed to thaw it must not be refrozen as it will severely affect the viability of the sperm.
(3) The straw should be removed from the liquid nitrogen just before it is required, and placed in a beaker of water at 37°C for 7 seconds.
(4) It should be removed, dried, the tip with plug cut off with clean scissors and inserted into the Cassou pipette (Fig. 5.19).
(5) Using a clean, conventional transrectal approach, the pipette should be carefully introduced through the cervical canal so that its tip is just within the uterine body cranial to the internal opening of the cervix.
(6) The plunger should be firmly depressed to deposit the semen just into the uterine body.

Excessive manipulation and palpation of the genital tract and ovaries should be discouraged. Pregnancy rates of 55–60% should be obtainable if cows are inseminated at the correct time, using the correct technique, with good quality semen. However, in the UK pregnancy rates to AI are declining at about 1% every 3 years and now average 46% (Kossaibati and Esslemont, 1995). Poor results can

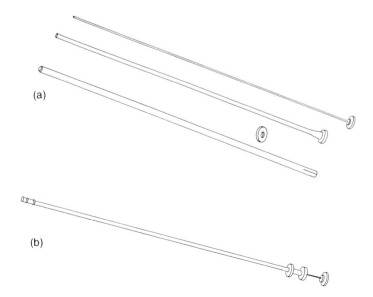

(a)

(b)

Fig. 5.19 Cassou insemination pipette, (a) dismantled and (b) assembled.

be associated with poor technique especially inexperienced DIY inseminators. The most likely faults are:

- Poor storage of semen
- Prolonged handling of stored straws
- Incorrect thawing technique
- Incorrect site of semen deposition
- Rough manipulation of the genital tract.

There is now considerable interest in depositing semen towards the tip of the uterine horn ipsilateral to the dominant pre-ovulatory follicle. With this technique the number of spermatozoa required for each insemination can be drastically reduced; however, with inexperienced operators, there will be a much greater chance of damage to the endometrium.

Embryo transfer

Embryo transfer has become an important technique in cattle breeding, mainly due to the use of multiple ovulation and embryo transfer (MOET). In this procedure, genetically superior females are superovulated using FSH-rich preparations such as porcine pituitary preparations. After multiple inseminations with semen from genetically superior sires, embryos are recovered by transcervical flushing at about day 7 and either frozen (and stored) or transferred fresh to donors. The recipients must be healthy, their oestrous cycles must be synchronised ± 1 day with that of the donor and they must be capable of giving birth to the calf naturally.

Embryo transfer is described in detail elsewhere (Hafez, 1993). In the UK it is covered by statute under the Bovine Embryo (Collection, Production and Transfer) Regulations 1995 and the Veterinary Surgery (Epidural Anaesthesia) Order 1992.

Heifer size and age at first service (see also pp. 40–43)

Rearing replacement heifers is expensive because, until they calve and start to produce milk, they are not generating income for the farm. Ideally, Friesian heifers should be calving for the first time at about 24 months of age; in seasonal calving herds they should do so about 1 month before the cows. Thus, dairy heifers should be served at about 13–15 months of age. However, it is also important that they should be capable of a normal calving; for this reason size at service or insemination is important. To ensure good conception rates, Friesian heifers should be about 325 kg and be growing at 0.7 kg/day. At the same time, a bull with an easy-calving record should be selected.

Oestrus synchronisation

One of the problems with using AI on dairy heifers is the difficulty associated with oestrus detection. For this reason, the oestrous cycles can be synchronised, which makes detection of oestrus easier since if several animals are in oestrus together, behavioural expression is more overt. Alternatively, a system of single or repeat inseminations can be performed at a fixed time in relation to treatment or the withdrawal of treatment. Details of the timings should be confirmed according to the manufacturer's instructions.

There are two basic methods available for synchronisation. The first involves the use of prostaglandin F2α or analogue which causes premature luteolysis of the CL of dioestrus. The second involves the use of a depot progestogen preparation which functions as an exogenous CL, thus suppressing cyclical activity until it is removed. PGF2α or analogues are used in two ways:

(1) The double injection regimen in which PGF2α is injected in two separate doses, 11 days apart, with a single or repeat AI at a fixed time after the second injection.
(2) A one-and-a-half regimen in which all animals are injected with a single injection of PGF2α, and observed for oestrus 2–5 days later. Any observed in oestrus should be inseminated as normal, any that are not observed should be injected 11 days after the first, followed by single or repeat AI. Provided that other aspects of management are satisfactory, acceptable conception (pregnancy) rates will be obtained, although if fixed-time AI is used they may be 5–10% less compared with AI at observed oestrus.

Progestogens are available in a variety of different preparations:

- As a progesterone-releasing intra-vaginal device (PRID) (Fig. 5.20), in the form of a stainless steel coil covered by a layer of inert silastic in which 1.55 g of progesterone is impregnated. Also attached to the coil is a gelatin capsule containing 10 mg oestradiol benzoate which is included because of its luteolytic action. The PRID is inserted into the vagina for 7–12 days and,

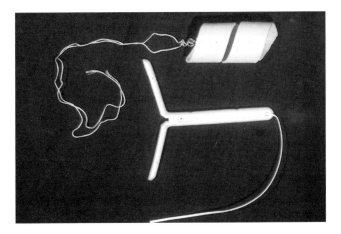

Fig. 5.20 Progesterone releasing intravaginal device (PRID) – note coiled structure, controlled internal drug release device (CIDR) which is Y-/T-shaped.

following its withdrawal, oestrus occurs 2–3 days later. Thus, if PRIDs are inserted into a group of animals for synchronisation and withdrawn at the same time there is a good level of synchronisation of oestrus so that fixed-time AI can be used. Better synchronisation can be achieved if PGF2α is administered on the day before withdrawal, particularly if the PRIDs are left in the vagina for 8–9 days rather than 12 days.

- As a controlled internal drug release device (CIDR type B) which comprises a 'Y'/'T'-shaped nylon spine covered with an elastomer containing 1.9g of progesterone, and a plastic tab to assist in its removal (Fig. 5.20). It functions in a similar way to a PRID, but requires the use of PGF2α or analogue either on the day of withdrawal or at any time from 6 days after insertion. When used in suckler cows, in which there is a possibility of true acyclicity (see 'Oestrus not observed'), then eCG (at a low dose rate) or oestradiol benzoate are sometimes used at the time of insertion to stimulate the onset of cyclical ovarian activity.

- As the potent synthetic progestogen 'Norgestamet' which is available as a subcutaneous polymer implant containing 3mg of the active substance. The implant is inserted subcutaneously in the outer surface of the ear and the animal injected intramuscularly with 2ml of a solution containing 3mg Norgestamet and 5mg oestradiol valerate. Nine to ten days later the implant is removed. In suckler cows, where there is a chance of some animals being acyclical, up to 500 iu of eCG can be given at the time of removal of the implant. Superovulation can occur in some animals. *Norgestamet cannot be used in dairy cows where milk is intended for human consumption.*

Oestrus synchronisation is expensive both in terms of the cost of prostaglandin F2α, progestogens, veterinary visits, AI and increased handling of stock, especially if repeat inseminations are used. In addition, conception (pregnancy) rates, if fixed-time AI is used, are generally lower than AI in relation to observed oestrus because the timing is a compromise particularly in cows as opposed to heifers. Several reasons have been proposed for this, such as abnormal oestrous cycles or a longer post-ovulatory refractory period for the CL. However, the most likely explanation is related to the stage of folliculogenesis at the time of the second PGF2α injection and hence the time required for the dominant follicle to reach the preovulatory stage. Various combinations of hormone treatments have been used, particularly GnRH analogues and oestradiol, to overcome this difficulty, with varying success. Careful consideration must be given in relation to the cost benefit and the likely management advantages of such a scheme.

The importance and cost of infertility in dairy herds
(see also p. 318)

The main objective of a dairy farmer is to produce milk of the desired quality as efficiently and as economically as possible. In addition, the cow will produce a calf which, if a heifer, can be reared as a herd replacement, or, if a male, can be reared as a potential sire if of sufficient genetic merit, or for meat. With the exception of high yielding cows (8000 kg/lactation and above) and first calvers, it is generally accepted that the optimum interval between successive calvings should be 365 days; in the former groups it is acceptable and desirable for the interval to be extended. Why is 365 days the optimum? There are a number of reasons:

- In the typical lactation curve of a dairy cow, milk yield declines progressively after peaking at 6–8 weeks after calving; thus although lactation can be extended beyond the accepted 305 days, average daily yields are reduced.
- There are fewer calves per year in the herd. There are also obvious advantages where the production system demands that cows calve at a particular time of the year, every year. The average calving interval in the UK is about 395 days.

Furthermore, if cows are being inseminated and not conceiving, then there are additional insemination costs. If cows are not becoming pregnant they will be culled and replaced with expensively reared or purchased heifers, at the same time restricting the numbers that can be culled for other reasons such as poor yield or health status. It has been calculated that the cost of an extended calving interval is £3.00 per day (Kossaibati and Esslemont, 1995).

Measuring infertility in dairy cows

Whilst herdsmen will usually have made a subjective assessment of the fertility of an individual cow and the herd, it is preferable to provide some definable quantitative figure or figures. Most are based on how close an individual cow, or the mean value of the herd, is to producing a calf every 365 days. Others are based on the number of times a cow is served/inseminated before she becomes pregnant or the probability of a cow becoming pregnant each time she is served.

In order to measure accurately the fertility of a cow or a herd it is imperative that accurate and permanent records are kept of certain reproductive events, and that the identification of each animal is accurate. The following details should be recorded:

- Cow identity
- Age or lactation number
- Calving date, preferably with details of the calving
- Dates of first service and repeated services
- Identity of the sire
- Result of examination for pregnancy.

Details of health, both general and reproductive, are important, as are dates of observed oestrus when the cow is not served, especially in the immediate post partum period. Given these details is possible to calculate the fertility of an individual cow and the herd as a whole. Readers are recommended to use the definitions listed in *Dairy Herd Fertility: Reproductive Terms and Definitions* (MAFF, 1984a).

Non-return rates to first inseminations have been used for many years, particularly in AI centres. They measure the numbers of cows or heifers that are not presented for a repeat insemination at a particular time interval after the first service, i.e. 30–60, 60–90, 90–120 days. Whilst this is a measure of fertility, in the case of the 30–60 day rate it is generally about 20% above the calving rate for a herd because no account is taken of the reasons why a cow has not been re-inseminated, viz. she may have been selected for culling after returning to oestrus, natural service was used or she may not have been observed to return to oestrus within the time.

The *calving interval* (for an individual cow) or the *calving index* (mean calving interval for the herd) should be, as stated above, 365 days. It is essentially a retrospective measurement of fertility.

Alternatively, a predicted value can be calculated on the assumption that the cow will calve after being identified as being pregnant. The calving index can be reduced if many non-pregnant cows are culled; hence the use of the calving index as a measure of fertility should always be accompanied by a statement of the *percentage culling rate* which should not be more than 15% in total and of which one-third should be for reproductive disorders and infertility.

The *calving to first service interval* should be about 65 days, by which time the reproductive system will have had plenty of time to recuperate after calving. If cows have a reasonable chance of conceiving at each service or insemination, a *calving to conception interval* of 85 days is achievable. A similar term is *days open* which simply means, for an individual cow, the number of days after calving before a new pregnancy is established (calculated to the date of the recorded service which resulted in the pregnancy). For the individual cow, if she becomes pregnant, then days open is identical to the calving to conception interval; however, if she fails to conceive, then days open can still be calculated even if she is sold barren. The *mean days open* for a herd will always include such animals and therefore will be longer than the *mean calving to conception interval* for the herd. The *predicted calving to conception* interval is a useful measure of fertility since with a relatively fixed gestation length of 280 days, a figure of 85 days will achieve a calving interval of 365 days.

Cows should not normally be served before 42 days after calving, because the genital tract will not have returned to normal. On many farms cows are not served before 55 days. This is the cow's earliest service date and within the next 24 days she should come into oestrus, be seen in oestrus and inseminated. This enables a *first service submission rate* to be calculated, which is defined as 'the number of cows or heifers served within a 21-day period expressed as a percentage of the number of cows or heifers at or beyond their earliest service date at the start of the 21 day period'. Ideally this should be 100%, but realistically, in a well-managed herd, a figure of 80% should be achieved.

In some herds a figure for the *oestrus-detection rate* is calculated. However, since it cannot be measured accurately, it can only be considered to be an estimate. A better way of assessing the efficiency and accuracy of oestrus detection is to examine the *percentage distribution of inter-service intervals*. These are divided into the following: 2–17 days, 18–24 days (a normal interval), 25–35 days, 36–48 days (2 × a normal interval) and >48 days. If oestrus detection is good and accurate, at least 50% of the intervals will be in the 18–24 day range; ideally there should be 100%. A large percentage in the 36–48 day group or >48 day group is indicative of a poor oestrus detection rate, whereas a large percentage in the 2–17 days and 25–35 days groups is indicative of incorrect detection with too many cows being inseminated during dioestrus, particularly if the sum of the consecutive short and long intervals is 36–48 days (see p. 35).

The ease with which a cow becomes pregnant can be measured in a number of ways:

- The number of services required for each pregnancy, a figure of 1.65 or less being very good.
- The *pregnancy (conception) rate*, which is the total number of cows that become pregnant (conceive) expressed as a percentage of the total number of services used. These are frequently divided into *first service pregnancy (conception) rates* where a figure of 60% is the target, and *overall pregnancy (conception) rates* where 58% is the target. The current figure to AI in the UK National Herd is 46%. These indices can be calculated only when pregnancy has been confirmed.

For many years, composite indices have been proposed to provide a broad assessment of the fertility of dairy herd. Reproductive Efficiency, Fertility Factor and Fertility Index are described elsewhere (MAFF, 1984a; Arthur *et al.*, 1996).

Investigating poor fertility in a herd

Before it is possible to investigate poor fertility, it will be necessary to:

(1) Determine the farm policy and objectives with regard to breeding practices and fertility
(2) Measure the fertility using the indices described above.

In the case of (2), where good records are available usually this is not too difficult, but where poor records are kept it can present a problem. However, even in the latter situation it is surprising what can be obtained from diaries, AI records and milk recording sheets. Even without records, information obtained at casual visits can provide a useful indication of the cause of the problem. For example:

- A large number of cows found not to be pregnant when presented for examination for pregnancy is indicative, in the first instance, of poor oestrus detection, since the reason for assuming that a cow is probably pregnant is that she has not returned to oestrus after service.

- A large number of repeat inseminations would suggest poor pregnancy rates.
- A large number of cows with a vulval discharge suggests the presence of a specific or non-specific agent causing a vaginitis or endometritis.

It will be necessary to determine the management practices on the farm in relation to oestrus detection, earliest service date, use of artificial insemination or natural service, identity of sires, health status of the herd, duration of the actual or perceived infertility, details of the feeding systems, the quality and source of feedstuffs and the source of advice on nutrition (if any). The general bodily condition of the cows should be assessed either subjectively or using a recognised condition-score system. If possible, body weight changes could be determined.

Signs of a fertility problem

Extended calving index

If the calving index is extended beyond 365 days, examine the values for mean calving to first service and calving to conception interval.

Extended mean calving to first service interval

If the mean calving to first service interval exceeds 65 days then it indicates that: (1) cows are not returning to oestrus after calving or (2) cows are returning to normal cyclical ovarian activity, but oestrus is either not being expressed or detected, or the cows are not being presented for service or insemination; therefore, there will be a poor first service submission rate (see below).
Examine the range of intervals for individual cows to determine whether the mean value is skewed.

Extended mean calving to conception interval

If the mean calving to conception interval exceeds 85 days and the calving to first service interval is close to 65 days, then this is indicative of two problems:

(1) Too many cows are not conceiving at insemination.
(2) An acceptable number of cows are conceiving at insemination (particularly first insemination), but those not conceiving are not being identified when they return to oestrus.

If (1) is the cause, pregnancy (conception) rates will be poor, whereas if (2) is the cause, pregnancy (conception) rates will probably be acceptable. In the latter situation pregnancy diagnosis is often performed infrequently at irregular times and too late.

Poor pregnancy (conception) rates or high services/conception rates

Poor pregnancy (conception) rates or high services/conception rates are an indication that either fertilisation is not occurring or that it has occurred but that there is early embryonic death. Separation into first service and overall pregnancy (conception) rates is useful, particularly since if cows are served too early for the first time after calving poor first service values will be obtained.

Whereas many factors can be responsible in an individual cow (see above), if it is a herd problem then the following causes are likely to be responsible:

- Incorrect timing of insemination, which can be confirmed by examining the distribution of inter-service intervals (see below).
- If DIY AI is used, poor handling of semen or insemination technique (see p. 130).
- If natural service is used, then the bull should be examined for fertility (see pp. 146–7) and freedom from venereally transmitted disease. The cows should be examined for the presence of the same infections.
- Inadequate nutrition. Assess body condition score and determine the nutrient intake of the cows especially in relation to energy and forage quality. Perform metabolic profiles (see Chapter 4).

Low first service submission rate

See page 138. Remember that mean values may give an erroneous impression if there is a skewed distribution of data or a long tail. Always examine the distribution of all values with numerical ranges.

Distribution of inter-service intervals

The distribution of inter-service intervals provides a valuable method of assessing the rate and accuracy of oestrus detection. Poor oestrus detection rates can be improved by increasing the frequency and duration of observation of cows, other than at milking times, to three 20- to 30-minute periods, with particular emphasis on the period after 22.00 hours when there is a greater evidence of overt oestrus behaviour. Alternatively, detection aids such as heat mount detectors can be used or routine $PGF2\alpha$ or progestogen therapy (see pp. 140–41).

If there is evidence of inaccurate timing of insemination with cows being inseminated in dioestrus, then there will be a large number (>15%) of intervals in the 2–17 day range with a comparable increase in the 25–35 day range. The measurement of milk progesterone concentrations with high values on the day of insemination will provide evidence, since if a cow is in oestrus then milk progesterone concentrations will be low, whereas if she is in dioestrus they will be high.

A large proportion of extended and irregular inter-service intervals can also be indicative of late embryonic or early fetal death; in the absence of a specific infectious agent it is unlikely to be a major problem.

Infertility in the individual cow or heifer

The fertility of the herd is a reflection of the fertility of the individual cows within the herd. As part of monitoring the fertility of the herd, individual cows will require clinical examination. What determines an infertile or sub-fertile cow? The answer must be any aberration of reproductive structure, function or behaviour which will result in the individual animal failing to satisfy the criteria required for the herd. Such aberrations can be classified as follows:

(1)   Oestrus not observed
(2)   Repeated, regular returns to oestrus
(3)   Extended and irregular returns to oestrus
(4)   Persistent or frequent oestrus
(5)   Abnormal vulval discharge
(6)   Abortion and stillbirth.

Oestrus not observed

Once a heifer has reached puberty, provided that she remains in normal health and is adequately fed, she will have repeated regular oestrous cycles into, and thoughout, adulthood. Pregnancy and the immediate post partum period will interrupt the pattern. Most dairy cows will ovulate 3–4 weeks after calving and although the first ovulation often is not accompanied by behavioural oestrus, the second and subsequent ones are. Thus, most cows should have exhibited one oestrus before the earliest service date. In all cases of cows not showing oestrus the absence of pregnancy must always be confirmed. Beef suckler cows generally have a longer interval to first ovulation, which may be genetically determined or due to the effects of suckling and/or weight loss.

A diagnosis, in the absence of pregnancy, can usually be made on rectal palpation of the ovaries, although it must be stressed that inaccuracies can occur on rectal palpation; for this reason transrectal ultrasonography or a concurrent milk progesterone assay are useful aids. Thus:

- Normal genital tract, ovaries with a palpable or ultrasonically imaged CL (Figs. 8a–15a,b) and high milk progesterone are indicative of non-detected oestrus either because of absence of overt signs, or short duration or poor observation. Administer PGF2α or analogue; perhaps in addition use some oestrus-detection aid such as a KaMaR or tail paint. If oestrus is not observed in 5 days, repeat the PGF2α treatment 11 days after the first with fixed-time AI.
- Normal genital tract with good tone, rounded ovaries, no obvious CL palpable or ultrasonically imaged and milk progesterone low; perhaps a clear vulval mucus discharge. The cow may be approaching the first post partum oestrus or subsequent oestrus, or she may be in oestrus or going out of oestrus. If the time interval from calving is less than 55 days then she should be re-examined in 7–10 days when she will have a CL. If after 55 days, then insert

a PRID or CIDR (Fig. 20) for 8 days, with the injection of PGF2α 24 hours before removal.

- Normal genital tract with small, smooth, flattened ovaries, no CL identified with transrectal ultrasonography and low milk progesterone concentration. The cow is probably acyclical (true anoestrus) particularly if she is in poor bodily condition and/or a high yielder. Confirmation can be made by a re-examination after 7 days or another milk progesterone assay performed at this time. If possible, increase the food intake and administer a PRID for 12 days, or a CIDR for 7 days, or a GnRH analogue.
- Normal genital tract with one or both enlarged ovaries containing one or more fluid-filled structures greater than 2.5 cm in diameter. The cow has an ovarian cyst which is probably a luteal cyst if thick-walled (>3 mm luteal tissue; Fig. 5.22) with a high milk progesterone; if so, treat with PGF2α and oestrus will occur in 2–3 days. If milk progesterone is low, with a thin-walled cyst (<3 mm luteal tissue) (Fig 5.21) treat with GnRH analogue, or hCG or insert a PRID.
- Enlarged, doughy uterus, perhaps with evidence, or history, of a mucopurulent discharge and a CL palpable or identified ultrasonographically on one ovary. This is a pyometra with a persistent CL; however, pregnancy must always be excluded. Treat with PGF2α which will result in the regression of the CL and evacuation of the uterus.

Repeated, regular returns to oestrus

The cow has returned to oestrus after at least three services at normal intervals of 18–24 days; these are sometimes referred to as 'repeat breeders' or 'cyclic non-breeders'. In many cases they are normal, and provided that inseminations are

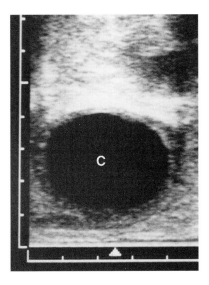

Fig. 5.21 Ovary with folliculcer cyst (C) greater than 3 cm in diameter, note the thin wall (*x–y*).

repeated at each observed oestrus they will ultimately conceive. Rectal palpation can be used to determine the presence of any gross pathological lesions, such as adhesions, which might explain the failure to conceive, but in many cases there are no obvious abnormalities present. Regular return indicates that either fertilisation is failing to occur or the embryo is dying before the maternal recognition of pregnancy has occurred (see pp. 127–8). Investigation of such cases can be time consuming and expensive, and in commercial dairy cows probably uneconomic, particularly if there is a long time interval from calving. Treatments to induce ovulation at the correct time (GnRH analogues or hCG at the time of insemination), a repeat insemination 24 hours after the first, and or GnRH analogues 11 or 12 days after insemination, to prevent luteolysis and subsequent embryonic death, or progesterone supplementation after service can be used. It is worthwhile using semen from a bull of known high fertility. The insertion of a donated embryo on day 7 after artificial insemination has been used to improve pregnancy rates with either the cow producing twins or a single calf (its own or from the donor cow).

Extended and irregular returns to oestrus

A normal genital tract with evidence of normal cyclical ovarian activity is usually indicative of an incorrect identification of oestrus associated with the non-detection of the previous or subsequent true oestrus. While in any dairy herd there will be a small number of such cows, if there is a substantial number, the procedure for oestrus detection needs to be assessed (see p. 139). If this occurs in a number of cows in association with a vulval discharge, and if natural service is used, the possibility of a venereally transmitted infectious disease such as *Campylobacter fetus*, *Tritrichomonas fetus* or genital bovine herpes (BHV1), or other non-venereally transmitted disease such as BVD should be considered.

Persistent or frequent oestrus

Indicated by a normal genital tract, perhaps with increased uterine tone and a clear mucoid vulval discharge, and with one or both ovaries enlarged and containing several fluid-filled structures >2.5 cm in diameter; milk progesterone concentration is low and on ultrasonography the wall of the fluid-filled structures will be <3 mm thick. The cow has true follicular cysts associated with nymphomania. Such cows will have depressed milk yields, may become injured and will disrupt oestrus detection in the herd. They are best treated by the immediate insertion of a PRID for 12 days which will result in suppression of aberrant behaviour in about 24 hours. Alternatively, luteinisation can be induced with hCG or GnRH therapy, perhaps followed by PGF2α 14 days later.

Abnormal vulval discharge

Abnormal vulval discharge may originally be from the urinary system, uterus or vagina. Rectal palpation and vaginal examination should enable identification of

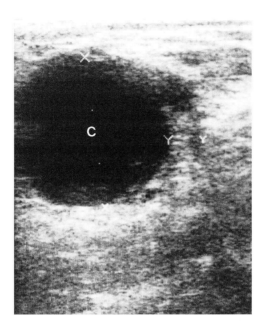

Fig. 5.22 Ovary with luteal cyst (C) greater than 3 cm in diameter. Note thick wall. (Scale: 6.5 mm.)

the source. Ovarian palpation will reveal normal cyclical ovarian activity. If the site of infection is the vagina or uterus then fertility will be compromised. In the former, it may be associated with infections such as genital BHVI and ureaplasmas or with pooling of urine in the vagina. In the latter, it will be associated with opportunist pathogens which have colonised the uterus. Frequently, mild uterine infections will be resolved spontaneously; however, if the cow is close to, or beyond, the earliest service date then treatment is indicated. If a CL is present, the luteal phase can be shortened by the use of PGF2α. If no CL is present, 3 mg of oestradiol benzoate in oil can be used intramuscularly, or the intrauterine infusion of a broad-spectrum antibiotic such as oxytetracycline at a therapeutic dose rate for the cow, followed by milk withdrawal or other licensed proprietary preparations.

Abortion and stillbirth

An abortion is defined as the expulsion of one or more calves less than 271 days after service or AI; they are either dead or live for less than 24 hours. A stillbirth is the birth of a dead calf, either spontaneously or following assistance, after 272 days. Between about 1 and 2% of cows will abort and whilst every case should be investigated thoroughly, this is accepted as being a normal level. When it exceeds 5% then there is cause for concern. Quantifying stillbirths is more difficult since most will occur intrapartum as a result of dystocia.

In the UK, under the Brucellosis Orders of 1979 (Scotland) and 1981 (England and Wales), a specific course of action must be followed after an abortion, although variations on this have now been made depending on the stage of gestation:

(1)   The Ministry of Agriculture, Fisheries and Food must be notified.
(2)   The cow that has aborted must be isolated together with the abortus and placenta.
(3)   The fetus, calf and placenta must be retained on the premises.

However, irrespective of such legislation good hygiene and isolation procedures are most important to prevent the lateral spread of infection, should it be present, from occurring. Once these initial measures have been implemented it will be necessary to carry out a thorough investigation; however, it is important to stress that in the UK the number of abortions in which a specific agent is isolated is low, viz. between 6 and 7%, either because of the true absence of specific infectious agents or a failure to isolate organisms that are present, or were present.

In pursuing an investigation into an abortion the following approach might be adopted:

• Details of herd history and of the affected cow
• Examination of the affected animal
• Examination of the aborted fetus and placenta
• Collection and submission of samples for laboratory investigation.

History: size and composition of the herd, the nature and source of any additions if it is not a closed herd, whether natural service and/or AI is used. Determine whether there are any other signs of reproductive disease, e.g. embryonic death, mummification, stillbirths, neo-natal deaths, dysmaturity, congenital defects, abnormal vulval discharges. Determine the vaccination status of the herd and obtain details of feeding, especially changes in feed and the quality of the food, e.g. silage, mouldy hay. If previous abortions have occurred then seasonal distribution and gestational age are important. The latter needs to be determined in the cow that has just aborted. Evidence of illness or other premonitory signs before the abortion, e.g. pyrexia, inappetance, milk drop, CNS signs, respiratory disease.

Examination of the animal: this will usually yield little additional information but can be used to confirm details provided in relation to the history of the case.

Examination of the aborted fetus and placenta: this can provide useful information about the likely cause. At the same time the fetus should be measured, weighed and thus aged (Arthur *et al.* 1996; Roberts, 1972) and compared with predicted gestational age for signs of dysmaturity.

The degree of autolysis of the fetus should be noted. In the case of abortion due to infectious agents such as *T. fetus, Actinomyces pyogenes, Salmonella* sp. and. *Leptospira* sp. there is usually advanced fetal autolysis at an early stage, whereas with infectious agents such as fungi, *Listeria monocytogenes* and *Bacillus licheniformis*, autolysis is not apparent.

Placental examination may reveal characteristic lesions which are common to several infectious agents; for example, bovine herpes virus 1, *L. monocytogenes* and *Leptospira* sp. produce a diffuse placentitis. *Brucella abortus*, fungal agents, *Bacillus* sp. and *Campylobacter* sp. result in thickened, leathery and necrotic cotyledons.

Collection and submission of samples: as soon as possible, placental tissue and the whole fetus should be sent to the laboratory. Where the latter is not possible, after careful necropsy of the fetus, the ligated abomasum, lungs and liver should be submitted. Blood samples should be obtained from the dam on the day of abortion and at least 3 weeks later for serological examination.

Frequently, in the investigation of the cause of fetopathies, no causal organism is identified. This may reflect the relatively low level of infection causing fetal death in cattle but is more likely to be due to the problems of identifying the presence of an infectious agent. The organism responsible may not be present at the time when the material is examined, incorrect samples may be submitted or there may be a delay in sending them to the laboratory. The frequency of isolation of particular pathogens will vary depending on the development of new techniques for identification and the emergence of new causal agents. This is illustrated by the frequency of identification in the UK of two relatively 'new' but important causes of abortion, viz. *Bacillus licheniformis* and *Neosporum caninum*. In addition, with the elimination of major infectious causes of abortion, for example *Brucella abortus*, other pathogens that were probably co-existing are now readily identified.

Infectious causes of fetopathy can be controlled by the introduction of vaccination, i.e. *Leptospira interrogans* serovar *hardjo*, *Brucella abortus*, bovine herpes virus 1, BVD virus; identification of asymptomatic carriers, i.e. *B. abortus*, *C. fetus*, *T. fetus*; good hygiene, i.e. all infectious agents. Such measures can form part of control schemes which can result in the elimination of a particular pathogen from the national herd.

Fertility control schemes

Even if the fertility of a dairy herd is good it can always deteriorate. The early identification of reduced fertility in a herd and the implementation of methods to correct the cause can prevent the enterprise suffering major financial losses. Thus, the routine monitoring of fertility using a control scheme can be cost effective in the same way that an insurance policy operates. Such schemes are based on the following:

(1) The keeping of accurate records as outlined in 'Measuring infertility in dairy cow' (p. 135) and the measurement of the various indices.
(2) The identification of cows whose reproductive performance is not satisfying the criteria for good fertility, or whose reproductive status needs to be determined.

(3)   Regular, routine visits to examine the cow identified in (2). Such a scheme requires good teamwork and thus the active and enthusiastic cooperation of farm staff, the owner and veterinarian. If any member of the team is not committed the scheme will probably fail.

It is important to agree on the targets for fertility that are achievable and are compatible with the overall farm policy. Once these have been established, then routine visits should be implemented, the frequency depending upon the size of the herd and the calving pattern. Analysis of the records before each visit will identify the cows that should be examined. In small herds this can be done using manual recording schemes, but in large herds computerised systems such as the DAISY system (National Milk Records) have much to commend them. The following categories of cows should be examined at each visit:

- Cows that have had parturient or periparturient reproductive problems at 3–4 weeks after calving
- Cows with an unnatural vulval discharge 3–4 weeks after calving
- Cows that have aborted (these will be under investigation)
- Cows that have not been seen in oestrus by 42 days after calving
- Cows that have not been inseminated by 60 days after calving
- Cows showing signs of nymphomania
- Cows that have not returned to oestrus by 42 days after insemination or service (pregnancy diagnosis)
- Cows that have been confirmed pregnant at a previous examination but subsequently have been observed in oestrus
- Cows that have returned to oestrus after insemination three or more times (repeat breeders).

Infertility in the bull

Semen purchased from reputable AI organisations, provided that it is stored and handled properly, can be assumed to be free from venereally transmitted pathogens and of satisfactory fertility. If natural service is used, there is obviously no guarantee of the bull's fertility unless he is a proven sire. Because the introduction of a new bull into a dairy herd could have a disastrous effect on fertility if he was infertile it is important that he is examined at the time of purchase and preferably at the start of the breeding season for reproductive soundness. However, in most cases, a request to examine a bull will usually follow evidence of infertility. This will be apparent because:

- The bull will have reduced or no libido.
- The bull will be incapable of serving cows because of impotence.
- The bull will have reduced ability or be incapable of fertilisation following normal service, resulting in cows failing to become pregnant and returning to oestrus.
- The bull may be suspected of having a venereal disease which may be infect-

ing animals that he has served, interfering with fertilisation or causing prenatal death. Cows may be returning to oestrus at a normal or extended irregular interval without any other clinical signs.

Reduced or complete absence of libido

A bull with good libido will normally respond to a cow or heifer in oestrus by mounting and serving within a few minutes of access. Age, breed and environment can exert an effect. Beef breeds usually have a poorer libido than dairy breeds, whilst a new or distracting environment can exert an influence. It is important to take this into consideration when a recently purchased bull is examined in unfamiliar surroundings with unfamiliar personnel. Libido can be quantified by measuring the time interval from introducing the cow in oestrus and the first mount, intromission and ejaculation, and also by the frequency of repeated services (see pp. 129–30).

Poor libido cannot be improved by the administration of exogenous gonadotrophins or androgens. Rest, a change in the environment, more sympathetic handling and attention to intercurrent disease, such as lameness, may help. Alternatively, the sight and smell of another bull might be tried.

Impotence

Impotence may be due to an inability to mount because of some locomotor disorder. Inability to perform intromission may be because of failure of erection of the penis, spiralling, deviations, ruptured *corpus cavernosum penis* or vascular shunts interfering with erection. The bull should be teased and the penis examined closely if and when it is protruded. Examination under general anaesthesia, deep narcosis or pudendal nerve block may be worthwhile. Finally, impotence may be associated with failure to ejaculate after intromission which is detected by the absence of the characteristic ejaculatory thrust. The cause of this latter problem is frequently difficult to determine and hence correct.

Reduced or complete failure of fertilisation

The bull may be observed to mount, perform intromission and ejaculate, but the pregnancy (conception) rates may be nil or very low. Some indication of the cause may be detected on clinical examination: for example, testicular or epididymal lesions or changes, or infections of the vesicular glands. However, confirmation will require the collection of semen preferably using an artificial vagina, and its examination for the normal parameters (see pp. 120–24). The presence of infection, low sperm concentrations, aspermia, poor motility, or a large number of dead or obviously abnormal spermatozoa can be assessed quite readily using conventional microscopy. However, some sperm defects require more sophisticated techniques and examination by an expert. If infection is the cause of the infertility then antibiotics may be used. However, defects in spermatogenesis rarely if ever respond to exogenous hormone therapy.

Spread of venereal disease

The presence of venereal disease can be detected in the cows that the bull has served using smears and cultures and serological tests, or directly from the bull. Semen can be cultured, or more usually preputial washings or the washings from a contaminated artificial vagina can be examined directly or following culture, or using fluorescent antibody techniques. Depending on the infection and the bull's genetic value, he could be culled, his use restricted to immune females or he could be treated. The latter can be difficult, particularly in older animals which frequently become asymptomatic carriers of the disease.

References

Arthur, G. H., Noakes D. E., Pearson, H. & Parkinson, T. J. (1996) *Veterinary Reproduction and Obstetrics*, 7th edn. W. B. Saunders, London.

Ashdown, R. (1986) Anatomy of male reproduction. In: Hafez, E. S. E. (ed.) *Reproduction in Farm Animals*, 5th edn. Lea & Febiger, Philadelphia.

Chenowith, P. J. (1986) Libido testing. In *Current Therapy in Theriogenology*, 2nd edn., pp. 136–42. W. B. Saunders, Philadelphia.

Foulkes, J. A., Cookson, A. D. & Sauer, M. J. (1982) Artificial insemination of cattle based on daily enzyme immunoassay of progesterone in whole milk. *Veterinary Record* **111**, 302.

Hafez, E. S. E. (1993) *Reproduction in Farm Animals*, 6th edn. Lea and Febiger, Philadelphia.

Hall, L. W. & Clarke, K. W. (1995) *Veterinary Anaesthesia*, 9th edn. W. B. Saunders, London.

Kossaibati, M. A. & Esslemont, R. J. (1995) *Wastage in Dairy Herds*. Report no. 4, DAISY – The Dairy Information System. University of Reading.

MAFF (1984a) *Dairy Herd Fertility: Reproductive Terms and Definitions*. Booklet 2476. HMSO, London.

MAFF (1984b) *Dairy Herd Fertility*, Booklet 259 HMSO, London.

Noakes, D. E. (1997) *Fertility and Obstetrics in Cattle*. Blackwell Science, Oxford.

Peters, A. R. & Ball, P. J. H. (1995) *Reproduction in Cattle*, 2nd edn. Blackwell Science, Oxford.

Pierson, R. A. & Ginther, O. J. (1984) Ultrasonography for detection of pregnancy and study of embryonic development in heifers. *Theriogenolgoy* **22**, 225–33.

Pieterse, M. C., Szenci, O., Willemse, A. H., Bajcsy, C. S. A., Dieleman, S. J. and Taverne, M. A. M. (1990) Early pregnancy diagnosis in cattle by means of linear-array real-time ultrasound scanning of the uterus and a qualitative and quantitative milk progesterone test. *Theriogenology* **33**, 697–707.

Roberts, S. J. (1972) *Veterinary Obstetrics and Genital Disease*, 2nd edn. Published by the author and distributed by Edwards Brothers Inc, Ann Arbor, Michigan.

Short, R. V. (1969) *Implantation and the Maternal Recognition of Pregnancy in Foetal Autonomy*. Churchill, London.

Trimberger, G. W. & Davis, G. K. (1943) *The Relationship Between the Timing of Insemination and Breeding Efficiency in Dairy Cattle*. Nebraska University Agricultural Experimental Station Research Bulletin 129. University of Nebraska.

Chapter 6
Lameness

A. David Weaver

Introduction

Lameness is assuming ever-greater importance in management of the dairy herd in the UK, Continental Europe and North America. This importance is inevitable when, on some farms, virtually every cow of a 150 milking herd may become lame at some time during the year. A cow may be lame more than once annually and the average in some parts of the UK may reach 1.4 incidents of lameness each year (i.e. 100 cows have 140 incidents). Curiously, some herds still have an incidence below 7%, a figure that corresponds closely to the veterinary-visited lameness incidence in a national survey in the 1970s. Little reliable information is available in other countries with intensive dairy operations. Beef cattle, including suckler herds, in contrast have a much lower lameness incidence.

This chapter emphasises treatment and control of some major lameness problems in British dairy herds (Table 6.1), but the control recommendations, both general and specific, are applicable to many intensive units worldwide. The key to a low incidence of lameness appears to be good management: careful observation, good quality accommodation, gentle handling, optimal diet composition and slow adoption of the seasonal and parturition-related dietary changes.

Digital lesions are the most common cause of lameness, accounting for about 80–90% of all incidents. Currently (1999), problems of the horny tissues appear to be more frequent than those of the digital skin.

Economics

Lameness is the third most significant cause of economic loss, after infertility and mastitis, in dairy herds. Lame cows lose farmers money through the cost of replacement following culling of a severe case, with reduced carcase value, through the infertility resulting from a prolonged calving to conception interval, owing to reduced milk yield, and withdrawal of antibiotic-contaminated milk, veterinary costs and staff time (Table 6.2). The lame dairy cow has an increased risk of infertility for various reasons (see Table 6.3 and p. 320 onwards).

Table 6.1   Major problems of lameness in British dairy herds.

Adults Digital lameness (85%)		Other lameness (15%)	Calves
Horny tissues	Skin		

Sole ulcer
White line disease
Laminitis including
   subclinical
Claw overgrowth
'Slurry heel'
	Digital dermatitis
	Interdigital phlegmon
	   including 'superfoul'
	
	Interdigital dermatitis
		Peripheral paralysis
		Degenerative joint
		   disease
			Neonatal polyarthritis
			Neonatal fractures
			Interdigital
			   necrobacillosis
			Vitamin E/selenium
			   deficiency
			Congenital
			   contracted tendons

Table 6.2   Economic losses owing to dairy cow lameness.

Major losses	Minor losses
Culling loss Replacement cost Prolonged calving interval	Reduced milk yield Milk withdrawal (antibiotics) Veterinary treatment Labour cost

Table 6.3   Causes of infertility in lame dairy cows postpartum.

Delayed return to oestrus Unobserved oestrus Lower body condition (negative energy balance) Conception failure Intercurrent disease (e.g. mastitis)

What figures can be given to these production losses? Accurate economic cal-culations for the UK clearly depend on the true annual incidence of lameness. Ten years ago it was quoted as 28% (Somerset data; Weaver, personal data). Such figures were considered reliable as they included herdsman- as well as veterinary-treated cows. It seems that only about one-quarter of lame cows are seen by the veterinarian. Both the Liverpool Survey (Clarkson *et al.*, 1993) involving dairy farms in the Wirral, Cheshire, mid-Wales and Somerset and a personal survey of 55 Somerset dairy farms, have shown that the average incidence is higher than in pre-1990 studies (Weaver, 1998).

Studies from the University of Reading (Esslemont and Spincer, 1992) suggest a range of £25–400 per lame cow, depending on the response to treatment, and assuming one or more veterinary visits; 1995-estimated real costs for a single inci-dent of interdigital disease, digital disease and sole ulcer in a typical UK cow were respectively £129, £244 and £392. Averaging these figures to £250, and with

1.1 incidents per lame cow and a conservative figure of 35% lameness incidence in the British dairy herd (though known to range from 7 from 100%), the cost to the dairy industry (2.6 million adult dairy cows) may be estimated. The annual loss must be about £250 000 000. Previous data (1984) did not exceed £75 000 000 primarily as a result of a grossly underestimated lameness incidence.

Despite the sporadic introduction of 'lameness scoring', subclinical lameness has been omitted from economic consideration as being impossible to quantitate. The use of 'no withdrawal time' antibiotics such as ceftiofur may cut the veterinary cost marginally, as the increased drug cost is more than balanced by the non-discarded 60–100 litres of milk (see also Chapter 11).

Welfare

The importance of welfare in dairy cow lameness is obvious. The cow is lame to a varying degree as a direct result of pain on weightbearing. If unable to bear weight due to the severity of the pathology, then the three-legged cow is still more handicapped and most liable to spend a considerable period recumbent, whether at pasture or in indoor housing where the animal is particularly liable to be bullied, to slip, and to have a severe decrease in feed intake.

Welfare issues extend to weight loss, to an increased risk of being culled (due to weight loss, delayed conception, humane considerations) and an increased risk of mastitis following enforced recumbency. The relative lack of approved anti-inflammatory and analgesic drugs suitable for pain relief [an exception being ketoprofen (Ketofen 10%, Merial) which has a nil milk withdrawal] has led to many individual cows having considerable periods of pain as a direct result of digital or other lameness. Hyperalgesia occurs in lame cows and may persist a long period after resolution of the lesion, causing lameness (Whay *et al.*, 1998).

Herd lameness programmes

Since one major problem has long been the lack of reliable data on the lameness problem on an individual farm, the recent introduction of herd health schemes has been a major advance since lameness may easily be recorded alongside reproductive and mastitis details. More widespread use of computerised records is anticipated in the next decade. The individual cow record (Table 6.4) should contain information such as the farm identification (ID), cow ID, agent ID, date, limb affected, lameness grade ('score'), and claw lesion or upper limb diagnosis. The condition of the claws should be recorded at the lameness incident, and also at claw trimming (see p. 176). A simple locomotion score system is shown in Table 6.5. An outline claw sketch can indicate the site of sole, heel, white line and interdigital skin abnormalities. Therapy should be simply recorded in four categories: medical, claw trim, surgery and other.

These records should be made in duplicate, one copy remaining on the farm (in the 'Lameness File') for potential entry into a dairy office computer (Fig. 6.1). The other copy should be filed in the veterinary practice. At a later stage the

Table 6.4   Individual cow record of lameness incident.

Farm ID
Cow ID
Agent ID
Date: day/month/year
Limb affected:
    LF   RF   LH   RH
Lameness grade:
    0   1   2   3   4
Claw lesion diagnosis:
Upper limb diagnosis:
Secondary lameness diagnosis (if any):
Condition of claws:
    0 = normal
    1 = bilateral overgrowth
    2 = unilateral overgrowth
    3 = unequal size
    4 = other abnormality
Therapy:
    1 = medical
    2 = claw trim
    3 = surgery
    4 = other
Lactation number*:
Last calving date*:

* Entered later.

Table 6.5   Simple locomotion or lameness scoring system.

Score	Definition
0	Normal
1	Slight abnormality: uneven gait, stiff, tender
2	Slight lameness: moderate consistent lameness
3	Obvious lameness affecting behaviour
4	Severe lameness, frequently recumbent

individual cow record can have details of lactation number and last calving date added.

As herd size continues to increase, and as culling decisions depend more and more on accurate recorded data of pregnancy status, milk yield and disease problems rather than on the herdsman's memory, incorporation of lameness details into DAISY-type record schemes (National Milk Records) is inevitable.

Differential diagnosis

While every cattle veterinarian will have occasionally made a mistaken diagnosis in a lame cow and applied the incorrect treatment, he or she will usually learn

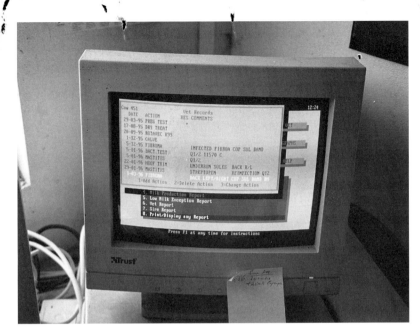

Fig. 6.1 Computer screen in dairy showing individual cow health data in 1995, including veterinary record of diagnosis of 'infected fibroma' on 5.12.95, and later 'hoof trim' and comment of 'under-run soles'. Information is readily retrievable from such records.

the lesson at the second visit to the lame cow, and, somewhat embarrassed, remove the interdigital foreign body. However, in a chapter on lameness in the dairy herd, it is vital that every veterinarian and stockkeeper remains aware of the possibility that foot-and-mouth disease may be the diagnosis in a group of lame cattle. Other causes of group lameness include BVD/mucosal disease, rarely malignant catarrhal fever, and in youngstock salmonellosis and, in parts of the USA, fescue foot. All except the last are accompanied by severe systemic signs.

Major problems of the digit

Problems affecting the hard horny tissues, sole ulcer, white line disease, claw overgrowth and subclinical laminitis today appear to outweigh skin disease, principally digital dermatitis and interdigital phlegmon including 'superfoul'. The Liverpool survey (Murray *et al.*, 1996) recorded sole ulcer (28% of total lesions) and white line lesions (22%) as making up exactly half of all claw lameness cases.

Sole ulcer (*pododermatitis circumscripta specifica*) (see also p. 39)

Focal weightbearing at the sole–heel junction, usually of the lateral hind claw, results in an aseptic laminar necrosis, originally elegantly described by a Swiss veterinarian, Rusterholz, in 1920. Although generally seen in second and third lactation cows, several 'outbreaks' have involved many, even a majority, of a group of first calf heifers aged 2–3 years. Sole ulcer was the major problem in a survey of 55 Somerset dairy herds (1995–1997) (Weaver, 1998).

Deep bruising and haemorrhage are the first stages of damage, often immediately distal to (below) the prominence of the flexor tubercle on which the deep flexor tendon inserts. Examination reveals a haemorrhagic area of horn at the 'typical site', somewhat towards the axial border of the sole–heel junction (Fig. 6.2). Paring away this horn reveals deeper necrosis, peripheral separation of horn, and necrotic and haemorrhagic pododerm (corium). More chronic cases have a 'strawberry-like' protrusion of granulation tissue in the horn defect. Cows with sole ulcer and swelling of the coronary band and pastern usually have deep infection.

Many cows with sole ulcer have a degree of claw overgrowth, which has a disputed aetiological role in the development of sole ulcer. The stance of sole ulcer cases is often unbalanced. The limb is rotated outwards, the hocks inwards, and therefore increased weight is taken on the lateral claw (e.g. ratio of lateral : medial = 60 : 40). The sole–heel junction and heel area has an excessive depth of

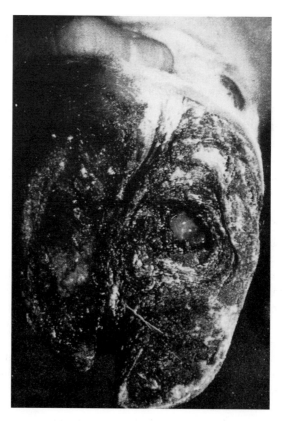

Fig. 6.2 Sole ulcer in lateral claw of hind leg. Typical site at sole–heel junction shows protruding granulation tissue.

horn which may extend axially as a wedge. Many cows have less severe changes in the corresponding claw of the other hind leg, which should therefore always be examined. In cubicle housing, affected cows may either stand on the back edge or with the hind limbs in the passageway in an attempt to relieve weight on the heel area. Cubicle length was not significantly shorter, however, in dairy herds with a major problem of sole ulcer compared with similarly cubicle-housed herds without this problem.

Cases usually peak in the period 6–12 weeks postpartum, suggesting a relationship to laminitis which also has an incidence peak in the early weeks postpartum. Not all animals with sole ulceration show lameness and especially if bilateral the gait may be slowed and cautious rather than lame.

Severe cases develop a localised osteomyelitis of the distal phalanx followed by a peripheral spread of sepsis through the soft tissues of the pododerm. In the absence of natural or surgical drainage, a septic infection can spread into the distal interphalangeal joint and navicular bursa, and then ascend along the deep flexor tendon sheath. Increasing swelling of the pastern region and marked lameness accompany any of these complications.

Treatment

Simple case: the limb should be elevated in a well-lit area under adequate restraint for thorough exploration to determine the absence of osteomyelitic changes. If the procedure is likely to be painful, digital analgesia should be induced, e.g. by intravenous regional anaesthesia (IVRA) (Fig. 6.3). The under-run horn is removed to expose normal surrounding tissue. Any granulation tissue is resected by sharp surgery. The depth of the defect is explored with a blunt probe. The absence of increased purulent drainage on exploration is a favourable sign, and conservative treatment is then appropriate.

Functional trimming (see p. 176 onwards) is performed. Briefly, the unaffected (medial) claw is minimally pared: the toe is shortened, but the sole and heel are left with a maximum depth of tissue to serve as a 'functional block'. Many cows with sole ulcer have unequal-sized claws, and often a ledge of sole–heel horn overlaps the interdigital space axially. Considerable paring of the lateral (sole ulcer) claw is then justified. The axial ledge is trimmed away together with an overall reduction of sole depth, in order temporarily to transfer more weight-bearing to the medial claw.

The white line must be checked for normality, i.e. absence of widening with impaction, especially the abaxial white line near the sole–heel junction. Often removal of the axial ledge of horn, reveals a double sole with impacted debris packed across towards the abaxial white line region. Movement of the weightbearing horn surfaces is liable to have caused some widening of the abaxial white line which predisposes to such impaction (see p. 176 for management).

Removal of the granulation tissue in the sole ulcer leaves a bleeding surface which may be controlled by an organic iodine pressure swab firmly packed into

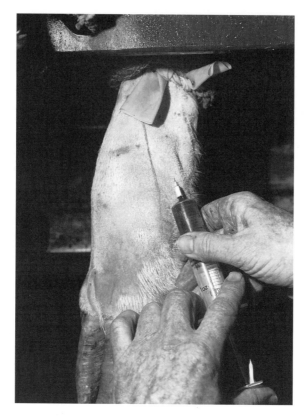

Fig. 6.3 Intravenous regional analgesia; 20 ml lignocaine hydrochloride is injected into the lateral plantar digital vein distal to a rubber tourniquet placed below the hock.

it for a few seconds. Bandaging is unnecessary, and may be contraindicated as it inevitably increases weightbearing by the diseased and painful tissues.

Ideally, the cow should be confined to a small strawed box between milkings, and not permitted to return to a cubicle yard. Even a few hours spent after treatment in a box helps an earlier recovery. No antibiotics are needed in uncomplicated cases.

Complicated case: complications invariably involve septic spread. Radiographic examination, underutilised in practice, can usefully determine the extent of bone destruction and the need for radical surgery. The possible structures involved in digital sepsis following sole ulceration are:

- Solar pododerm
- Distal surface of distal phalanx
- Distal interphalangeal joint
- Distal sesamoid (navicular) bone
- Navicular bursa
- Necrosis of deep flexor tendon insertion
- Ascending septic tenosynovitis of deep flexor sheath.

Treatment options include:

(1) Curettage and indwelling drainage system
(2) Curettage and plaster cast
(3) Resection of distal interphalangeal joint
(4) Digit amputation.

Options (1)–(3) have the ultimate aim of joint ankylosis.

The details of these surgical techniques are available elsewhere (Weaver, 1986; Greenough & Weaver, 1996; Desrochers & St Jean, 1997) but their merits are briefly considered here.

(1) Curettage and an indwelling drainage system is limited to cases where infection has not extended proximal to the level of the coronary band. It is very labour-intensive in terms of aftercare, and therefore costly, but the digit is preserved. The prognosis is doubtful at the start of this surgery.
(2) More radical curettage, irrigation and immediate plaster/resin casting of the digit including pastern and fetlock for several weeks involves minimal aftercare. It may result in an ascending infection and generalised septicaemia, and usually results in gross digital deformity.
(3) Resection of the distal interphalangeal joint is technically demanding and surgical experience is largely limited to specialist clinics. The rapidity of recovery, when compared with digit amputation, is disputed. Prolonged aftercare is again needed. Several surgical approaches have been described:
    • A vertical plantar incision starting distal to the accessory claw and extending to the sole–heel junction
    • A horizontal incision around the heel
    • Two arthrostomies proximal to the coronary band, dorsally and abaxially.
(4) Digit amputation, either at the coronary band, through the proximal interphalangeal joint or through the distal one-third of the proximal phalanx, depending on the extent of infection and surgeon preference, is a rapid and inexpensive procedure, with an early return to milk production. However, many animals are culled due to poor long-term adaptation (heavy bodyweight with soft tissue breakdown, discomfort in housing system).

Prevention

Prevention involves avoidance of the various suspected predisposing factors:

• Subclinical laminitis (predisposing to haemorrhages)
• Insufficient exercise (predisposing to overgrowth)
• Sudden introduction postpartum to winter housing (predisposing to claw trauma).

These general measures are discussed later in this chapter (see 'Laminitis').

- Preventive (functional) claw trimming, routine in most UK herds, should be introduced carefully, especially in first calf heifers. If performed incautiously, shortening of the toe and appropriate thinning of the sole and heel may result in several animals with subclinical laminitis becoming lame. The trimmed sole proves to be inadequate to prevent pain developing from pressure at the typical sole ulcer site on the thin and already microtraumatised pododerm (see 'Claw trimming').

Digital dermatitis (dermatitis digitalis)

Digital dermatitis (DD) is an important cause of lameness in dairy cows, especially in the first three lactations. DD, first described in northern Italy (hence 'Mortellaro disease') in the early 1970s, has now been recognised in many other countries of Western and Central Europe, North America and Asia (Japan). It assumes epidemic proportions in some herds.

The classical site is the plantar skin immediately proximal to the heels. Less common sites include the coronary band and the dorsal skin above the interdigital cleft. Often both hind limbs are affected to a varying extent. The early stage presents as a moist circumscribed eczematous area about 1 cm in diameter. The hairs are unusually erect, and the lesion enlarges with a central area of superficial necrosis, and ulceration, accompanied by a foul odour. The margin is pale and slightly elevated. The lesion is hyperaesthetic and lameness is obvious. The cow may occasionally lift and stretch or shake an affected limb at this time. At a later stage the lesion is more proliferative with papillomatous processes up to 3 cm long developing in the ulcerative area (Fig. 6.4), which in rare cases extends proximally towards the dew claws. Lesions rarely involve the heel horn. Some cows develop discrete focal lesions on each side of the interdigital cleft (so-called kissing lesions) (Figs. 6.5 and 6.6). In some countries severe erosive lesions present as several square centimetres of smooth red raw skin surrounded by a whitish border. Untreated cases take months to resolve, as the papilliform fronds break off following iatrogenic abrasion and further proliferative masses develop. Lameness in these more chronic cases is less severe. Sometimes lesions also involve the interdigital space where interdigital hyperplasia may co-exist (Fig. 6.7).

The aetiology of DD remains uncertain. Histopathology of proliferative US cases (papillomatous digital dermatitis or 'footwarts') shows a lesion indistinguishable from a true fibropapilloma. UK material reveals suppurative epidermal inflammation, superficial necrosis and hyperkeratosis. Some cases have mild inflammatory changes extending into the dermis. Other descriptions (Ireland) refer to epidermal thickening with numerous mitoses in the basal layer and acanthosis and pseudoepitheliomatous hyperplasia. Further aetiological confusion arises from the recognition of many DD cases in the UK as seropositive to *B. burgdorferi*, the significance of which is doubtful. Spirochaetes have been repeatedly seen, both on the surface and deep in the epidermis of typical cases. The identity of the spirochaetes is unknown, but they may be a *Treponema* species, one appearing to be *Treponema denticola*.

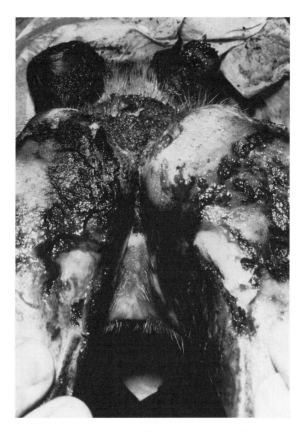

Fig. 6.4 Digital dermatitis with 'strawberry-like' sagittal lesion of volar skin. Mild interdigital dermatitis is evident between the bulbs of the heel though dorsal interdigital skin is unaffected.

Current studies include the examination of biopsy material by immunofluorescence and immunoblotting techniques for this organism. A DNA papillomavirus or papovavirus has not been confirmed as the cause, despite the apparent contagious nature of DD. Neither inclusion bodies nor viruses have ever been identified. Immunoperoxidase assay on biopsy material has consistently been negative. Autogenous vaccines have been unsuccessful in control measures.

Most affected herds are cubicle-housed (in free stalls), and the peak incidence is in the winter. Some cases arise during summer months at pasture, but dairy management dictates that such herds intermingle twice daily in collecting yards before and after milking. A DD-free herd has frequently become infected following the purchase of in-calf or calved heifers from an infected herd. Such purchased heifers have often not shown any DD lesions or lameness at purchase.

Diagnosis of DD is no problem at the typical plantar site. Difficulties occur with:

- Solitary lesions at an abnormal site, e.g. dorsal to interdigital cleft, coronary band
- Failure to examine the contralateral limb and the forelimbs for similar but less extensive lesions

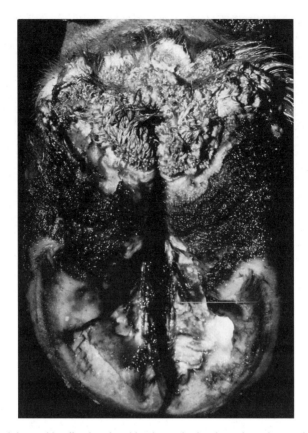

Fig. 6.5 Digital dermatitis affecting the skin above the heels and contiguous heel horn. Papilloma formation is marked. Note prominent hairs to right and more ulcerative nature of lesion proximally.

- Failure to recognise the onset of a herd problem. All herds should have a sample of dairy cows checked for DD when the first cases are diagnosed.

Differential diagnoses should include:

- Interdigital dermatitis (a milder and non-proliferative interdigital lesion; Fig. 6.8)
- 'Slurry heel' or heel horn erosion
- Plantar eczema, a mild and very superficial non-proliferative and non-ulcerative dermatitis
- Interdigital hyperplasia with papilloma formation (solitary lesion): compare with Fig. 6.7.

Treatment

Sporadic cases may justifiably undergo surgical resection to remove potentially infectious material. However, surgery is an impractical and uneconomic control

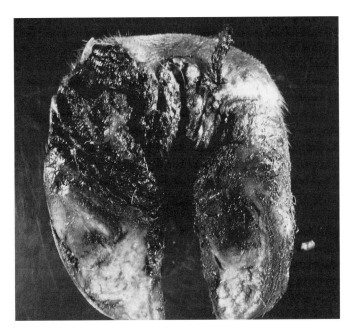

Fig. 6.6 Digital dermatitis showing typical 'kissing lesions' to each side of sagittal plane. Relatively chronic changes.

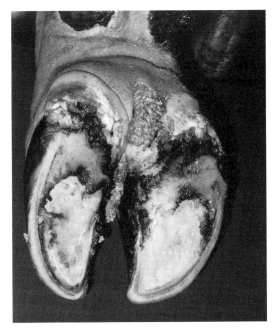

Fig. 6.7 Digital dermatitis at two sites, both in the plantar skin and also in the interdigital skin hyperplasia. Both sites show chronic papillomatous changes. The interdigital mass has been traumatised by contact surfaces.

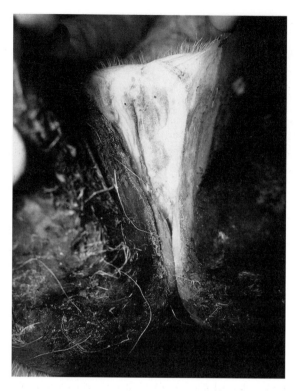

Fig. 6.8 Interdigital dermatitis. Superficial circumscribed lesion of skin only (compare with Fig. 6.9).

method in a herd problem. A circumferential incision should be made into normal tissue around the lesion, and should extend only through skin, avoiding subcutaneous tissues altogether. The ensuing wound may be dressed with a topical antibacterial aerosol (e.g. oxytetracycline), or a sulphonamide paste may be applied, and covered by a light dressing. Medical treatment of small solitary lesions has never been consistently successful. Topical oxytetracycline aerosol, applied twice on successive days to a washed, dried and gently curetted lesion appears the best approach today. No residues have been detected in milk following this topical therapy.

Multiple cases of DD require a different approach to reduce labour and drug costs inevitable with individual treatment of perhaps 20 cows. Some farmers use a knapsack and pressure spray system in the parlour where the long neck and nozzle increase personal safety. A footbath containing either oxytetracycline (5–6 g/litre) or 150 g of a mixture of lincomycin and spectinomycin in 200 litres of water is suitable both for group therapy and prevention. A minimum volume footbath can further reduce drug costs. The herd should be put through the bath, preferably after going through a pre-treatment wash bath, twice daily for 3 days on exiting the parlour. The routine is repeated in 10–14 days. The success rate is reported to be high. Resistant cases should have topical oxytetracycline sprayed on each lesion twice at successive milkings. For prevention alone, the concentration may be reduced from 0.75 to 0.37 g/litre monthly, after milking, on four occasions.

An alternative water-soluble product is tiamulin hydrogen fumarate which is used in a footbath as a 12.5% solution (2 ml/litre or one 250-ml bottle/125 litres for treatment or half this concentration for prevention). The feet should be pressure-hosed before walking through the footbath at six consecutive milkings for therapy. For preventive purposes the dairy cows may be put through the bath once or twice weekly. None of these topical products is licensed for use in cattle. Further, drinking of footbath fluid is likely to result in detectable amounts of antibiotic in blood and milk.

Except in general trials (where a different organism has consistently been isolated from cases of DD), no success has been reported following vaccination of dairy cows with an autogenous vaccine. General hygienic measures to improve removal of slurry from yards and cubicle houses (e.g. twice, not once daily), to improve the quality of tracks to reduce trauma to the skin of the coronary band and pastern, and putting cows out to grass (reducing the concentration of the infectious agent per unit area and the incidence of accidental cow-to-cow spread) can help to reduce the magnitude of a problem.

Ideally, bought-in calved heifers should be kept as a separate group for 4–6 weeks before joining the herd, to permit latent DD lesions to develop without the risk of immediate spread to homebred stock. However, few farms have such quarantine facilities.

Other potential sources of transmission include infected knives and ropes used in claw-trimming.

Heel horn erosion ('slurry heel')

Heel horn erosion (HHE) is an irregular loss of bulbar horn, initially manifest as multiple pit-like erosions, and later as deep oblique grooves which in severe cases lead to flaps of ragged horn. The horn itself is discoloured. The changes affect several claws, predominantly hind, and the effects are fairly symmetrical.

Clinical features

Lameness is not usual except in complicated cases (see below). Many cattle, especially adult cows both beef and dairy, have non-significant lesions. It is favoured by warm humid conditions (damp straw yards, winter housing, overcrowding). Often HHE is combined with lameness resulting from solar ulcerative or white line disease. It has been allegedly associated with extension from or predisposal to interdigital dermatitis. The absence of interdigital dermatitis in cases of HHE, or vice versa, strongly suggests that the two conditions are separate entities.

Sequelae to extensive chronic HHE include sole ulcer, possibly as a result of forward extension of infection through foreign material becoming lodged in a deep fissure and seriously affecting digital loading. Other sequelae include sole abscessation, septic laminitis and white line abscess.

Diagnosis and differential diagnosis

The appearance is characteristic. The possible spread to the interdigital space (interdigital dermatitis) must be considered. Deep infection such as abscessation in the heel should be eliminated as a possible complication. Some cases of HHE have a simultaneous sole ulcer.

Treatment and prevention

Treatment in mild cases is unnecessary towards the end of the winter housing period, as spontaneous resolution is generally seen following turnout to pasture. Severe cases, with undermined flap formation, and milder cases seen in early winter which are likely to deteriorate, should have abnormal horn trimmed off. This trimming should be carefully done to maintain even (50:50, lateral:medial) weightbearing. Some cows with chronic HHE require general paring following generalised overgrowth and long toes which force the heels and heel–skin junction to have greater ground contact. Following heel paring the area should be lightly dressed with an antibiotic (e.g. oxytetracycline) aerosol. Subsequently, prophylactic footbathing with 3–5% formalin hardens the horn and may inhibit bacterial activity. If practical, treated cows should spend a few days in a straw yard on clean dry bedding.

Prevention is important and effective. At-risk herds are characterised by excessive exposure to slurry in cubicle systems and yards, and to a lesser extent to mud in tracks and gateways and feed mangers. Slurry should be removed from passages in yards three times rather than once or twice daily. The cubicle usage should be checked. Cows standing with their rear feet in the passage may have too short or otherwise uncomfortable standings (narrow, inadequate bedding). Cows may be overcrowded and restless, constantly using and standing in passageways. Careful observation over several days may determine the precipitating factors (see also Chapter 10). Cows standing in slurry and fallen silage at a silage face is a precipitating factor which requires preventive steps.

Regular claw trimming, preferably at the beginning of the indoor housing period, when the extent of HHE can be checked, is the second most important preventive step. Apart from footbathing, which can be carried out at four successive milkings every 2 weeks, and has proved beneficial, a further preventive step is the use of lime in cubicles. Lime is put down and the cubicles then bedded with conventional straw.

White line disease

White line disease is one of the most common lameness diagnoses in many UK dairy herds (along with sole ulcer, interdigital phlegmon and digital dermatitis). The plethora of contributory factors often makes investigation and identification of the precise aetiology very difficult.

White line (zona alba) is the specialised horn tissue visible at the junction between the distal border of the claw wall and the sole. The horn is softer and looser in texture than that of wall and sole. The white line has an important function in establishing and maintaining the attachment of the wall to the sole. Of its two components, the inter-digitating or 'terminal horn' is continuous with the sole horn tubules, while the laminar horn is continuous with the wall horn. The visual effect is a striated appearance, which is further easily distinguished on microscopy. The interdigitating horn is produced by the epidermis overlying the distal surfaces of the dermal lamellae. The white line horn has a vital role in weightbearing as weight is transferred to the wall horn. It must also protect deeper structures, withstanding penetration, excessive wear and physical forces resulting from locomotion. Locomotion and weightbearing necessitate a degree of elasticity in the interdigitating horn. This elasticity depends on the fibre orientation within squames (stratum corneum).

The area particularly exposed to injury is the abaxial border of the lateral hind claw near the sole–heel junction. Sometimes the white line near the toe is involved. White line disease develops when its integrity is impaired by poor quality horn production and by impaction with foreign material such as stone particles. Normal white line horn resists this insult. However, predisposing factors include a widened white line following claw overgrowth, excessive wear including abrasive concrete, and awkward sudden turns which may relate to evasive action (bullying by other cows), rough tracks and walkways, and nutritional factors leading to subclinical laminitis.

White line disease causes lameness only when pressure is abnormally exerted on its sensitive laminae as a result of impaction, or subsequently when infection develops deep to such impaction. Pus can then track proximally, to burst eventually above the coronary band. Potential septic sequelae at this point include osteomyelitis of the distal phalanx, distal interphalangeal sepsis and septic navicular bursitis.

Investigation of a herd problem should always include examination of several other cows to discover whether white line disease is extensive, widespread and aetiologically significant. Hind limbs must be lifted, and claw soles lightly pared! Factors to check include:

* Claw conformation:
    Dorsal angle (hind <55° poor, fore <45° poor)
    Overgrowth, including axial rotation of abaxial wall
    Width of white line
    Quality of white line horn (haemorrhages, softness)
    Quality of sole (haemorrhages, softness)
    Quality of wall (rings, cracks)
* Environment:
    Outdoor tracks (stone chips, flints)
    Distance to pasture
    Yard concrete
    Slurry removal
    Cubicle quality

- Behaviour:
    Lying-in facilities
    Social grouping (bullying)
    Route to parlour and housing/feeding areas
- Nutrition:
    Composition and intake (in kilograms) of concentrate
    Concentrate:roughage ratio
    Roughage quality, texture and intake.

Since white line disease is often related to previous episodes of laminitis, which may have been recognised as 'soreness' or may have been clinically inapparent, the diet during the previous months should be checked in terms of possible rumen acidosis. This metabolic upset is prone to occur close to parturition either in increased concentrates proffered in the last prepartum weeks, or in the first 4 weeks postpartum. These physiological and behavioural stresses are particularly great for first-calf heifers. While white line problems do not have a higher incidence in this age group (unlike some herd 'outbreaks' of sole ulcer in freshly calved heifers), the cumulative damage in terms of claw conformation and specifically of the white line may result in clinical problems of white line disease following the second or third calving.

Clinical features

The white line may show areas of new (reddish) or old (dark grey or black) haemorrhage, which do not result in lameness. Loss of white line horn with separation and impaction of the defect by dirt or other foreign bodies may cause mild lameness. Infected lesions can only be recognised following paring out of the foreign material: pus exudes. Such animals are lame to a varying degree. The typical cow with an abaxial white line problem tends to abduct the leg, placing more weight on the medial claw. Sometimes impaction or infection in the white line leads to an underrun sole ('false sole'). Unless this sole in turn is filled with debris, the cow may not be lame, and a new light-coloured sole horn forms. The white line sepsis may alternatively track proximally along the line of least resistance, i.e. the laminae, to discharge at the coronary band as a coronary sinus. Others discharge at the heel or penetrate the navicular bursa, causing a septic bursitis.

Diagnosis

Diagnosis depends on careful paring and examination of the white line along its entire length if the common site (abaxial, at the sole–heel junction) appears normal. Any black spots in the white line should be followed down to normal horn. It is particularly easy to miss penetrations of the toe and axial white line. Gentle pressure with hoof testers over a suspect area of distal wall and sole may aid localisation of the lesion.

Differential diagnosis includes foreign body penetration of the sole, vertical fissure, especially one involving the coronary band, fracture of the distal phalanx and distal phalangeal osteomyelitis.

Treatment

Treatment involves the drainage of pus and removal of debris from the infected site. To avoid repeated impaction, an inverted V- or U-shaped area of wall should be removed proximal and adjacent to the focus. Since this paring can be painful, but must be precise, local analgesia can be helpful (IVRA). Where infection has resulted in development of a discharging coronary sinus, the entire undermined wall will probably require removal. The coronet should be preserved otherwise horn production will be inhibited.

Animals with extensive joint swelling accompanying the white line abscessation should be investigated to determine the extent of deeper digital pathology. Radiography may assist diagnosis in revealing the degree of osteomyelitis of the navicular bone and distal phalanx. In some such cases of bone involvement, successful management may involve curettage through an abaxial window in the claw wall, followed by prolonged irrigation and placement of an irrigation drainage device. A low-speed electric drill also is effective in creating an uninfected cavity, the final result being a deformed but ankylosed and weightbearing claw. Claw amputation is the radical alternative to this claw-paring technique in cases of deep infection and osteomyelitis (see p. 157).

Both claws should be pared in all cases (see p. 176 onwards). It is often helpful, following conservative surgery of infected white line lesions, to apply a block to the sound claw for several weeks. Systemic (tetracycline, ceftiofur) and local (tetracycline aerosol) antibiotics should be given for 4–5 days to cows following surgery for deep infection following white line abscessation.

Prevention

Prevention and control depend on:

- Breeding for good conformation, i.e. a steep (>55°) dorsal angle to obtain compact claws
- A nutritional programme that avoids sudden dietary changes (excess starch and protein) and which includes trace mineral (e.g. Zn) supplementation
- Adequate exercise to ensure optimal horn wear and growth, which is stimulated by a good intra-ungular blood flow
- Maintenance of good quality tracks and gateways to pastures (see Chapter 10)
- Maintenance or construction of correctly sized and designed cubicles, permitting easy movement in the shed and to and from the dairy (see Chapter 10)
- Avoidance of areas of pooled slurry where cows, potentially standing for hours, develop soft horn

- Avoidance of sudden steps up or down, and awkward tight corners around which cows could slip, thereby seriously and regularly abrading the sole and white line
- Maintenance of an attitude of caring herdsmanship in which cows are encouraged to move around and out to yards and pastures at their own pace, along good quality tracks
- Prophylactic use of a footbath, placed under cover, and preceded by a wash bath, containing 5% formalin to harden the horn, to be used four times weekly every 2 or 4 weeks, the contents of which are replaced between usage periods
- Regular claw trimming to maintain normal claw shape, and specifically to control dorsal overgrowth and axial overgrowth of the abaxial wall (double sole formation)
- In herds still subject to white line disease despite adoption of such preventive measures, consideration should be given to major changes such as winter housing in a large straw-bedded yard (to reduce abrasion by concrete) and adoption of a summer calving pattern (avoiding the simultaneous dual stress of parturition and entry to winter housing).

Interdigital phlegmon (UK 'foul-in-the-foot')/interdigital necrobacillosis (US 'footrot')

Although interdigital phlegmon was once considered the most common cause of digital lameness in a dairy cow, its significance now appears to be less than sole ulcer, white line disease and on many farms digital dermatitis. The incidence may have remained unchanged, while that of other problems has increased. The infection occurs at all ages, but is less commonly seen in young cattle. While sporadic cases are possible, mini-outbreaks may follow common traumatic incidents (e.g. turnout onto stubble or meandering among clippings of thorn hedge), as well as passage along sharp-stone tracks and gateways.

Interdigital phlegmon is an acute or subacute necrotic infection of the interdigital space. Infection starts in the subcutis, following skin trauma and performation, with swelling and cellulitis causing pain, mild pyrexia and partial anorexia. The claws are separated and an oedematous swelling is evident over the heels. The skin is erythematous and within 24 hours a longitudinal fissure develops with mild exudation of necrotic foul-smelling tissue. This fissure extends towards the axial borders, and skin may slough leaving an irregular necrotic wound which may be contaminated by secondary invaders (Fig. 6.9). *Fusobacterium necrophorum*, together with *Bacteroides melaninogenicus* appear to act synergistically in the pathogenesis. *Actinomyces pyogenes* is a frequent secondary invader. The role of several saprophytic bacteria isolated from characteristic lesions is not clear.

In 1993 a more severe form of interdigital phlegmon ('superfoul') was first recognised in the UK. Peracute in onset and refractory to conventional therapy, rapid development of interdigital swelling and fissure formation is followed by extensive necrosis and granulation tissue formation, swelling of the coronet and pastern, and rapid development of a severe septic pedal arthritis which has often

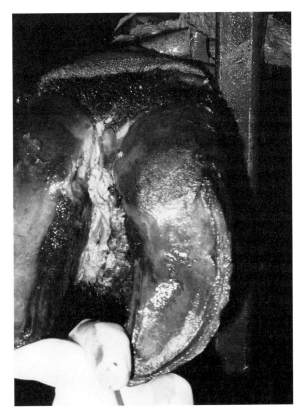

Fig. 6.9 Interdigital phlegmon or interdigital necrobacillosis with severe slough of skin and subcutaneous tissues.

necessitated emergency slaughter. As in the classical syndrome, both *F. necrophorum* and *B. melaninogenicus* have been recovered. Anecdotal evidence suggests that the severe syndrome tends to be seen on farms with a digital dermatitis problem.

Diagnosis is easily made on the characteristic signs of sudden lameness, mild pyrexia, digital and interdigital swelling with separation of claws, and the typical malodorous interdigital lesion. The most important differential diagnosis is an interdigital foreign body, and other possibilities include severe interdigital dermatitis or digital dermatitis.

Treatment and prevention

Both systemic and local therapy is recommended. Conventional cases respond well to ceftiofur, oxytetracycline or ampicillin by injection. Superficial necrotic material should be removed by gentle swabbing. The ulcerated area is best sprayed with an oxytetracycline aerosol or dressed with sulphanilamide/copper sulphate (4:1) ointment. Bandaging is not recommended so as to avoid further sloughing tissue remaining in contact with the wound surface. The patient should preferably be placed onto a dry surface (e.g. in a loose box) for several days.

Treatment of 'superfoul' must be particularly aggressive. Early cases respond well to 6000 mg oxytetracycline. More advanced cases require 8000 mg tylosin followed by 4000 mg for 3 days, together with debridement under local analgesia and a local antibiotic dressing (Cook and Cutler, 1995).

Of potential but still unproven benefit is the adoption of regional intravenous antibiosis by which a high local concentration of penicillin G or oxytetracyline can be achieved and maintained in the diseased tissues for up to an hour before the proximal tourniquet is released (by the farmer). The antibiotic dosage rate is about one-tenth of that given as a normal systemic injection. Severe thrombophlebitis has occasionally been reported following high dose rates.

Animals with interdigital phlegmon, including 'superfoul', are actively shedding infection. Such cattle should therefore be isolated. Improved drainage and walking surfaces may be urgently considered in concentrated and infected traffic areas. The herd may require removal to a 'clean' dry pasture, or be prematurely and temporarily housed.

Prevention involves avoidance by the herd of any potentially traumatic material (e.g. stubble, rocky tracks), improved hygiene in cubicle houses to reduce the wet and damp underfoot conditions and possibly use of a copper sulphate (5%) or zinc sulphate (7–10%) footbath (see p. 182) as a regular prophylactic measure during high risk periods. In 'superfoul' herds with concurrent existence of digital dermatitis, the latter requires additional measures (p. 158).

Laminitis (pododermatitis aseptica)

Laminitis is a common non-infectious circulatory disturbance of the bovine claw. The wall and sole both undergo degenerative changes at the dermal–epidermal junction resulting in abnormal horn production, manifested initially in softening and haemorrhage of the dermis. Later effects include gross ('ulcerative') defects in the sole and heel, double sole formation, white line separation and ridging and loss of periople from the claw wall.

Until some 20 years ago the forms of laminitis were classified as acute, subacute and chronic. Today the preferred classification is acute, subclinical and chronic, their incidence being respectively low, high and high.

Pathogenesis

Despite increased awareness of different forms of laminitis in cattle, confusion still surrounds the pathogenesis. Predisposing factors are numerous: systemic conditions both normal (e.g. parturition) and abnormal (acute metritis, displaced abomasum), lactic acidosis following excessive ingestion of carbohydrates or protein, secondary endotoxaemia, and mechanical factors (walking surfaces, either excessive or limited exercise, overgrown claws, breed size and weight). The significance of these factors is discussed under 'Prevention'. Particular controversy surrounds the use of the term subclinical laminitis.

Pathology

The term laminitis is a misnomer, since the condition is non-inflammatory. The primary insult of a locally impaired blood supply to digital horn results in a degree of haemostasis while blood is shunted over into the venous circulation through vessels proximal to the coronet. The intradigital sludged blood causes hypoxic damage to the walls of arteries, arterioles and capillaries. Histamine release adds to the vasodilation and congestion in the stratum vasculosum. Large haemorrhages develop following diapedesis, and as the vascular walls become permeable, exudation causes a generalised oedema of the dermis. A vicious cycle develops as the oedema increases the intra-ungular pressure, causing a further reduction of blood flow, thrombus formation, the manifestation of pain, and the appearance of lameness.

Histopathology

The critical area of change is the interdigitating dermal–epidermal junction of the wall lamellae, which slide distally past the laminae towards the ground contact surface. Normal weightbearing is transferred from hoof wall to the laminar–lamellar interface, then to the fibro-elastic dermis (corium) and hence onto the periosteum of the distal phalanx and the appendicular skeleton. Laminitis results in damaged lamellar germinal cells, some loss of the onychogenic substance (tonofibrils) and loss of keratohyalin granules from the matrices of the soft horn (e.g. periople). A mild inflammatory cell response of lymphocyte infiltration develops in the damaged tissues.

The poor keratin production resulting from the reduced blood supply, damaged germinal cells and loss of tonofibrils lead to structurally poor horn and gradual separation of the close lamellar–laminar link. The failure of support results in potential sinking of the distal phalanx within the claw horn capsule. Continuing compression of the dermis (corium) of the sole and heel leads to further vascular damage, haemorrhage, oedema, ischemic necrosis and thrombosis. Severe pain in the acute laminitic phase often manifests itself as marked lameness and later recumbency. No visible abnormalities may be evident in the claw at this time. This is a later step in the acute syndrome.

Later changes follow after several weeks (chronic laminitis). The coronary band becomes rough and irregular, the perioplic sheen is lost, horizontal grooves develop on the dorsal wall which tends to become somewhat concave, and the white line becomes wider than normal. The sole also shows chronic changes as layers of dark grey or black staining (blood; Fig. 6.10) or a yellow discoloration in soft flaky horn (as in subclinical laminitis). The foreclaws may show similar changes to the hind limbs (Fig. 6.11). Paring of the abnormal horn often reveals a double sole, sole ulcer or impaction of the widened white line. In very severe cases dropping and rotation of the distal phalanx occasionally can result in its potential perforation through the damaged sole horn.

Histopathology of chronic laminitic claws reveals chronic scar tissue formation

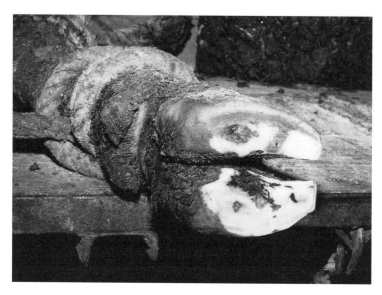

Fig. 6.10 Chronic laminitis, with multiple areas of long-standing damage to sole and white line.

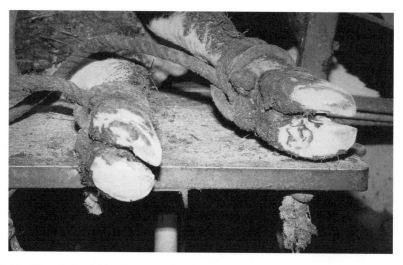

Fig. 6.11 Chronic laminitis. Cow stood with forelegs crossed. Claw examination reveals several areas of old solar haemorrhage, predominantly in medial claws, thereby accounting for stance. Similar stance is seen in some cows with acute laminitis.

in the thin corium. Sclerosis of vascular walls replaces the necrotic process. At this stage the dorsal wall is somewhat concave and obviously ridged, the sole is flattened, and the white line enlarged and possibly impacted with debris. These changes are seen in all eight claws, but are often more marked in the lateral hind claws (e.g. white line and solar 'ulcerative' changes). The abaxial wall may to a variable extent have overgrown axially to form a weightbearing sole.

Clinical signs and diagnosis

Acute laminitis: the majority of cases develop in the first postpartum weeks. Heifers may be affected as often as older cattle. Lameness affects two or four limbs, classically presenting a gait 'like a cat on hot bricks' with obvious generalised digital soreness. There may be reluctance to rise. Forelimbs may be extended or crossed (Fig. 6.11) and hind claws advanced under the body. Cows have an arched back and turn reluctantly. Palpation of the claws reveals increased heat and pain is evident on percussion or pincers pressure. The digital vessels, in thin-skinned cows, may be unusually prominent and sometimes distal arterial pulsation is exaggerated. Paring is unlikely to reveal any lesions in early acute laminitis. Later lesions are similar to the picture in subclinical laminitis.

Subclinical laminitis: by definition the animal is not lame. All ages may be affected and diagnosis depends on determination of the previously described digital horn lesoins. The suspicious signs include most of the following: soft wax-like solar horn and extensive subsolar haemorrhages in several claws, tenderness to pincers pressure, incipient sole ulcer formation, a hesitant gait (lameness score 1; see Table 6.5), possible widening of the white line and a tendency to claw overgrowth due to limited wear.

Chronic laminitis: most cows show intermittent or persistent lameness (score 2), in part largely mechanical due to claw overgrowth. Visible features include the parallel and horizontal horn ridges, which may develop into fissures (Fig. 6.12), the flaky half-powdered appearance of the periople near the coronet, and flattening and broadening of the wall which becomes rather concave. Changes involve several or all claws.

Radiography of the digit in a horizontal plane reveals a variable degree of downward rotation of the distal phalanx. Other features of chronic laminitis have been described under the section on histopathology, page 171.

Treatment and control

This section discusses both individual and herd control of different forms of laminitis.

Acute laminitis: acute laminitis in a freshly calved heifer or cow is an emergency which requires prompt medication with analgesics, transfer to soft bedding or to pasture, and encouragement of limited exercise. The associated precipitating condition is usually not apparent but if identified (e.g. acute metritis) requires appropriate intensive therapy. Suggested analgesics in such cases include aspirin (50–100 mg/kg b.i.d. orally) after an initial dose of flunixin meglumine (2 mg/kg iv). Alternative analgesic drugs in acute laminitis include butorphanol (0.05 mg/kg iv) and ketoprofen. Only flunixin and ketoprofen are currently licensed for use as analgesics in dairy cattle. The benefits of antihistamines and

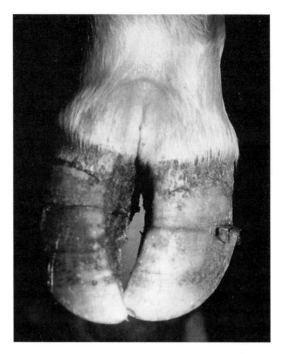

Fig. 6.12 Chronic laminitis showing horizontal fissures at same position in each claw.

corticosteroids are disputed. Anecdotal reports state that digital analgesia by ring nerve block in the recumbent acute case can lead to dramatic improvement as the animal stands and moves about in comfort.

Cattle with ruminal (lactic) acidosis causing signs of acute laminitis (e.g. following gorging on concentrates – high carbohydrate or high protein) require prompt medical therapy and occasionally emergency rumenotomy. Treatment to correct the metabolic disturbance should include intravenous fluids, e.g. lactated Ringer's solution, with added sodium bicarbonate, and intravenous calcium (do not mix solutions!).

Chronic laminitis: lameness in chronic laminitic cows may be alleviated but rarely abolished. The steps involve repeated claw trimming at approximately 3-month intervals. Where 'thimbles' result from deep horizontal grooves and increasing mobility of the distal section of wall, resulting in increased pressure on the sensitive corium, the loose 'thimble' should be removed as early as possible. Prevention of chronic disease depends on avoiding predisposing factors leading to subclinical laminitis.

Subclinical laminitis: control of subclinical laminitis depends on management changes related to:

(1) Nutrition (e.g. concentrates: roughage ratio)
(2) Environment (e.g. housing)
(3) Genetics.

Nutrition – some rules (see also pp. 83–4)

- Avoid sudden feed changes of any type in the 4 weeks before and after parturition. There is often a tendency to attempt (lead feeding) to boost cattle, particularly freshly calved heifers, to reach peak milk yield within 3 weeks.
- Avoid a high risk of clinically apparent or subclinical rumen acidosis by:
  - buffering rumen pH against sudden swings towards excessive acidity (pH <5.5);
  - including grass or lucerne-based feed (e.g. nuts) in concentrates;
  - including 1% sodium bicarbonate;
  - increasing the daily period of access to concentrates by thrice daily feeds (if the ideal of complete diet feeding cannot be adopted). Permit unrestricted access to iodised or rock salt licks to increase saliva production.
- Do not permit the concentrate : roughage ratio to exceed 60 : 40 in the first 6 weeks postpartum. Concentrate intake may be increased at 0.25 kg (multiparous cows) or 0.20 kg (heifers) per day from 1 week postpartum. This regime will keep the ratio under 60 : 40 even at 6 weeks postpartum, as long as roughage access remains unrestricted. Plenty of roughage (whether hay, grass or maize silage, or straw) should be long-stemmed, as this form increases rumination time and therefore saliva production. If grass silage is a staple ration, it should not only be of good quality but also have a high dry matter content.

  A relationship has been suggested between feeding of excess protein and subclinical laminitis, but neither convincing research nor a convincing mode of action has yet been apparent.
- Do not allow more than 4 kg concentrate feed to be consumed at one time. The advantage of computerised feeding systems is obvious in that an individual will regulate concentrate intake to 'little and often'. If concentrates must still be fed in the parlour, potentially resulting in a sudden drop in rumen pH, such cows should have immediate access from the parlour exit to *ad libitum* long-stemmed roughage. Otherwise the initial subclinical rumen acidotic environment may not only cause the development of laminitis from the release of various mediators, including endotoxins, from ruminal microbes; the same microbes, destroyed by the low pH, can lead to hepatic abscessation, caudal vena cava thrombosis and abomasal ulceration.

Environment including housing

- Accustom down-calving heifers to concrete yards several weeks before parturition. A combination of concrete yard and straw yard is better still.
- Ensure cubicles are comfortable with plenty of bedding or effective mattresses or mats, that cubicles have the correct dimensions (height of kerb <20 cm) and that their number is sufficient. In larger dairy units it may be advantageous to keep both lactating heifers and cows in a straw yard for the first 8 weeks postpartum, and only then to transfer them to a cubicle system.

- Permit yarded or cubicled cows plenty of loafing space and encourage exercise by positioning hay and silage feed bunks distant from the cubicles and straw yards. Social interactions less marked than frank bullying of younger and smaller cows may contribute to the predisposing factors for subclinical laminitis and indeed other forms of injury to the digital horn. Behaviour involving long periods of standing in slurry rather than lying in a comfortable cubicle, of scurrying along a slippery alley and turning several corners, of forcing the head and neck between other cows to gain access to a feed bunker or silage face: all these activities, stressful in themselves, can lead to claw and especially hoof horn micro-trauma hundreds of times daily. A good quality environment ensures happy cows. Careful long-term observation (and note-taking) brings quick rewards in ascertaining the necessary steps for enhanced cow comfort.
- Herd cows along farm tracks at their own natural pace, avoiding the use of a dog, tractor or stick.
- Keep tracks and especially gateways in good physical condition, correctly crowned and well drained along the sides. If considerable costly improvement is needed, consider the installation of a narrow synthetic cattle-only track. In any event discourage movement of tractors and other farm machinery along cow tracks.
- Consider regular prophylactic use of a footbath to remove dirt, and to disinfect the interdigital skin and harden the claw horn which is likely to be soft in cases of laminitis (see p. 170 onwards).

Genetics

- Note the claw shape of cows with a good lameness record and consider seriously further use of those bull lines.
- Avoid breeding from cows with long small-angled claws (<45°), a characteristic which in US Holstein studies was associated with decreased longevity. Less convincing was a correlation of longevity with straight hind limbs (higher hock angle). It has also been reported that serous tarsitis (bog spavin), spastic paresis and degenerative arthritis are more liable in straight-legged cattle, so advice is confounded by two sets of contrary trends.

General considerations: A random group (early, mid and late lactation) of cows totalling 9–12 should have their claws examined at 1- to 2-monthly intervals to track the development of subclinical laminitis. One foreleg and one hindleg should be examined. The presence of any lesions (e.g. old solar haemorrhage) should necessitate lifting and examination of the contralateral claws. The findings should be simply recorded (see pp. 151–2 and Table 6.4), and the current herd management reviewed at this opportunity.

Claw trimming

Functional claw trimming is frequently essential to maintain normal function of the limb. With some herds recording all cows being lame at one or more times during the year, awareness of the value of this procedure has increased.

One personal survey carried out in 1995 (Weaver, 1997) revealed that digital lameness was a major problem on two-thirds of Somerset farms, and a minor problem in the remainder. With one exception, all farms practised claw care by trimming, usually done by farm personnel, only a few of whom had been on a recommended training course. Most had been taught by their veterinarian, or had just 'picked it up'. Major recommendation follow.

Time of trimming

Ideally trimming should be carried out at drying-off, but this time is often inconvenient. Spring turnout is also a suitable time when, following winter housing, claw neglect is relatively more prone to exist. Since the whole herd is potentially involved, this time may also be practical for the most severe cases. It is rare for a cow to abort in late pregnancy as a result of struggling during restraint for claw trimming.

Where should claw trimming be done?

The crush should be indoors, with easy entry and exit, and well lit, and with surroundings easily cleansed. A purpose-built crush is preferred as it reduces the labour requirements (i.e. time) and is less dangerous. This crush has fitments for holding hind legs (Fig. 6.13). A Velcro-equipped broad nylon hobble is less traumatic and easier to apply than the usual rope. The main features of a claw-trimming crush are summarised in Table 6.6. As herds continue to increase in size more farmers will realise the advantages of an appropriately designed trimming crush or a tilting crush incorporating belly straps (Fig. 6.14). The WOPA crush (Fig. 6.15), either the simple model or the electric hydraulic type, is specifically designed for claw trimming and is increasingly popular owing to its ease of operation. This crush can involve a team of two, though a single experienced individual can also work unaided.

What equipment is needed?

Left- and right-handed hoof knives of best quality steel, a narrow-bladed search knife, and single- or double-action hoof pincers (nippers), preferably supplemented by a mechanised sander, are required. A guillotine cutter (also made by WOPA) is an optional choice. This equipment (excluding electric-powered sander) should, between cows, be put through a bucket containing disinfectant to avoid possible spread of digital diseases (e.g. digital dermatitis).

What is the technique?

Weight distribution should be even between claws, in other words medial and lateral claws should carry similar loads. The major problem is usually overgrowth and overloading of the lateral hind claw, which needs careful correction. The dorsal wall of the medial hind claw is briefly trimmed first: the length of its dorsal wall is reduced to about 7.5 cm (normal length) by vertical trimming at the toe

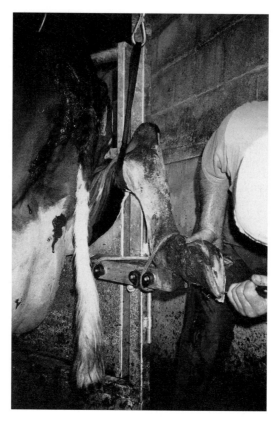

Fig. 6.13 Claw trimming in a standing crush. Right leg is raised by soft webbing above hock, and foot is fixed by soft rope onto angled wood block with quick release catch. Note lateral claw has long toe and a high heel, both of which require correction.

Table 6.6 Requirements for a claw-trimming crush.

Site	Equipment
Under cover	Suitable for one-person operation
Well lit	Non-slip corrugated wood base
Easy approach and exit, preferably holding pens	Wooden rests for hind and fore claws
Area easily cleansed by pressure hose to drain	Padded nylon hobbles with Velcro-type closure
	Pulley system or hydraulic for easy lift
	Quick release catch on rope

(hoof cutters or guillotine). The sole is not trimmed at this stage. The lateral claw is then trimmed to the same length. The sole is trimmed to the same level as in the still untouched medial claw sole. Specifically the heel height of the lateral claw should be reduced to that of the medial claw. The middle part of the sole is trimmed to be slightly concave towards the axial border.

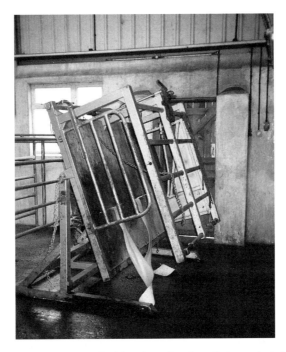

Fig. 6.14 Tilting table recently installed for claw trimming. Swing gate is brought to contact right rear vertical bar for entry of cow, which is restrained by yoke (far end) and supported by two belly bands. Note exit door immediately in front of cow.

The handle of the pincers may be laid transversely across the medial and lateral heels to confirm that they are the same height, and that therefore weight distribution should be equal. In cows with sole ulcer (see p. 153) trimming should be specifically concentrated on the appropriate sole depth and heel height of the lateral claw to transfer more weight to the medial claw and the toe region of the affected lateral claw.

Problems

Attention should be paid to abnormalities revealed during claw trimming. These tend to be concentrated in the lateral claw:

- Haemorrhage or ulceration at the sole–heel junction (see p. 153)
- Black spots in the white line, especially abaxially in the lateral claw (see p. 164)
- Overgrowth of the abaxial wall of the lateral claw.

If there is such pathology in the lateral claw, weightbearing may advantageously be transferred to the medial claw (see above). This step is a simple method of promoting natural healing of sole or white line lesions in the previously overburdened lateral claw.

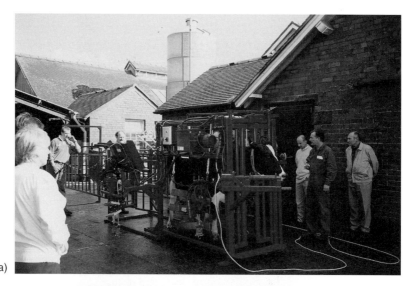

(a)

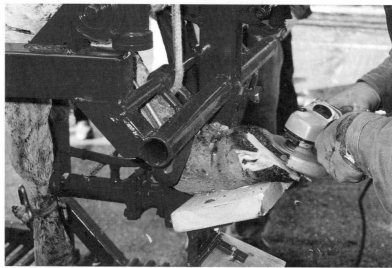

(b)

Fig. 6.15 The WOPA (Danish-built) crush specifically designed for ease of claw-trimming (a) and close-up of sander in action (b). Note exposed abaxial white line defect.

The result of abaxial wall overgrowth of the lateral claw is naturally increased weightbearing by the wall, formation of a false (double) sole, and further localised pressure over the sole–heel junction favouring sole ulcer formation. Any over-lapping ledge of horn is first removed with hoof pincers, impacted debris is then pared out, and the abaxial white line and sole–heel junction of the bearing surface carefully examined. Damaged areas are appropriately managed.

Constant quality control of claw trimming is vital. While the farmer perceives the cost of veterinary trimming to be excessive, resulting in professional routine trimming being rare, he or she should be competent to instruct, advise and correct para-professional trimmers, dairy personnel and managers.

Prosthetics

Some cows have painful sole and wall lesions which require minimal weight-bearing for some weeks to reduce unnecessary suffering and maintain appetite, locomotion and production. Artificial plastic devices may be fitted to the non-diseased claw (usually medial) so that the diseased claw has no weightbearing function. Three possibilities are:

(1)   Wood block fixed to claw by methyl methacrylate resin or a metal or rubber shoe nailed to claw.
(2)   A plastic shoe ('Cowslip') into which liquid methyl methacrylate is poured before the device is applied over the cleaned and trimmed sound claw, elevating it about 2 cm.
(3)   A plastic slipper, with one distal (sole) surface thicker than the other, into which both claws are inserted. The slipper ('Shoof') is held in place by strapping laced tightly round the pastern of the fully extended leg.

Neither the 'Cowslip' nor 'Shoof' should be left on the cow for more than 4 weeks. A hammer and chisel aid removal of the acrylic resin-adhesed wood block or the 'Cowslip'. These prosthetic devices have a firm place in permitting the natural repair processes of the digital horn to continue without chronic trauma from weightbearing. They may also be used on cows where accidental overtrimming has resulted in the exposure of sensitive laminae. Bandaging of such cases is inadvisable. The ability of cows to move around with such a prosthesis on a claw varies with bodyweight, location of prosthesis, distance travelled and under-foot conditions.

The risks associated with use of a mechanical claw grinder have been exaggerated. Certainly prolonged continuous contact of a sander (>5 seconds) leads to heat production in horn, just as overenthusiastic paring can expose sensitive laminae and lead to soreness or lameness. However, careful manipulation, bearing in mind the structures that are being restored to a normal shape, leads to minimal side-effects. A lay claw-trimmer should be warned of these risks and have at least 1 day's experience with a skilled teacher.

All veterinarians should be competent to advise on improvement of paring facilities and equipment, technique and the steps required to reduce the amount of claw work needed on a particular premises.

A number of countries including Denmark, Sweden, the USA and in 1998 the UK have established formal groups of farrier associations. The UK group of claw trimmers includes some veterinarians. The aim is to establish a register of qualified personnel through formal courses and examinations, to discuss recurrent and difficult problems, and to be of mutual benefit through health insurance and accident prevention. Their work throughout the world is aided by a biennial meeting of veterinarians and claw trimmers where the latest meeting (Lucerne, Switzerland, September 1998) emphasised problems in digital dermatitis, subclinical laminitis and locomotion scoring of cattle. Increased liaison between hoof trimmers and veterinarians on the farm will aid lameness prevention and improve animal welfare.

Footbaths

Routine use of a footbath aids the control of infectious interdigital and digital skin disease. It has little or no effect on reducing diseases of the horny tissues but does make horn hard and less flexible. A footbath therefore aids in some reduction of the environmental bacterial count, which is important in intensively housed dairy herds. The bath has been recommended for both treatment and control of digital dermatitis, interdigital phlegmon and interdigital dermatitis.

The bath should be placed near the exit from the milking parlour and should preferably be under cover to avoid dilution by rainwater. A pre-wash bath or trough, or a power water spray device to remove mud and manure, reduces the rate of contamination of the bath contents. While previously permanent installations were common, the market now offers several varieties of durable portable non-slip baths which can be incorporated into an existing chute or race. The conventional size is 3m minimal length, 1m minimal width and 10–12 cm working fluid depth. A plastic minimal solution bath has also been developed. Its advantages include lower running costs for chemicals (volume 10–15 litres compared with 125–200 litres), and fewer problems in disposal of exhausted solutions.

Products used in cattle footbaths include formalin (2–5%), copper sulphate (5–10%), zinc sulphate (10%) and antibiotic powder preparations including oxytetracycline, a lincomycin/spectinomycin mixture and tiamulin (not licensed in the UK). Use of a footbath is not without hazards:

- Higher concentrations of formalin (10% or more) cause skin irritation around the pastern and coronary band.
- Accidental splashing of formalin into the eyes and inhalation of its fumes are hazardous to human health.
- Ingestion of fluid from antibiotic footbaths can lead to detectable levels in blood and milk (e.g. oxytetracycline).
- The correct disposal of exhausted fluid can be difficult.

General recommendations for prevention of digital lameness

This chapter has discussed several specific problems of the digit. There is obvious overlap in the control measures suggested for several, such as white line problems and subclinical laminitis, since some common factors are important in the aetiology. These risk factors are confused by the different methods of assessment of a disease, whether by the existence of lesions (as in subclinical laminitis) or by clinical lameness. One Dutch study of over 2000 cows, for example, revealed only 1.2% to be clinically lame, but 83% of all cows had interdigital dermatitis and 75% had lesions allegedly associated with laminitis (pododermatitis aseptica).

Five main groups of risk factors are evident:

(1) Behaviour
   • Inadequate lying time
   • Poor cow comfort (cubicles)
   • Social confrontation (bullying)
   • Insufficient exercise
   • Stress
(2) Building facilities
   • Poor floor surfaces (abrasive, slippery)
   • Inadequate space, poor cubicle design
   • Poor slurry disposal
   • Excessive moisture
   • Poor management (little observation time, impatience)
(3) Genetics
   • Poor claw conformation (small toe angle)
   • Poor hock conformation ('cow-hocked')
(4) Infection
   • Poor hygiene (greater infectivity)
   • Micronutrients (poor resistance, poor immunity)
(5) Nutrition
   • Fibre, its quantity, quality and physiochemical form (starch, fibre)
   • Protein quantity (excess volume and percentage of total DMI)
   • Buffers (poor supply, little saliva)
   • Excess fertiliser
   • Pasture management

These factors have all been considered elsewhere is this chapter. The above headings may serve as a checklist *aide-mémoire* when investigating a complex digital lameness problem.

Bone fractures and physeal separations

It is a common misapprehension that bovine fractures are rare. Whilst adult cattle are rarely affected, calves more commonly develop iatrogenic fractures or physeal separations during manual extraction during or soon after dystocia. Common fractures involve the metacarpal and metatarsal shaft and distal physeal separations (usually Salter-Harris type 2) and the femoral shaft. Most such fractures are attributed to the dam standing on a calf limb. Rarely is this so. Physeal separations are less common in calves over 2 months and rare in stock over 1 year old (but see Fig. 6.16).

   The aetiology of the metacarpal/metatarsal trauma is grossly excessive traction, often with obstetrical chains placed on the limbs, fore or hind, proximal to the fetlock. Misdirected traction (usually with inadequate downward direction of the limbs, i.e. towards the hocks of the dam) is an additional inciting factor. In the femoral fracture, occurring in either anterior or posterior presentation, misdirected traction is again the main error.

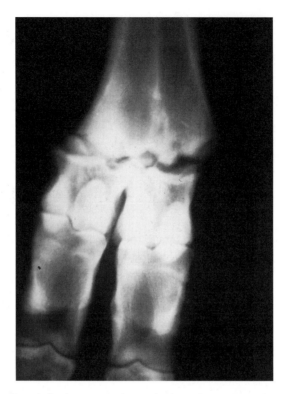

Fig. 6.16 Separation of distal metatarsal growth plate of metatarsus in 14-month-old steer. Cranial-caudal radiograph. Successful treatment included reduction of the separation following traction and 4 weeks immobilisation of the fetlock in a cast.

A common and significant sign in neonatal long bone fractures and physeal separations is an inability to stand. This sign is often initially and incorrectly attributed to exhaustion. The problem is clearer when the calf stands up weight-bearing on three limbs. Such calves are very liable to be colostrum-deficient following a failure to suck in the first 8 hours, and this effect compounds a serious problem. An accurate history (time of birth, evidence of having sucked or having been given colostrum) is vital for optimal management.

While distal fractures (e.g. metacarpal) are more liable to be open due to the lack of overlying muscle, the special problems and poor prognosis of neonatal femoral fractures are related to the weak and thin cortex, which often results in severe comminutions.

Many lower limb fractures undergo a limited and relatively superficial examination firstly by the owner and then by the veterinarian. The result of failing to detect an open fracture before applying external immobilisation and fixation for 3 weeks is usually veterinary embarrassment as osteomyelitis and a non-healing fracture are revealed on cast removal (Fig. 6.17). At this stage euthanasia is often the only option. The skin should therefore be clipped over all such fracture sites to check for perforation and the likelihood of subcutaneous infection (Fig. 6.18).

Radiographs may be useful to determine the best method of fixation, hence it

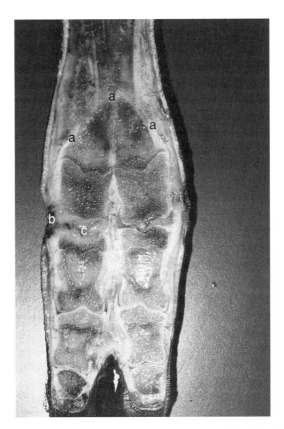

Fig. 6.17 Vertical section through distal extremity of 7-week-old calf which originally had a diaphyseal fracture of the metacarpus (a). A skin wound (b), overlooked originally, was detected when the plaster cast was removed after 4 weeks' immobilisation. Spread of infection has led to sepsis in the fetlock joint (c). Note that the metacarpal fracture had healed.

is often better to have such calves referred to the practice hospital facilities for a few hours. In moving a calf or adult bovine for examination and treatment of a fracture, the site should be temporarily immobilised by a splint (e.g. polyvinyl gutter pipe, broom handle), by a modified Robert Jones bandage or possibly a Thomas splint. This measure reduces further soft tissue damage, the possible development of an open fracture, and minimises patient discomfort.

The prognosis in calfhood fractures is related to several factors (better > worse):

Site	:	Distal > proximal
Type	:	Closed > open
Type	:	Simple > comminuted
Duration	:	<12 hours > 12 hours
Time of occurrence	:	Postpartum > peripartum
Immune status	:	Immune competent > colostrum deficient

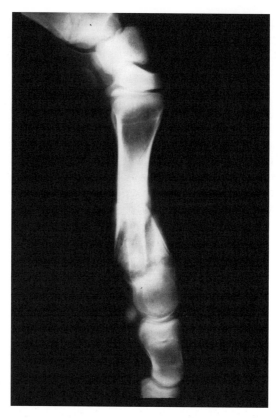

Fig. 6.18 Comminuted fracture of distal metacarpal diaphysis 3 weeks after external immobilisation (plaster cast) showing signs of severe osteomyelitis. Open nature of fracture was
overlooked at original examination. Lateral-medial radiograph.

Methods of management depend on patient size, age and temperament, economic
factors, the site and conformation of the fracture, and surgical experience and
facilities.

Fracture of distal phalanx

Sporadic fracture of the distal phalanx can be associated with trauma (e.g.
sudden turnout onto hard roadways and pasture in springtime), osteomyelitis
following penetration by a foreign body (pathological fracture), or fluorosis
(from ingestion of high fluorine-containing compound feeds or contaminated
pasture), but most cases have an unestablished aetiology (Desrochers & St
Jean, 1996).

Clinical features

Lameness usually has a sudden onset and is severe. Rare cases have bilateral fractures of the foreleg medial claws, resulting in a cross-legged stance. Slight heat

and mild swelling of the coronary band is evident. Compression of the claw with hoof testers or percussion are resented. Lateral radiographs using an interdigitally positioned non-screen film confirm the diagnosis. Most fractures are intra-articular extending to the distal surface of the phalanx.

Diagnosis and differential diagnosis

Diagnosis is based on the sudden onset of severe lameness which can be localised to pain within the claw by hoof testers, confirmed by radiography. As major differential diagnoses include solar foreign body penetration and abscessation, and severe bruising, the sole horn should be carefully pared during examination. The white line area should not be ignored.

Treatment and prevention

Although the severity of lameness is reduced after some days, healing of this minimally displaced fracture is very slow. Treatment should relieve pain and reduce potential distraction by the flexor tendon and is easily achieved by placing a wood block on the adjacent sound digit for 4 weeks (see p. 181). Clinical healing takes 4–8 weeks.

Cases of pathological fracture and osteomyelitis often necessitate digit amputation (see p. 157). If the osteomyelitis and pathological fracture are limited to the toe area, amputation of the claw tip may be successful. Occasional cases have alternatively responded to radical curettage and frequent dressing changes along with follow-up radiography. Such measures are limited to valuable breeding stock.

Prevention in an incident involving several cases in a few days involves examination for possible fluorine toxicity and for traumatic traps along tracks and roadways.

Metacarpus and metatarsus

Simple closed mid or distal shaft fractures respond well to casts of fibreglass (light, expensive, water-resistant) or plaster of Paris (heavier, cheap, softens on exposure to water). Deep sedation and analgesia, or general anaesthesia are generally necessary for optimal and efficient manipulative fracture reduction. Considerable traction may be required in growing cattle weighing 200–400 kg to effect reduction of physeal separations, as in Fig. 6.16. Following reduction the fibreglass or plaster cast should extend from the coronary band to the mid-radius (forelimb) or mid-tibia (hindlimb), to ensure that the joint on either side of the fracture is immobilised. A few millimetres' depth of padding is first wrapped round the leg, and down over the coronary band. A piece of obstetrical wire encased in some plastic intravenous tubing can be placed below the plaster to facilitate later removal of the cast. Bony protuberances should be well padded as they are at most risk from pressure necrosis. Calves tolerate this form of cast well. A walking bar may be included in the cast, passing under the foot, and in locomotion transfers weight to the top of the cast, so reducing concussion.

The first check of the healing process should be at 2–3 weeks, preferably again under xylazine sedation. Poor prognostic indicators at this time include evidence of osteomyelitis and the presence of pressure sores. Common initial errors include failure to detect an open fracture, failure to appreciate multiple comminution, and poor fracture reduction. Later errors include failure to detect sequestrum development at follow-up examination, even when this check includes radiography.

Open fractures of the metacarpus/metatarsus are a major challenge. The wound should be cleansed, debrided, and the site explored with sterile instruments to remove foreign material (soil, grass). The wound should be irrigated with sterile physiological saline. If the fracture is recent (<12 hours), it is probably satisfactory to apply a cast over the limb including the wound, and to give systemic antibiotics for 5 days. In older cases or where the wound is extensive, an indwelling catheter may be placed for twice-daily irrigation. A cast may be put on and a window (e.g. a cross-section of a 5- to 20-ml polypropylene syringe case) placed over the infected site. Systemic antibiotics should be given for at least 10 days.

Some metacarpal/metatarsal fractures, characterised by long oblique fracture lines, are liable to override following external support alone, and transfixation pinning, with or without a hanging cast, has been very successful for over 40 years. The technique can be used in the field under certain conditions. A minimum of two Steinmann pins are placed through both cortices proximal and distal to the fracture site following manual reduction. The simplest and very adaptable pin fixators comprise flexible 1-cm-diameter polypropylene tubing which is placed over the pins in a longitudinal direction. One end of the tubing is occluded by a cork, and the interior is then filled with freshly mixed methyl methacrylate which acts, after setting, as a strong bar. The pin and tubing are lightly wrapped to avoid iatrogenic trauma to the pins, which are removed, again in an aseptic manner, after clinical healing of the fracture. An alternative method of transfixation pinning involves attachment of the proximal pins to a 'hanging cast' which extends distal to the claws and on which the calf bears weight.

Femoral fractures

Femoral fractures are comparatively common in calves, especially if <7 days old, and rare in older cattle. This section primarily discusses calves. The forms include diaphyseal, distal, metaphyseal or physeal fractures and proximal physeal separation. The first two are the common forms in dairy calves. Clinical signs include severe lameness, swelling due to haematoma formation and crepitus. Usually considerable overriding of the fragment ends results in an apparent shortening of the leg. The differential diagnosis includes coxofemoral luxation, acute septic gonitis and proximal fractures and physeal separation of the tibia.

Most fractures are comminuted and spiral or oblique. Radiography is essential if correction is desired and economically viable.

Treatment

Femoral fractures do not respond favourably to box rest or Thomas splintage as immobilisation and stabilisation of the fracture ends are impossible. Transfixation pinning is also unsuitable due to the overlying depth of muscle and the potential medial situation of the pin ends. Internal fixation is probably the method of choice for most femoral shaft fractures in calves. Open reduction via a lateral approach is used to reduce the fracture, followed by stabilisation with bone plates and screws (4.5- to 5.5-mm cortical screws) or retrograde intramedullary stack pinning (4.8 or 6.35 mm diameter).

The major problem with internal fixation with screws is the inherently soft and thin cortical bone of the neonatal femur, leading to pullout in the early days after the calf stands. Distal intramedullary migration of the pin into the stifle is a major risk in the stack pinning technique. Other failures commonly result from infection (osteomyelitis or septic arthritis), the signs including localised pain and swelling, reluctance to bear weight, and sometimes a septic exudate from the surgical wound. Distal femoral physeal separations can be treated by Rush pins inserted in a cruciate pattern.

The prognosis for femoral fractures in young calves is very guarded, but is better than in adult cattle where the mechanical limits of all available fixation methods are exceeded. Clinical stability and radiographic evidence of callus formation in calves should be present in 4–6 weeks in calves, though radiographic bone union may be delayed till 8–10 weeks.

In adult cattle femoral diaphyseal fractures tend to be oblique or spiral. Conservative treatment (box rest) may occasionally result in clinical union after some months of chronic lameness. Some cases develop lameness and breakdown of the contralateral leg. The prolonged period of pain is incompatible with the concepts of animal welfare.

Tibial fractures

The incidence (12%) of tibial fractures as a percentage of all bovine fractures is lower than that of the metacarpus/metatarsus (about 50%) and femur (20%). The signs resemble those of femoral fracture, but swelling and mobility at the fracture site are more evident (Fig. 6.19). Most are comminuted and many are open, as the medial tibial shaft lies in subcutaneous tissues. The mid or distal shaft fractures are often successfully managed by external coaption techniques, but proximal shaft and proximal physeal fractures and separation are unlikely to be stabilised without internal fixation. Discussion is again directed towards fractures in calves.

Treatment

Methods of tibial fracture immobilisation have included Thomas splint and splint–cast combinations, transfixation pins, intramedullary pins and bone plates. The difficulty of immobilisation of the proximal joint (stifle) is a major problem

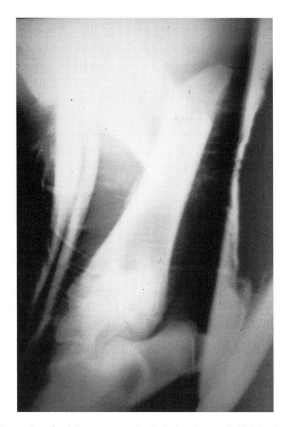

Fig. 6.19 Radiograph of oblique comminuted fracture of tibial shaft (lateral-medial projection).

in proximal fractures of the tibia. The use of casts and splints in tibial fracture management has been reviewed (Adams and Fessler, 1996).

Rapid production of callus is desirable in healing following external immobilisation. Disadvantages of this callus proliferation include possible impingement on joints (tibiotarsal), leading to undesirable ankylosis, adhesion to surrounding soft tissues such as nerves and muscle bellies, poor alignment of the fracture ends, pain during healing, persistent lameness and disuse atrophy resulting in bowing of the contralateral hind limb.

The modified Thomas splint–cast combination is recommended for external immobilisation of most midshaft or distal tibial fractures handled on the farm and considered unsuitable, for economic reasons, for referral to a clinic for possible internal fixation. Cast material is preferably light and strong, e.g. fibreglass or polyurethane-impregnated resin and fibreglass. It is placed over a waterproof stockinette bandage or a foam bandage. The cast should be applied following optimal fracture reduction (traction!) and, if possible, both hock and pastern should be slightly flexed to shorten the overall limb length.

Four layers of fibreglass bandage may be needed for adequate cast strength in a calf. The cast extends over the claws which are kept separated by padding. The toes or heels may be wired to maintain traction, and the cast material is run over the wire. Methyl methacrylate (e.g. Technovit) padding may be placed on the bearing surface to avoid wear and tear of the fibreglass component. The cast should extend just proximal to the tibial crest where padding should be carefully first positioned to avoid the development of pressure sores.

In open tibial fractures the wound should be carefully cleansed, debrided and irrigated (see p. 187 onwards) before cast application. A window may be left in the cast for later daily irrigation.

Thomas splints can usefully supplement hind limb casts. Steel rods (e.g. 0.5-inch or 12-mm diameter) are ideal material, but welding equipment is necessary. A well-padded ring, proximally located in the inguinum, is essential to avoid pressure necrosis. The precise dimensions (proximal ring, cranial and caudal longitudinal bars) must be initially determined to ensure a good fit. The splint is attached to the cast by further fibreglass-resin tapes from the mid-tibial region distally, especially at the level of the hock joint, fetlock and claws, where a small ring may have wires incorporated from the toes.

Thomas splints may be applied to some younger calves with simple comminuted distal tibial shaft fractures without an additional cast. If immobilisation proves to be inadequate, then additional management may include transfixation pinning. Such external transfixation with Steinmann pins and methyl-methacrylate bridges, performed in one clinic under image-intensified fluoroscopy resulted in a 65% recovery rate (35/55). The reasons for failure included failure to support the fractured leg (10 cases), poor weightbearing (6) and refracture (4) (Martens *et al.*, 1996).

Further surgical methods of tibial fracture fixation include bone plating and intramedullary pinning, often with cerclage wiring to maintain smaller fragments in apposition.

Humeral fractures

Humeral fractures are rare in cattle. They are infrequently diagnosed in calves in which distal epiphyseal fractures tend to be Salter type I or II. Considerable force, due to the protective musculature overlying the bone, is needed to produce a fracture. The configuration is usually spiral, comminuted and closed. Signs of a humeral fracture include dragging of the leg and a 'dropped elbow' appearance, considerable local swelling and palpable crepitus. Differential diagnoses include radial nerve paralysis without fracture and an olecranon fracture.

Humeral fracture may involve radial nerve damage since the fracture line often lies in the musculo-spiral groove located immediately below the nerve. Pain from the fracture site may render it difficult to demonstrate integrity or otherwise of the radial nerve. Care should be taken in manipulation to avoid further soft tissue damage.

Treatment

Management is controversial. Box rest for calves may result in satisfactory healing, albeit with malunion, in 6–10 weeks. Complications include severe weight loss, carpal deformity (contracted tendons), non-union, as well as angular limb deformity and marked fetlock overextension in the contralateral limb.

Use of the Thomas–Schroeder splint is not helpful in stabilisation of humeral fractures. Intramedullary fixation (Steinmann pins, Rush pins) is technically often easier than bone plating through a cranial or lateral approach. Stack pinning, combined with cerclage wiring, increases the stability at the fracture site.

Infectious arthritis

Infectious arthritis is a major problem in calves, especially in the first month of life, but is sporadic in adult stock. The syndromes are discussed separately.

Infectious arthritis ('joint ill') in calves – neonatal polyarthritis

Infectious agents are predominantly *E. coli*, *Salmonella* sp. and *Streptococcus* sp. *A. pyogenes* is an early secondary invader. The condition tends to be neonatal and polyarthritic. The classical route of entry is blood-borne infection via an infected umbilicus. Some cases also have meningitis and deteriorate rapidly. The likelihood of infection is related to the environmental pathogen load and the immune status of the calf.

Clinical signs and diagnosis

The neonatal calf with infectious arthritis is pyrexic, septicaemic, depressed and acutely lame or reluctant to rise. Nervous signs such as head tremors, opisthotonus extension, blindness and iridocyclitis are possible. The joints most commonly involved are the hock, carpus and stifle. All major limb joints should be palpated. Several joints may be affected simultaneously though bilateral symmetry is rare. For the first 24 hours post-infection, joint heat and swelling are absent, though pain is apparent on joint flexion and extension unless the calf is semicomatose. The swelling results from the increased synovial fluid volume, synovitis and peripheral oedema.

In slightly older calves sporadic cases of septic physitis are encountered in the distal radius and distal tibia following haematogenous spread. Diagnosis is difficult and radiography usually is needed.

The umbilicus may show signs of sepsis. Deep transabdominal palpation of the umbilical structures may reveal pain and thickening of vascular remnants or urachus. Arthrocentesis following a sterile scrub (3-cm 18-gauge needle attached to a 5-ml sterile syringe) can disclose initially serofibrinous and later purulent synovia. Analysis of such synovia reveals a very elevated total white cell count (>50 000 leucocytes/µl), a high percentage of neutrophils (>90%), and elevated protein (>3 g/dl) and glucose levels.

Samples of synovia should be collected into appropriate tubes: plain or blood culture medium sterile tube for microbiology, heparinised and EDTA tubes for general examination and cell count, and into sodium fluoride for glucose estimation. Bacterial culture of synovia may prove valuable, however, until results of sensitivity tests are available after 48 hours, empirical therapy is given.

Radiographic examination, carried out routinely in two planes, is valuable in differentiating infectious joint disease from septic physitis, fractures or other iatrogenic conditions. Radiographic changes in very early neonatal polyarthritis are limited to soft tissue swelling, but after a further 24–48 hours subtle changes of subchondral osteolytic erosion and a widened joint are evident. Early periosteal new bone formation is also possibly detectable. The rate of development of such radiographic changes varies considerably. Serial radiographs (e.g. days 1, 3 and 7) are invaluable in reaching an early prognosis.

Diagnosis is based on thorough clinical examination (including the umbilicus and CNS), radiography if available and in doubt, and gross examination of synovia obtained at arthrocentesis.

Treatment

Neonatal polyarthritis should have both systemic and local therapy. If the calf is considered immune deficient, blood or plasma transfusion from a healthy cohort is helpful. The umbilicus should be cleaned of septic material. Systemic antibiotics (current first choice ceftiofur, second choice enurofloxacin or oxytetracycline) at a high dose rate should be given for 7–10 days depending on the clinical response.

In acute infections, essential management includes repeated joint lavage. Affected joints (polyarthritic case) should be surgically prepared and irrigated by a through and through system with two 14-gauge needles and lactated Ringer solution daily, and preferably twice daily. The joint initially is maximally distended and then drained through the second needle. The incorporation into the lavage solution of antibiotics is unhelpful. The joints are lightly bandaged between treatments.

In certain circumstances such as late diagnosis of acute monarticular infectious arthritis, arthrotomy and joint curettage may be justified. In older cattle similar results may be achieved by arthroscopy, though this technique is more awkward due to joint size and anatomy than in the equine species. Recently, experimental therapy of monoarticular septic arthritis in calves has involved the insertion of gentamycin beads and gentamycin-impregnated collagen sponges.

Infectious arthritis in older cattle

In older calves and adult stock infectious arthritis is usually monarticular and non-umbilical in origin, but may follow iatrogenic injury (extension of periarticular cellulitis, pressure sore, puncture wounds) or intestinal (e.g. *Salmonella* sp.) or respiratory (*Haemophilus* sp-) pathogens. Adult cattle occasionally have haematogenic spread into a joint from a septic focus in another organ (hepatic or pulmonary abscessation, digital sepsis, etc.). Organisms isolated almost always include *A. pyogenes.* Mycoplasma infection (*M. bovis*) is rarely confirmed but may be underdiagnosed due to laboratory technical problems of isolation.

Secondary flexor tendon contracture develops in some calves that spend much time recumbent.

Diagnosis is not different from the disease in young calves, and may be easier due to the relative absence of systemic signs. Since the disease process is often more advanced in the older calf or adult, and may indeed be chronic, rigorous joint irrigation is again essential. Therapy should also be directed towards the control or elimination of the primary septic focus, and the institution of high level systemic antibiotics for a minimum of 1 week. Surgical arthrodesis has been successful in a limited number of calves (radio-carpal, metacarpal-phalangeal joints).

Degenerative joint disease or degenerative arthritis

Degenerative joint disease (DJD) is a chronic progressive non-infectious and initially non-inflammatory condition. DJD involves a primary degeneration of cartilage. Differentiation between a primary and secondary DJD is largely arbitrary and theoretical since at the time of clinical presentation the distinction has been blurred.

Articular cartilage softens, fibrillates and becomes eroded to expose subchondral bone, which in turn becomes eburnated or 'marble-like'. Simultaneously the joint is remodelled by osteophyte formation at the joint margin where the joint capsule is attached, by thickening of the lamina propria, chronic villous proliferation of the synovial membrane, low grade synovitis and an accumulation of cellular and tissue debris within the joint cavity.

Aetiology

It has long been claimed that, as in the human, bovine DJD is a 'wear and tear' phenomenon. However, sudden trauma almost certainly plays a part in some cattle in which femorotibial stability results from partial or complete rupture of the cranial cruciate ligament. In one series of cattle in which one or both hind limbs were condemned for disease, frequently 'atrophy' or 'arthritis', most cows had severe changes in the stifle or hip joints, but never in the hocks (Weaver, 1977). Cranial cruciate damage (complete or partial rupture) was frequently seen, usually with severe DJD and meniscal injury. It is speculative to consider that the cranial cruciate rupture was primary, leading to secondary meniscal damage and progressive degenerative changes of the weightbearing articular cartilage. Medial and lateral collateral ligamentous injury appears to be rare. Medial collateral ligamentous damage to the stifle may occur as a downer cow, with legs abducted, attempts to stand. Hip dislocation is also a risk. The volume of synovial fluid in stifle DJD varies from near normal (<20 ml) to greatly increased (100–240 ml).

Sometimes mild lameness and stifle joint effusion in young cattle 6–18 months old are due to subchondral bone cyst formation. Most such cysts are nevertheless asymptomatic. The aetiology of development of such cysts, which may

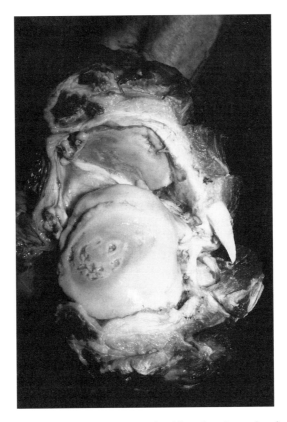

Fig. 6.20 Osteochondrosis dissecans in the shoulder of a steer, showing loss of articular cartilage and eburnation and pitting of joint surfaces.

measure 1–2 cm in diameter, is unknown. Some cases progress to develop DJD. Clinical lameness is occasionally seen in growing cattle affected with osteochondrosis dissecans of the hock, stifle or shoulder joints (Fig. 6.20).

Incidence and clinical signs

The incidence is higher in older cattle of both sexes and involves the larger weightbearing joints. The onset of lameness is usually insidious. An A1 stud bull may slowly become less willing to mount for natural service. In other cases some cows experience a sudden deterioration after some weeks of stiffness, lose considerable weight and spend much time in recumbency. The salient signs are reduced weightbearing, localised muscle atrophy leading to unusual prominence of bony landmarks, joint swelling, possible crepitus on flexion and extension of the affected joint and (in the hip joint) crepitus on rectal palpation. Hydroarthrosis may be appreciated in some cases of stifle and hock DJD.

Ancillary aids to diagnosis include radiography, ultrasonography, arthroscopy, arthrocentesis and punch biopsy. Of these five aids, arthrocentesis is most valuable in providing a rapid differential diagnosis from an infectious arthritis. At the same time, if doubt persists as to the site involved, 10–20 ml plain lignocaine hydrochloride may be injected into the joint to produce local anaesthesia and a potential temporary abolition of the lameness.

Other differential diagnoses include small chip fractures, ligamentous injury and, in younger animals, nutritional osteoarthropathy, osteochondrosis dissecans, rickets and osteoporosis.

Treatment and prevention

Treatment can only be palliative involving analgesics and anti-inflammatory drugs. Cows with DJD can be nursed along if confined to straw yards close to the milking parlour and kept on high quality feed to slow the progressive weight loss. Other forms of treatment such as intra-articular corticosteroids, antibiotics, arthrotomy or arthroscopy with joint curettage have been unrewarding.

Treatment of subchondral bone cysts of the stifle (often the medial femoral condyle) has been successfully resolved either following prolonged rest and analgesic therapy or, when this fails, by surgical curettage.

Contracted flexor tendons

Contracted flexor tendons (CFT) is the most frequent congenital anomaly in calves. It is rarely an acquired condition. CFT affects all dairy breeds, is usually bilateral and generally involves only the forelegs. Mild cases have slight flexion of the fetlock and tend to knuckle over, damaging the dorsal skin of the fetlock. Severe cases are recumbent and have marked contracture of both fetlock and carpus. Occasionally one sees calves with generalised contracture (arthrogryposis), but this section deals only with the classical calfhood bilateral flexure. Severely affected calves, being unable to stand, cannot nurse and are liable to be colostrum-deficient, and need to be bottle-fed within 8 hours.

Clinical examination reveals excessive tension in superficial (SFT) and/or deep flexor tendon (DFT). In only very severe cases is radical surgery needed. Mild cases can self-correct the knuckling-over, while slightly more severe cases should be splinted from proximal radius to the fetlock distally, using an appropriate length of polyvinyl chloride (PVC) gutter tubing over a protective bandage and cotton wool. More severe cases may require a cast. Such supports should be removed after 1 week to assess improvement.

Severe cases require tenotomy of SFT and usually also DFT, after which the degree of extension is determined. In some cases the suspensory ligament and carpal joint capsule must be cut. Strict asepsis is needed in this surgery which is usually performed under sedation and local anaesthetic infiltration. Occasional cases fail to have a return of normal extension despite transection of the above structures.

Since CFT is considered to be inherited though the mode is not known, attention should be paid to genetical factors.

Nutritional osteopathy ('rickets') (see also p. 26)

Rickets is seen occasionally in young growing calves, especially early-weaned and rapidly growing stock. The cause is a severe calcium:phosphorus imbalance and deficiency of either element and/or vitamin D. Clinical problems tend to develop in calves either outside and fed P-deficient rations or inside without adequate exposure to sunlight. The signs include stiffness, a reluctance to move, an arched back and joint swelling (most obviously fetlock, carpus and tarsus). An angular limb deformity [outward (varus) bowing of carpus] may occur. Appetite and growth rate are poor. Furthermore, dental and jaw abnormalities can severely impair feeding ability.

The main clinical problem is the failure of bone mineralisation. Radiographic features include cortical thinning, enlarged and wide epiphyseal plates, increased metaphyseal bone density, a radiolucent line at the metaphyseal–epiphyseal junction, and epiphyseal 'lipping'. Samples taken from the costochondral junction for histopathology can be diagnostic. Serum alkaline phosphate is elevated above normal values for growing calves, but blood calcium and phosphorus may be within normal limits. Bone ash ranges from 1:2 to 1:3 (normal 3:2). Diet analysis is usually needed to confirm the clinical diagnosis.

Differential diagnoses include septic arthritis or polyarthritis, copper deficiency, epiphysitis, selenium/vitamin E deficiency, hyperparathyroidism and, in some regions, fluorosis.

Treatment and prevention

Adequate calcium and phosphorus should be ensured. Suitable supplements include dicalcium phosphate (23% Ca, 18.5% P), bone meal, or limestone with added phosphorus. Vitamin D is often given by injection but is ineffective without an adequate Ca and P intake. Most calves, unless very severely affected, make a prompt recovery. Advanced cases have severe chronic joint changes, persistent lameness and remain unthrifty.

Prevention depends on a balanced diet. The increasing use of home-mixed rations in groups of rapidly growing Friesian crossbred beef calves is a potential hazard, avoidable by precautionary feed analysis and by supplementary minerals.

Nerve paralyses

Introduction and diagnosis

The major peripheral nerve paralyses are suprascapular and radial in the fore-limb, and femoral, obturator, ischiadic (sciatic) and peroneal in the hind limb. Table 6.7 gives the spinal origin of these nerves, the aetiology, clinical signs and major differential diagnoses of these six conditions.

Table 6.7 Major peripheral paralyses in cattle.

	Origin	Aetiology	Clinical signs	Differential diagnoses
Supras-capular	C 5–7	Severe trauma (crush, yoke); vertebral or spinal abscess	Shortened stride, abduction and circumduction of limb on weightbearing; shoulder atrophy	Spinal trauma, scapulo-humeral luxation or subluxation
Radial	C 7–8, T 1	Humeral fracture, prolonged recumbency on hard surface, trapping of distal limb	Distal injury: dropped elbow, flexed fetlock and carpus; proximal injury, also decreased flexed elbow, carpus and digit, analgesia over dorsum of metacarpus	Humerus, rib or elbow fracture
Femoral	L 4–6	Dystocia in (beef) heifers	Reduced weightbearing, flexed stifle, patellar luxation laxity, discrete quadriceps atrophy	Primary patellar luxation, septic gonitis, pelvic/-femoral fracture, hip luxation
Obturator	L 4–6	Intrapelvic trauma in dystocia; secondary following adductor rupture	Abduction of hind legs, 'downer cow', often with ischiadic damage	Pelvic fracture, femoral fracture
Ischiadic	L 5–S 2	Severe coxofemoral or pelvic trauma, iatrogenic from injection	Limb dragged, stifle extended, fetlock flexion, total analgesia distal to hock	Tibial or peroneal paralysis, pelvic fracture, proximal femoral fracture
Peroneal	L 5–S 2	Trauma over lateral aspect of stifle joint	Hock overextended, fetlock flexed and weightbearing	Tibial paralysis, gastrocnemius rupture, distal limb fracture

Vertebral column bones: C, cervical; T, thoracic; L, lumbar; S, sacral.

The history is vital: whether the onset was slow or sudden and the existence of known trauma. Gait and posture are the major signs investigated in possible paralysis and its differential diagnosis from musculoskeletal damage. Neurogenic atrophy may be seen after 5–10 days, being particularly marked following neonatal femoral paralysis. Flexor reflexes should be checked and also the only reliable extensor reflex, the patellar. Electromyography can be applied in clinics for valuable stock.

Treatment

Early treatment of a bluntly traumatised nerve may be attempted with anti-inflammatory drugs (e.g. NSAID) to reduce the oedematous and serous swelling which can lead to a secondary anoxia and nerve degeneration. Drug regimes include dexamethasone (10–40 mg im), phenylbutazone (4–8 mg/kg im on day 1, then 2–4 mg/kg every second day), flunixin meglumine, carprofen or ketoprofen, or aspirin (50–100 mg/kg b.i.d. by mouth). Many of these are not licensed in the UK.

The prime necessity is the provision of soft bedding, in relative confinement (to avoid skin abrasions) and plentiful feed and water. In limited cases splinting or casting the leg may be an improvement on simple bandaging. All cases should be reassessed on a daily basis.

Prevention and control

- Radial paralysis: reduce risk in cattle subject to prolonged lateral recumbency by using a minimum 6-cm padding under dependent shoulder. Also place inflated tyre round limb so that shoulder rests on it to reduce pressure on brachial plexus. Avoid potential trauma from feeding yokes in growing cattle by having sufficient number to eliminate competition for a feeding space and the associated potential excitement and stress.
- Femoral paralysis: avoid excessive traction in dystocia cases.
- Obturator paralysis: as for femoral. Also avoid moving calved cattle, especially heifers, along slippery passages and yards for the first 24 hours postpartum if calving has been difficult. Meanwhile keep calf with dam.
- Ischiadic paralysis: take care with site for intramuscular injection, which should normally be into neck region if the subcutaneous route is contraindicated.
- Peroneal paralysis: supply adequate bedding to provide soft non-traumatic flooring, especially at parturition.

The limb must be protected from iatrogenic damage resulting from the abnormal gait. In radial and peroneal damage the dorsum of the fetlock is at risk and should be bandaged. In exceptionally valuable animals (pedigree calves) in which the cause of paralysis, usually ischiadic, is an accidental intraneural injection, the site may be investigated surgically. This suggestion applies to oil-based compounds as aqueous injections should only result in a temporary paresis. Surgical exploration of the musculospiral groove could also occasionally be justified in radial paralysis following a midshaft humeral fracture. In horses, suprascapular nerve decompression by a technique of scapular notch resection has been successful in animals non-responsive to conservative treatment for some months (Adams, 1985). A similar procedure has not yet been reported in cattle, but such exploratory surgery could be justified in valuable breeding stock.

Management of the 'downer cow syndrome'

Management of the 'downer cow' should be both specific, directed at treatment of the primary aetiological condition (Table 6.8), and non-specific or general.

Table 6.8   Selected diagnoses of 'downer cows'.

Traumatic	Metabolic	Neurological	Toxic infections
Sacroiliac luxation or subluxation	Hypocalcaemia	Lymphosarcoma infiltration	Septic metritis
Bilateral or unilateral coxofemoral luxation	Hypokalaemia	Abscessation in spinal canal	Acute coliform mastitis
Pelvic or proximal femoral fracture	Other mineral imbalance	BSE	Peritonitis
Gastrocnemius rupture	Starvation		
Uterine trauma	Hypothermia		
Internal haemorrhage	Hypophosphataemia		
Obturator or ischiadic paralysis			

Specific management

Certain diagnoses that carry a hopeless prognosis necessitate early slaughter on humane and economic grounds. Examples include severe sacroiliac luxation, with signs of severe spinal cord injury, bilateral coxofemoral luxation, femoral fracture, complete gastrocnemius rupture at muscle–tendon junction, spinal lymphosarcoma or abscessation, massive intra-abdominal haemorrhage and peracute severe coliform mastitis.

Specific treatment is directed towards the diagnosis. In most cases parenteral minerals (Ca Mg, PO_4) are beneficial, even when the cow is not a non-responsive milk fever case. Intravenous fluids such as dextrose saline and Hartmann's solution aid fluid balance at a time when oral fluid intake is likely to have been minimal.

General management

- The cow should be made as comfortable as possible, preferably in a straw yard or box, where she will not be disturbed by other herd members. Ensure a solid, non-slip surface. If warm enough, another suitable site is an easily accessible field to which the cow is taken on a front-end loader.
- If hypothermic, the cow is covered with a thick dry blanket.
- Feed and water are kept in front of the cow at all times.
- The cow is turned at least four times per 24 hours.
- The udder and rectal temperature are checked twice daily. It may be possible to relieve udder congestion.
- If the cow struggles and keeps placing the hind legs in abduction ('spread-eagled'), they may be hobbled together above the fetlocks with about 50 cm of rope between them.
- If labour is available, regular daily attempts should be made to raise the cow using a hip sling (Bagshawe hoist), placed and tightened, for a maximum of 5 minutes' application, over the external angle of the ilia while a rope is attached to a front-end loader. The device is very liable to cause ischaemic

skin and muscle necrosis if left tightened on the cow for a longer period. Nets and slings are also popular as mechanical aids, but require more people.

- While inflatable rubber bags may have occasionally been used for additional comfort, the best aid to standing is the water tank, a metal tank ('Aqualift') about 3.5 m long, 1 m wide and 1.8 m high into which the cow is dragged. The open ends are then closed and the tank gradually filled with warm water, enabling the cow to stand and half-float for some hours daily. The circulation is markedly improved and some spectacular successes have been reported, but availability is the major problem.
- Supportive drug therapy has included corticosteroids (e.g. dexamethasone), analgesics (e.g. ketoprofen, carprofen, fluxinin meglumine), analeptics, vitamin E and selenium, and additional phosphorus salts.

Prevention

Certain predisposing factors can be controlled:

- Downer cows resulting from severe dystocia caused by fetal oversize or maternal immaturity indicate the need for improved genetic selection, careful obstetrical care, earlier veterinary consultation in dystocia and possibly induced parturition in other cows pregnant to the same bull.
- Downer cows resulting from failed therapy for milk fever should stimulate veterinary advice on prepartum nutrition, and early recognition of clinical signs.
- Downer cows resulting from slipping in yards and passageways require to have deep straw-bedded calving boxes in which cows can be kept till 24–48 hours postpartum. Some concrete areas may need to be regrooved.
- Downer cows following dystocia related to over-fat maternal condition (body score >3.5) mandates advice on feeding during the dry period, when a straw diet may be the appropriate solution.

References

Adams, O. (1985) A surgical approach to treatment of suprascapular nerve injury in the horse. *Journal of the American Veterinary Medical Association* **187**, 1016–18.

Adams, S. B. & Fessler, J. F. (1996) Treatment of fractures of the tibia and radius-ulna by external coaption. *Veterinary Clinics of North America: Food Animal Practice* **12** (1), 181–98.

Clarkson, M. J., Downham, D. Y., Faull, W. B., *et al.* (1993) *An epidemiological study to determine the risk factors of lameness in dairy cattle.* Report, Veterinary Faculty, University of Liverpool, Liverpool.

Cook, N. B. & Cutler, K. L. (1995) Treatment and outcome of a severe form of foul-in-the-foot. *Veterinary Record* **136**, 19–20.

Esslemont, R. J. & Spincer, I. (1992) *The Incidence and Costs of Disease in Dairy Herds.* Report no. 2, DAISY – The Dairy Information System. University of Reading.

Martens, A., Steenhaut, M., Gasthuys, E., Vlaminck, L., Desmet, P. & De Moor, A. (1996) Conservative and surgical treatment of tibial fractures in cattle. *Cattle Practice* **4** (2), 127–34.

Murray, R. D., Downham, D. Y., Clarkson, M. J., *et al.* (1996) Epidemiology of lameness in dairy cattle: description and analysis of foot lesions. *Veterinary Record* **138**, 586–91.

Weaver, A. D. (1977) Slaughterhouse condemnations for hind leg disease in cattle. *Veterinary Record* **100**, 172–5.

Weaver, A. D. (1997) Claw trimming: what farmers think! *Cattle Practice* **5** (1), 23–5.

Weaver, A. D. (1998) Analysis of some epidemiological factors in lameness on 55 Somerset (England) farms. In Proceedings of the 10th International Symposium on lameness in ruminants, Lucerne, Switzerland, 7–10 September 1998.

Whay, H. R., Waterman, A. E., Webster, A. J. F. & O'Brien, J. K. (1998) The influence of lesion type on the duration of hyperalgesia associated with hind leg lameness in dairy cattle. *Veterinary Journal* **156**, 23–9.

Further reading

Desrochers, A. & St Jean, G. (1996) Surgical management of digit disorders in cattle. *Veterinary Clinics of North America Food Animal Practice* **12** (1), 277–98.

Esslemont, R. J. (1990) *The costs of lameness in dairy herds*, pp. 237–51. Proceedings of the 6th International Symposium on diseases of the ruminant digit, Liverpool, 16–20 July 1990. Department of Veterinary Clinical Science, Leahurst, Neston, South Wirral.

Greenough, P. R. & Weaver, A. D. (1996) *Lameness in Cattle*, 3rd edn. W.B. Saunders, Philadelphia.

Rusterholz, A. (1920) Das spezifisch-traumatische Klauensohlengeschwür des Rindes Schweiz. *Archiv für Tierheilkunde* **62**, 421 & 505.

Ward, W. R. (1995) Lameness in British dairy cows. *State Veterinary Journal* **5** (4), 7–11.

Weaver, A. D. (1986) *Bovine Surgery and Lameness*, p. 176. Blackwell Scientific Publications, Oxford.

Chapter 7
Mammary Gland Development and Function

Chris H. Knight

Biology of mammary gland development

At birth the mammary gland comprises a rudimentary ductular arrangement of epithelial cells lying in a subcutaneous fat pad. By the time the heifer is first bred the duct system will have increased considerably in length and complexity, but no true secretory tissue will yet have formed. Most of this ductular growth is isometric (i.e. equal to whole body growth), but during several months around puberty there is an accelerated phase of allometric development. Since the secretory tissue will eventually proliferate at the extremities of the ducts, any disturbance of this growth can have profound and long-lasting deleterious effects. Such is the case in rapidly reared heifers. Overfeeding prior to puberty increases the fat content of the developing udder, but reduces the amount of ductular tissue. A reduced amount of secretory tissue in adulthood is at least partly responsible for the poor lactation yield usually associated with rapid rearing. For Friesian Holstein heifers, it is suggested that daily weight gains in excess of 600–700 g/day should be avoided during growth between 100 and 300 kg liveweight.

Mature secretory tissue has the general appearance of clusters of grapes attached by stalks to the branches of a vine. A vat placed underneath the vine with a tap for collecting and then releasing the wine would complete this rather inaccurate analogy! The grapes are secretory alveoli, hollow spherical sacs comprising a single layer of secretory epithelial cells surrounded by a collagenous membrane and a network of contractile myoepithelial cells. The stalks are fine milk ducts, and the branches are larger ducts. The two differ in that the single cell layer of the fine ducts has secretory capability, the double cell layer of the larger ducts does not. The ducts lead into storage sinuses, the gland cistern being separated from the smaller teat cistern by a sphincter arrangement of smooth muscle. Groups of alveoli drained by common ducts comprise a lobule of secretory tissue; groups of lobules are termed a lobe. The name lobuloalveolar tissue is thus often used to describe the secretory tissue. The stromal components include adipose cells (devoid of fat during lactation) and elastic and fibrous connective tissue. The lactating gland is very highly vascularised, and the whole structure lies in a 'glue' of extracellular matrix materials which help to regulate both structure and function.

Secretory cells are polarised, with an outer-facing basolateral membrane and a milk-side apical membrane. Substrates are taken up across the basolateral membrane and milk is secreted across the apical membrane into the hollow lumen of the alveolus. Neighbouring cells communicate with each other through gap junctions in the lateral membranes, whilst tight junctions prevent leakage of molecules between cells from plasma to milk.

The majority of secretory tissue proliferation (mammogenesis) occurs during gestation. It follows an exponential pattern, doubling monthly in primigravid goats (Fig. 7.1) and approximately 3-monthly in cattle. The necessity to quote goat data (obtained using magnetic resonance imaging *in vivo*) reflects the difficulty of obtaining accurate data in cows, for which serial slaughter is the only option. Probably for this reason it was believed for many years that secretory cell proliferation ceased at parturition in dairy species. We now know that this is not true, certainly for goats and probably for cattle. Exponential proliferation continues during the first week or two of lactation and a potential for growth is maintained throughout lactation.

Maturation or differentiation of secretory cells into the fully functional state is termed lactogenesis, and this process occurs in two main stages. During the latter third of pregnancy individual cells gradually acquire the necessary enzymatic and other machinery to synthesise milk constituents, but bulk secretion does not occur and synthesis is held in check. This is lactogenesis stage 1. Stage 2 is the onset of copious secretion and this happens at or around parturition in response to the changing endocrine environment. Having said that some proliferation of secretory tissue does continue, post-partum mammary development is mainly characterised by very marked increases in cell differentiation, which reach

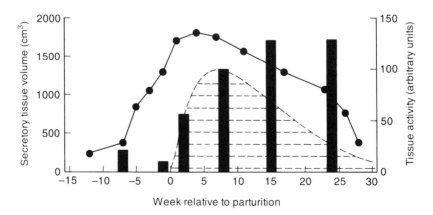

Fig. 7.1 Partly diagrammatic representation of caprine mammary growth. The *dotted line area* represents a typical lactation curve. Tissue volume data (*solid line*) were obtained using magnetic resonance imaging. Tissue activity data (*histograms*) are derived from several mammary enzyme activities measured in biopsy samples. The goats were dried off in week 25 post-partum.

a maximum at around peak lactation and account for most of the increase in milk yield during this period (Fig. 7.1).

Declining lactation, at least in the goat, is a time of gradual loss of secretory tissue. Gross measurements of udder size suggest that the same is true of the cow, but definitive data do not exist. Determination of key mammary enzymes in biopsy samples has revealed that cell differentiative state is just as high in late lactation as it is at peak. In other words, most if not all of the decline in milk yield can be attributed to loss of cells; remaining cells retain all of their synthetic capability (Fig. 7.1). Changes in cell number are necessarily a result of imbalance between cell proliferation and cell death. Non-pathological cell death is termed apoptosis, and in the ruminant mammary gland apoptosis has been detected in early lactation but is more prevalent during later lactation and most abundant in the recently dried-off gland. Clearly, in the pregnant animal mammary cell proliferation exceeds apoptosis, but during late lactation the reverse obtains.

The fact that the lactating mammary gland does retain a growth potential has relevance to mastitis. Severe clinical mastitis can often result in complete loss of one quarter; indeed it is relatively commonplace to see three-quartered cows. Many farmers claim that individual glands will compensate by increasing their own production, and there is experimental evidence to support this. Furthermore, we have shown in lactating goats that hemimastectomy causes a compensatory growth response, so it would appear that the udder is 'aware' of its correct size and will try to restore it when it is perturbed.

Mammary involution is usually thought of as the degenerative process that occurs after drying off or weaning. It should now be apparent that a gradual and slow involution of the gland occurs essentially from peak lactation onwards. The rate of involution is then greatly accelerated once milking ceases, although this process is highly variable between species. With the corollary that data are scarce, postlactational involution does seem to proceed less rapidly and to a less extreme endpoint in cows than in most other species. This is reflected in the cow's ability to 'rescue' lactation after even 2 or 3 weeks of temporary non-milking of individual glands, compared to the equivalent number of days in laboratory species.

When considering redevelopment of the gland between lactations it is important to take into account the animal's reproductive state. The desired norm is for the cow to be dried off when she is in the late stages of the next pregnancy, so the udder is in a state of multiple flux. Previously differentiated lactating cells are undergoing apoptosis, but at the same time the hormonal milieu of pregnancy is stimulating other non-differentiated cells to proliferate. It is likely, but not totally proven, that the mammary gland possesses a population of stem cells which never differentiate, remain pluripotent and are responsible for initiating regrowth of the gland. Other tissues have stem cells which are not only morphologically distinct but also spatially localised to specific regions, but this is not the case in the mammary gland. Here, putative stem cells appear to be dispersed throughout the epithelia. Udder redevelopment is actually a rather remarkable phenomenon and certainly contradicts a few dogmas; if proliferation does not happen during lactation (dogma) and if involution is at all complete (dogma) then the cow's mammary gland must do in 2 months what it previously did in 9, and, furthermore, it must do it better, since udder size increases incrementally between the first and subsequent lactations. In goats it is evident that involution does not totally revert the gland to its virgin state and the same is almost certainly true of cows, so some tissue is 'carried over' from one lactation to the next, although the amount is impossible to quantify. However, it is also true that redevelopment begins long before the lactation has finished; we have observed higher cell proliferation in the udders of concurrently pregnant lactating goats than in non-pregnant goats at an equivalent stage of lactation. Finally, there is also evidence (again in goats) of flexibility in the growth exponent, doubling time being less during the last few months of the second pregnancy than the first. In short, redevelopment is remarkable primarily for its adaptability; the mammary gland has at its disposal a number of mechanisms for ensuring that its developmental state is appropriate to the needs of the newborn young.

The amount of secretory tissue correlates very closely with milk yield. This is true both within species and across species, and also holds between breeds and within breeds of dairy cows. We recently analysed mammary characteristics in Holstein Friesians from two carefully defined genetic lines. The two lines were similar in body weight, but the high line produced 30% more milk from udders that were 30% larger but had equivalent secretory activity per gram of tissue. The amount of cisternal storage tissue is an important secondary determinator of yield. For a given mass of secretory tissue, cows with large cisterns will produce slightly but significantly more milk, for reasons that will become apparent later. Little is known about the development of the cistern. It is an elastic structure whose compliancy (ease of filling) changes during the course of lactation (more compliant in late lactation), during the lifetime of the cow (more compliant in older cows) and in response to different milking frequencies (less frequent milking increases compliance), but we do not know whether these alterations are due to growth responses or to physical changes in elasticity.

Endocrine control of mammary gland development and function

The essential features of endocrine control of mammary development have been understood for half a decade, but much of the detail is still to be unravelled. Classic endocrinectomy and replacement therapy established that oestrogen, progesterone, growth hormone (GH), prolactin and adrenal steroids are major elements of the mammogenic complex of hormones. Ductal outgrowth is stimulated by oestrogens, GH and adrenal steroids in combination, the further addition of progesterone and prolactin stimulates true lobuloalveolar development and if all but prolactin and adrenal steroids are then removed milk secretion will result. More recently, placental lactogens have been discovered, and it is now recognized that these largely replace the requirement for prolactin and GH during pregnancy. As a result, gestational mammogenesis has been shown to correlate with fetal number or mass in a variety of species, including cattle. In the absence of pregnancy, it is possible to induce mammary development and ultimately lactation with combinations of steroid injections (typically 60 mg oestrogen/day and 150 mg progesterone/day for 7 days) and milking to stimulate endogenous prolactin release. However, the response is rather variable, particularly in nulliparous cattle, and our own data (goats) indicates that only one-quarter of the total growth response actually occurs during the steroid treatment, the remaining three-quarters being attributable to the milking that follows. Other factors that have an influence on udder growth *in vivo* include nutrition and photoperiod. Mammogenesis is reduced by nutritional insufficiency or inadequacy, protein content of the diet being particularly important. It is not known how much of this is direct substrate limitation and how much is indirect, through endocrine changes for instance. The effect of photoperiod is quite small (although biologically significant) and most probably mediated by prolactin.

More detail has been added through *in vitro* experimentation, which is often the only way of demonstrating a direct action of a putative mitogen. Unfortunately the conclusions are not always clear cut, oestrogens being a case in point. For some time it was believed that oestrogens were not mitogenic, because addition to tissue cultures did not always induce cell proliferation. Subsequently it was shown that a dye present in most culture media possessed oestrogenic properties which could mask the effect of the added oestrogens, and in the absence of this dye most workers obtained consistent effects. Cell culture also threw up red herrings; insulin proved to be an absolutely obligatory requirement *in vitro* but has only a non-regulatory or permissive role *in vivo*. There have, however, been some major advances, none more so than in the field of growth factors. Growth factors, and there are a great number of them, are produced either locally or distally to the site of action usually in response to an endocrine signal and then act directly on the cell to either stimulate or inhibit proliferation. The stimulatory factors of most relevance to the mammary gland are epidermal growth factor (EGF), transforming growth factor alpha (TGFα) and the insulin-like growth factors, particularly IGF1. This latter was previously known as somatomedin-C, which gives a clue to its major proposed mode of action, namely mediation of the effects of GH. Other mammary mitogens include platelet-derived growth factor (PDGF), hepatocyte growth factor (HGF) and mammary-derived growth factor (MDGF), whilst still others such as fibroblast growth factor (FGF) will stimulate proliferation of particular cell types within the gland. Mammary-derived growth inhibitor, as its name suggests, is a growth factor of mammary origin which inhibits proliferation (but stimulates differentiation); TGFβ is the other major growth-inhibiting factor with mammary activity.

Whilst all of these factors have demonstrable activities in tissue culture, not all have been conclusively shown to have a regulatory role *in vivo*. One which has, and is arguably the most important growth factor in the bovine, is IGF1. This has been shown to stimulate udder development *in vivo* and to be mitogenic *in vitro*. Its main site of production is the liver, but it is also produced by several cell types in the mammary gland. Its systemic levels are influenced by GH and by energy status, such that high GH normally equates with high IGF1 but when high GH coincides with energy deficit IGF1 is low. During bovine pregnancy energy status is positive and treatment with recombinant bovine somatotrophin (BST, equivalent to GH) increases mammary growth, an effect that can be mimicked by IGF1 administration. GH certainly stimulates IGF1 production in the liver and most probably also increases local production in mammary stromal cells. Since IGF1 is directly mitogenic *in vitro* but GH is not, it is proposed that the mammogenic action of GH is indirect, mediated by IGF1. Since placental lactogen is not mitogenic but will increase IGF1 production, the same mediatory mechanism may apply here also.

Pregnancy is characterized by high levels of progesterone, which is responsible for preventing lactogenesis stage 2. At parturition progesterone falls precipitously and prolactin increases, and the net result is terminal differentiation of mammary tissue and the onset of milk secretion. If prolactin secretion is inhibited then lactogenesis does not occur. In many species prolactin is responsible not only for initiating lactation (lactogenesis) but also for galactopoiesis, the maintenance of established lactation. In dairy cows and goats this is not the case, since prolactin depletion during lactation reduces milk yield only by a small amount and supplementation generally has no effect. The major galactopoietic hormone in dairy species is GH, and it is now abundantly clear that GH (otherwise known as BST) can be used to increase milk yield. Curiously, there is no evidence to show that depletion of endogenous GH reduces yield; indeed our own work in goats and one experiment in beef cattle suggest that it does not. Corticosteroids and thyroxine are also galactopoietic, and prolactin cannot be totally discounted. Nevertheless, the crucial role of GH makes it worthy of special mention.

Bovine somatotrophin and milk yield

In November 1993 Posilac (Protiva) was approved for use as a lactation stimulant in US dairy herds. Posilac is recombinant bovine somatotrophin or growth hormone (BST) in a delayed release vehicle presented as 500 mg of product for subcutaneous injection (by the farmer) once every fortnight. Milk yield is increased by 10–15%, the maximum response being obtained in the second injection cycle and milk yield thereafter fluctuating slightly during recurring cycles, in direct correlation with the cyclical pattern of BST uptake into the systemic circulation. Gross milk composition is largely unaffected by BST, although there will initially be changes in the fatty acid profiles of milk fat. This is because the early stages of the BST response are achieved by depleting body reserves, hence more of the fat is preformed triglyceride. This stage lasts only for 2 or 3 weeks, after which appetite is increased. Long-term BST treatment does not deplete body reserves; treated cows have essentially identical body condition to untreated controls. The effect of BST is to redirect a greater proportion of ingested nutrients towards the mammary gland (in the lactating cow, to muscle in growing meat animals), a process known as homeorhetic repartitioning.

The overall energy balance of the cow is maintained at normal values, hence homeorhesis.

In one crucial respect the biological action of BST is still not understood. Driving extra substrate to the udder explains very adequately how the extra milk yield is supported, but not why it happens in the first place. In well-fed ruminants, infusion of substrates directly into the mammary arterial supply does not usually increase milk yield. Does BST have a direct action on the secretory cell? Almost certainly not, since receptors for GH are not present (receptors are proteins on the cell membrane to which the hormone binds in order to exert its action). Is IGF1 involved? Systemic infusion of IGF1 to mimic the increase caused by BST does not increase milk yield, but some have suggested a paracrine mechanism whereby BST acts on non-secretory cells in the lactating gland, causing them to release IGF1 which then stimulates the secretory cells. At this point the story becomes extremely complicated, due to the existence of IGF binding proteins (at least six, maybe more), which may either inhibit or enhance the action of IGF1 depending on a variety of individual circumstances. A number of these binding proteins have been identified in mammary tissue, but their precise role remains to be elucidated.

BST also affects mammary development. The IGF1-mediated mitogenic response seen in the pregnant animal does not occur during lactation; rather, long-term treatment with BST reduces or prevents the gradual post-peak involution referred to earlier. It is likely that this is due to decreased apoptosis, and the precise mechanism probably also involves prolactin, IGF1 and one of its binding proteins, IGFBP5. We believe that local IGF1 release is stimulated by BST and acts to maintain cell viability, i.e. it is a 'survival factor' as well as a growth factor. IGFBP5 is also produced locally and blocks the action of IGF1, leading to apoptosis. Prolactin inhibits IGFBP5 production, so IGF1 effects cell survival only in the combined presence of BST and prolactin. The consequence of reduced involution is that BST administered long term not only increases absolute milk yield but also increases lactation persistency. This is already causing American dairy farmers to rethink rebreeding strategies, and it is likely that many will move to 18-month lactations or longer.

Local control of the mammary gland

Farmers are very well aware that thrice-daily milking increases milk yield, typically by about 10%, but the biological mechanism is less well known. Experimentally, if only half of the udder is milked more frequently, the other half does not show a yield increase. This indicates that the mechanism is a local one operating within the udder, and does not involve a systemic endocrine stimulation. As milk accumulates in the udder between milkings pressure will slowly increase and in some cases will become sufficient to cause physical disruption of the secretory epithelium with a concomitant fall in secretion rate. This mechanism operates at drying off, but careful measurement has shown that pressure certainly does not reach inhibitory levels during normal milking intervals and may not during extended intervals of up to 24 h. So, something else must explain the stimulatory effect of thrice-daily milking. Chemical feedback inhibition was the proposed mechanism, and after two decades of research it has recently been proven. Mammary secretory cells produce and secrete into milk a variety of minor proteins. We have shown that one of these, a small molecular weight, glycosylated protein, downregulates further secretion, so we have named it FIL (Feedback Inhibitor of Lactation). Increasing milking frequency leads to FIL being removed more often, so secretion is maximal for a greater proportion of the time and yield increases. Opposite effects are produced by less frequent milking. Intraductal injection of FIL into a single gland reduces secretion reversibly in that gland only, diluting stored milk by infusion of inert solutions increases yield and immunoneutralisation of FIL increases secretion rate and reduces the yield-depressing effect of once-daily milking. *In vitro*, addition of FIL to mammary explant or cell culture reduces casein secretion in a concentration-dependent fashion. All of these observations support the hypothesis. At the cellular level, FIL acts at an early stage in the protein secretion pathway by disrupting membrane trafficking. Areas for further exploration are to determine exactly how this cellular action results in the observed gross effect of equal reduction in protein and fat secretion, and to determine the mechanics whereby the necessary reduction in FIL concentration is achieved post-milking.

Milking frequency actually has a number of effects on the udder. The immediate effect on secretion rate occurs very quickly (within a few hours) and in the shorter term the increased yield is achieved through altered activity of the existing secretory tissue. When thrice-daily milking is maintained for longer than a week or two a growth response is initiated, such that the slow involution of the gland referred to earlier is decreased or even prevented. A further consequence is an alteration in the gland's ability to respond to endocrine stimulation. The number of prolactin receptors on the secretory cell surface are increased by more frequent milk removal, and it may be that the longer-term developmental changes are achieved through this mechanism.

In practice, thrice-daily milking does not achieve a maximum milk yield response. In a collaboration with an Israeli group we showed that six-times-daily milking increased yield by 20% over and above thrice-daily milking. This may not be so esoteric as it sounds; robotic milking could offer the opportunity to milk much more frequently than thrice daily. There has been debate over the welfare implications of robotic systems, with some claiming that more frequent milk removal will improve cow welfare by avoiding udder pressure. Clearly, the increased metabolic load caused by the elevated milk yield must also be taken into account. In the Israeli experiment the very frequent milking was done only for the first 6 weeks of lactation, yet when the cows were returned to thrice-daily milking their yield did not drop completely to that of the control cows, but remained significantly elevated for the duration of the lactation. The treatment had caused a growth response which had long-lasting effects. Very recently we have also obtained evidence that more frequent milking will also change the actual shape of the lactation curve and reduce the rate of decline in milk yield, i.e. increase lactation persistency. Whilst more frequent milking increases yield, less frequent milking decreases it. Once-daily milking typically causes a 20% reduction in yield, and if maintained over a long period will accelerate lactational decline.

The udder of dairy ruminants is adapted by the possession of elastic sinuses such that milk storage can be tolerated for considerable lengths of time. It was pointed out earlier that large cisterned cows produce more milk per gram of secretory tissue, and the reason is now apparent. For FIL to be effective it must be in contact with the secretory cell; hence that milk which has moved away from the secretory epithelium into the cisternal sinus has no secretion inhibiting activity. Therefore, large cisterned cows are less affected by FIL. Not only is their secretion efficiency greater, but also they are less influenced by infrequent milking. On the other hand, they are also least responsive to frequent milking, so if some farmers introduce robotic systems whilst others extensify, the choice of cow may become crucial. Finally, since cisternal compliance is worst in early lactation and improves with parity, the peak lactation heifer is likely to be the most 'at risk' of yield problems associated with milking frequency or efficiency.

Oxytocin, the milk ejection reflex, mammary tight junctions and mastitis

The milk ejection reflex is a classic of neuroendocrinology. Stimulation of sensory nerve endings in the teat triggers a nervous input to the paraventricular nucleus of the hypothalamus and release of oxytocin from the posterior pituitary. Back at the mammary gland, oxytocin causes contraction of myoepithelial cells, resulting in simultaneous constriction of alveoli and dilatation of small ducts. Milk is thus expelled from alveoli and forced by positive pressure into the storage sinuses, from whence it is removed by the calf or milking machine. This is the let-down with which farmers are so familiar. Given good management the majority of cows will require no stimulation for milk ejection other than that provided by the milking machine; indeed some will start to let-down as a conditioned reflex even before they get into the milking parlour. However, the reflex is inhibited by stress and this can lead to problems in young heifers or when management is poor. Prestimulation is recommended practice in some European countries, but whether this reflects an animal problem or a man problem is uncertain. It should also be noted that the endogenous reflex does not remove all milk from the udder. Residual milk is that portion which remains after a normal milking but which can be removed following treatment with exogenous oxytocin at a supraphysiological dose. It is often 10% of the total milk volume and can in some cows be as much as 20%, a significant amount, but still quite normal. Since some farmers are starting to use oxytocin as a mastitis therapy it may be that they will witness residual milk and come to suspect milk ejection problems where none actually exists. Oxytocin does not in itself affect milk secretion; what one gains in residual milk at a single oxytocin-assisted milking one loses at the next milking. However, where a milk ejection problem does exist the FIL mechanism will come more into play and secretion rate will be reduced.

We have shown using a *Staphylococcus aureus* challenge model that oxytocin does indeed aid bacterial clearance. The most obvious rationale is that more efficient milk removal will equate with better 'flushing' of pathogen. This may indeed be the case, although it is not the only possibility. At high doses, oxytocin also has the effect of 'opening' tight junctions, the 'gaskets' between neighbouring secretory epithelial cells which prevent paracellular flux of small molecules from plasma to milk. This is something that happens normally during mastitis; indeed, the change in electrical conductivity which is the basis of automated mastitis detection is caused by a redistribution of Na and K ions as tight junctions become leaky. This could be a pathological change, but it could equally be a physiological response to the infection, designed to aid recruitment of immune-competent cells from plasma into milk. Oxytocin levels appear to be elevated during mastitis, and this probably accounts for the leakiness.

Suggested reading

Mammary gland development

Enright, W. J., Petitclerc, D. & Politiek, R. D. (eds) (1993) *Biology of lactation in farm animals*. Proceedings of the Joint EAAP/ASAS Workshop, Madrid, Spain, 1992. Livestock Production Science **35** special issue. Elsevier, Amsterdam.

Endocrinology of the mammary gland

Cowie, A. T., Forsyth, I. A. & Hart, I. C. (1980) *Hormonal Control of Lactation*. Springer Verlag, Berlin.

Local control of the mammary gland

Wilde, C. J., Knight, C. H. & Peaker, M. (1996) Autocrine regulation of milk secretion. In *Progress in Dairy Science* (ed. C. J. C. Phillips), pp. 311–32. CAB International, Oxford.

Chapter 8
Mastitis and Milk Production
Frank H. Dodd and James M. Booth

Introduction

Mastitis, an inflammation of udder quarters, must have been one of the first observed diseases of farm animals when cattle were domesticated over 5000 years ago and since that time it will have been an ever present problem for those who kept and milked cattle. When books on cattle husbandry were first published in the seventeenth century its importance was stressed and its association with poor management and particularly with 'leaving cows half milked'. From 1800 there has been a constant stream of papers in the agricultural and veterinary literature on its causes and control. Scientific research followed Pasteur's demonstration of the germ theory of disease in 1860 and by 1900 it was established that most mastitis followed microbial infection.

In 1938 Munch-Petersen in his comprehensive review of the mastitis literature was able to cite over 2000 papers dealing with the importance and complexity of udder diseases. It was evident that all herds were affected and in most it was a serious problem. There were several common pathogens causing mastitis and therefore it was not a single disease. Although clinical mastitis was readily detected by stockmen during milking this was only the tip of the iceberg; sub-clinical infection was much more common and caused greater financial losses. It is clear from Munch Petersen's review that by 1938 there was a basic under-standing of not only the microbiology of mastitis but also its epidemiology and aetiology.

In spite of the wealth of information in the 1938 review the attempts that had been made to control mastitis by immunisation and the available therapy had failed and the general view was that the solution to the problem would be found by improved cattle management. Little or no progress had been made in reducing the levels of infection on farms. Many key factors had been discovered that in due course would be invaluable in controlling mastitis, but it was difficult to distinguish these from other information, much of it incorrect, coming from field observation and inconclusive research. In fact it was probably impossible at this time to devise a control because there was no means of eliminating infections other than by culling cows with obviously diseased udders. Nevertheless, there was optimism that progress was possible because it had been demonstrated on a small scale in both the USA and UK that the most common type of mastitis, infection caused by *Streptococcus agalactiae*, could be eradicated from individual herds by segregation, culling and hygiene. Major schemes were started in New York State and Connecticut in the USA to apply this information on a wide scale, but the costs were high and the results inconclusive.

A breakthrough came in 1945 with the introduction of penicillin for mastitis therapy. At last it was possible to eliminate the most common mastitis infections from infected quarters. This proved to be a most important advance in controlling mastitis, but it was soon found that on its own therapy was not enough and it took another 25 years before an effective economic control was devised based on therapy, hygiene and improved dairy cattle management.

The effect of mastitis on lactation

Mastitis may completely destroy the secretory tissue of an affected udder quarter, but usually the changes are much less severe, with a reduction in the milk yield and changes in milk composition that can be detected only by laboratory tests (Table 8.1). The changes in composition are similar in many ways to those occurring normally with advance in lactation and drying off. Initially they are small and due to the inflammation increasing the diffusion between milk and blood. If the inflammation increases there is involution and destruction of secretory tissue and eventually the secretion can have a similar composition to blood plasma. The milk yield is reduced because there is an increased rate of involution, a temporary impairment of cell function and the inflammation blocks the ducts preventing the removal of milk. The changes in milk composition are due in part to impairment of the secretory process; for example the reduced fat content. To a greater extent they reflect the changed permeability of the secretory tissue. The main result is a diffusion of lactose and potassium from the milk into the bloodstream which is matched by an increased transudate of blood plasma into the milk, raising the sodium and chloride content. There are also increases in the milk constituents that normally diffuse from the bloodstream, such as blood proteins and enzymes.

The effects of mastitis on milk yield and composition are economically important to the dairy farmer. On average a quarter infected with a major pathogen will yield about 30% less milk than an equivalent uninfected quarter of the same cow and the fat and lactose contents are each depressed by about 0.2 percentage units. Infected cows are culled more quickly either because they are repeatedly clinically affected or because of low milk yields. Mastitis reduces the price the farmer receives for his milk because of the lower concentration of fat and lactose and because of its raised total bacterial count (TBC) and somatic cell count (SCC) (p. 320).

If an infection is eliminated from an udder quarter, either by therapy or spontaneously by the cow's natural defence mechanisms, there is an immediate partial recovery in the yield and composition of the milk, but it is by no means complete during the lactation in which it occurs. Depending on the degree of structural damage to the udder there is usually a considerable, sometimes complete,

Table 8.1 Effect of mastitis on composition of milk. In all cases extent of change is proportional to degree of inflammation. (From Kitchen, 1981.)

Main constituents	Normal level	Change
Fat (%)	3.45	–
Protein (%)	3.61	–
Lactose (%)	4.85	–
Fat components		
Free fatty acids (mEq/l)	0.6–0.8	++
Fatty acid pattern (mg/g fat)		
C4–C12	126.4	+
C16–C18	708.4	–
Protein fractions (mg/ml)		
Total casein	27.9	– –
Total whey protein	8.5	+++
Caseins (mg/ml)		
α-s$_1$-casein	13.3	– – –
β-casein	10.6	– – –
κ-casein	1.6	++
Whey proteins		
β-lactoglobulin	4–4.25	– – –
α-lactalbumin	1.03–1.22	– – –
Serum albumin	0.08	+++
Total immunoglobulin	0.25–0.3	+++
Anions and cations (mg/100 ml)		
Na	57	++
K	172.5	–
Cl	80–130	+++
Total Ca	136	– – –
Total Mg	18	– – –
P	26	– – –
Conductivity (mM NaCl)	<53	+(+)
Enzymes		
Most milk enzymes		++(+)

+ up to 10-fold increase   – up to 10% reduction.
++ up to 100-fold increase   – – up to 25% reduction.
+++ up to 1000-fold increase   – – – up to 75% reduction.

regeneration during the following dry period if the quarter remains uninfected (Table 8.2).

Aetiology

Mastitis can be caused by trauma or a physiological disturbance, but the disease of economic importance is always the result of microbial infection. The infections are nearly always bacterial, but yeasts, fungi, mycoplasma, viruses and even parasites are occasionally the agents.

Table 8.2 Examples of average depression in milk yield, fat % and solids not fat % of quarters infected with *Staphylococcus aureus* compared with uninfected quarters of the same udders. (From Kingwill *et al.*, (1979, p. 237.)

Classification	Milk yield	Fat %	SNF %
During infection	30.7%	0.29	0.27
Following cure, same lactation	34.7%	0.13	0.08
Following cure, next lactation	10.8%	−0.09	−0.02

There is not a normal intramammary flora; if microorganisms are established within an udder this is an infection. Although mastitis can be caused by many different types of bacteria, over 95% of cases are associated with fewer than ten bacterial species. For convenience these are often classified as *major* and *minor* pathogens on the basis of the severity of the intramammary reaction to infection. The common major pathogens are *Staphylococcus aureus*, *Streptococcus agalactiae*, *Streptococcus dysgalactiae*, *Streptococcus uberis*, *Escherichia coli* and *Actinomyces pyogenes*. The common minor pathogens are coagulase negative staphylococci (also called *Staphylococcus* species or micrococci) and *Corynebacterium bovis*. These minor pathogens are the most common cause of infection, but the resulting inflammation is usually small, clinical mastitis is uncommon and in most mastitis control work they have been ignored.

The bacterial contamination of the skin of the teat is the initial stage of the infection process, the pathogens subsequently entering the udder through the teat duct (Fig. 8.1). Entry from the blood circulation is possible and is the likely route in tuberculous mastitis and with a variety of serious cattle diseases when viable organisms are excreted into the milk, e.g. leptospirosis, brucellosis, foot-and-mouth disease and anthrax.

There are wide differences between herds in the prevalence of infection with the various pathogens and in the overall levels of infection. Before the introduction of penicillin the predominant pathogen was *Str. agalactiae*, but this responded to antibiotics and is now much less common. With its decline and possibly the coincidental change from hand to machine milking there was a rise in *S. aureus* infection. This responds poorly to antibiotics and became the most common cause of infection. After 1970 the widespread adoption of modern methods of control resulted in a marked decline in infection with *S. aureus*, *Str. dysgalactiae* and to a lesser extent *Str. uberis*. In many herds *Str. agalactiae* was eradicated. As a consequence there has been a proportionate increase in coliform and *Str. uberis* infection. These trends are important in relation to devising improved methods of control although the variation between herds in the patterns of infections continues to be an important factor.

The reasons why only a few of the many microorganisms that can infect the udder are common causes of mastitis infection are complex. All common mastitis pathogens grow well in milk, a medium with readily available sources of carbon and nitrogen. The pathogens differ in infectivity which in part is

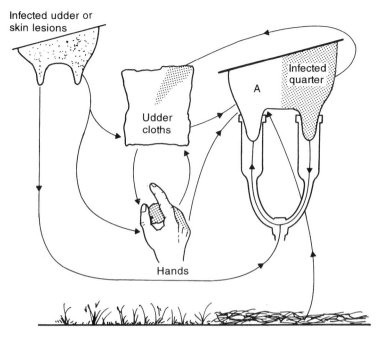

Fig. 8.1 Exposure of uninfected udder quarter (A) to pathogens from infected quarters, colonised teat lesions and contaminated bedding.

associated with their ability to survive phagocytosis. If pathogens adhere to epithelial surfaces they may be less readily flushed from the udder during milking. Virulence factors are associated with certain species, e.g. *S. aureus* and coliforms, and the strains of individual bacteria can show marked differences that are associated with their toxin and enzyme production. However, as we shall see, a most important factor influencing the success of a pathogen is its ability to maintain a high level of contamination of the teats. All successful mastitis pathogens are able to do this.

The udders and teats of all dairy cows in all herds are almost certainly exposed constantly to mastitis pathogens and yet intramammary infections occur infrequently. This is not surprising for in the course of their evolution cows have developed a high resistance to intramammary infection. Only cows that could resist the constant challenge of mastitis pathogens would lactate successfully and be able to nourish their progeny. The main component of this resistance is the ability of the teat duct to prevent bacterial penetration. This can be illustrated by a simple comparison. Even in herds where there is little or no hygiene and where exposure to pathogens is constant and at a high level the probability of an uninfected quarter becoming infected in a single milking interval is less than 1 in 200. However, if only ten colony forming units (cfu) of these pathogens are infused experimentally beyond the teat duct the probability increases to about 1 in 2. Supporting evidence for the importance of the teat duct is that intramammary infection usually follows damage to the duct and removing part of its keratin lining increases the chances of infection. Also, cows with patent ducts that are fast milking are more prone to infection. The effectiveness of the teat duct barrier is partly physical, due to its structure and keratin lining, and partly biochemical, the keratin inhibiting bacterial growth.

It is possible that during milking small numbers of microorganisms penetrate the teat duct without causing infection because they are immediately flushed out as the milk is removed. There is good evidence that the regular removal of milk at milking time is important in preventing infection. This has been demonstrated in experiments investigating the high rates of infection that occur immediately after the last milking of lactation.

Other factors provide resistance to mastitis infection that are not connected with either bacterial exposure, the teat duct or milk removal. Several cellular and immune defences operate within the udder and phagocytosis, killing of bacteria by polymorphonuclear leucocytes (PMN), is probably the most important. Phagocytosis is much less efficient in milk than blood because the leucocytes ingest milkfat and casein which decreases their efficiency against pathogens. The levels of immunoglobulin (IgG) transported from the blood to milk increase considerably during infection and the mammary gland synthesizes antibodies of the type IgA and to a lesser extent IgM. These mechanisms can give a degree of protection or reduce the severity of infection.

Several non-specific bactericidal and bacteriostatic systems occur in lactating and dry udders. They include lactoferrin, the lactoperoxidase system and lysozyme. There is evidence that they inhibit some mastitis pathogens particularly *E. coli* in the non-lactating udder and although they are potentially important their role in preventing mastitis is unproven. Under most conditions these internal defence mechanisms do not appear to be effective in preventing infection once the bacteria have penetrated the teat duct. They are, however, important in controlling the severity of the disease and in the spontaneous recovery of infections.

The marked differences in susceptibility to mastitis infection of cows in the same herd must in part be genetic; the patency of the teat duct has a high heritability and there will be other inherited factors. Physiological factors are also important. Susceptibility increases with the age of the cow and declines with advance in lactation.

Intramammary infection

Information on the most common intramammary infections is listed below.

Staphylococcus aureus

In many countries *S. aureus* is the most common cause of subclinical infection but not necessarily of clinical mastitis. It does not often cause peracute mastitis, usually producing a chronic disease with occasional occurrences of clinical mastitis.

Because the response to antibiotic therapy is poor it is the most persistent of infections, frequently lasting for several months and even years. The main primary sites of the bacteria are infected quarters, but the bacteria readily colonise skin lesions on the teat and at the orifice of the teat duct. Transmission is from the hands of the milker, udder cloths and milking machines. *S. aureus* infections can be eradicated from individual herds, but the high cost of establishing and maintaining this freedom makes it prohibitive as a general policy.

Streptococcus agalactiae

The sources and transmission of *Str. agalactiae* are similar to *S. aureus* and it also readily colonises lesions. Because sites other than the udder are rare and over 90% of treated infections are eliminated, its eradication from herds is practical. The disease may be seen as acute clinical cases or as persistent chronic infections.

Streptococcus dysgalactiae

The prevalence of *Str. dysgalactiae* infections in herds is usually low, but it causes a more acute disease than both *S. aureus* and *Str. agalactiae* although its epidemiology is similar. Primary sites of *Str. dysgalactiae* are the gut and the milk of infected quarters, transmission between cows is mainly during milking and teat lesions are readily colonised. Its association with lesions is particularly important and herd outbreaks of clinical *Str. dysgalactiae* mastitis are usually associated with cows that have many teat lesions and grossly soiled udders. Infection occurs frequently in dry cows and heifers indicating independence from milking. Over 90% of these infections are eliminated when treated with penicillin, but, unlike *Str. agalactiae* infections, it probably cannot be eradicated from herds because extramammary sites on cattle are more common.

Streptococcus uberis

Str. uberis has some similarities with *Str. dysgalactiae*; it is a common cause of infection in dry cows, resulting in acute clinical mastitis in early lactation, and has extramammary growth sites, but there are important differences. The most significant of these is that *Str. uberis* does not usually colonise damaged teat skin and the response to antibiotic therapy is much less than that of *Str. dysgalactiae*. As with all mastitis pathogens there is transmission from milking equipment, but the important sources are environmental particularly organic bedding materials, e.g. straw yards. Eradication is almost certainly impossible.

Coliforms

Several coliform species cause mastitis, in the UK principally *E. coli*. It is a frequent cause of acute and peracute clinical mastitis in early lactation particularly with housed cattle. Subclinical coliform mastitis is uncommon and microbiological tests on samples from a herd may not detect a single case even if clinical coliform mastitis is the main cause of mastitis in the herd. The reason for this is that coliform mastitis has a short duration. Infections usually become clinical within a day or two and unless they become peracute the infection is rapidly eliminated during the inflammatory process. A proportion of animals with the peracute disease die of endotoxaemia or are so debilitated that they are culled even when given antibiotic and other supportive therapy. The important transmission is not from milking equipment but from soiled organic bedding materials particularly when sawdust and shavings are used. Coliform infections rarely occur in the dry period, nor if they are present at drying off do they persist until calving. They do not colonise teat skin.

'Summer mastitis' (see also p. 43)

The acute and peracute mastitis that occurs in non-lactating cows and calves in the late summer is given the general name of summer mastitis (or heifer mastitis). It occurs in various forms in most countries but is best known as a serious problem in northern Europe. Its incidence is variable from year to year and is associated with particular farms and fields, often damp and near woodland. It is usually caused by a mixed infection of two or more pathogens and it is not possible to be certain of the cause of the infection from a clinical examination. If the mastitis is peracute with a foul-smelling secretion it is usually a complex infection associated with *Actinomyces pyogenes*, *Peptococcus indolicus* and *Str. dysgalactiae*. With this type of summer mastitis the transmission of the pathogens to the teats is via insects, which in Europe is the sheep head fly, *Hydrotaea irritans*. This sucking fly is seen, often in large numbers, on the backs and teats of cows in late summer. The pathogens are sensitive, *in vitro*, to the commonly used antibiotics, but therapy is rarely successful because the antibiotic cannot penetrate the grossly affected tissues and exudate. Some success has been reported with early infusions of oxytetracycline, but often treatment is restricted to salvaging the cow. Even when there is a clinical cure most affected quarters do not subsequently secrete economic amounts of normal milk.

Less common major pathogens

Of the less common types of infection, *Pseudomonas aeruginosa* occurs infrequently in most herds and may cause a herd outbreak. It is widespread in contaminated water, soil, faeces and bedding materials. The isolation of *Pseudomonas* from samples of milk from known infected quarters is intermittent. Acute and peracute infections occur and therapy is usually ineffective.

Mycoplasma bovis infections are rarely found in Europe but are reported to be a problem in North America. The disease is highly infectious and spreads rapidly by milking machines and contaminated antibiotic. The clinical disease is characterised by a sudden fall in milk yield of all four quarters; it is rarely systemic. Antibiotic therapy is ineffective and infected cows are usually culled.

Infection by 'minor pathogens'

The most common intramammary infections of dairy cows are caused by *Corynebacterium bovis* and *Staphylococcus epidermidis* (micrococci), which are often referred to as 'minor pathogens' because the inflammation is normally slight and clinical mastitis uncommon. In herds not using post milking teat disinfection and drying off therapy, infection with *C. bovis* frequently exceeds 60% of quarters. The pathogens are both part of the normal teat skin flora. They are common contaminants in milk samples and in routine mastitis control work are usually ignored. Herd outbreaks of clinical mastitis have been associated with *S. epidermidis* infections though this is infrequent. Nevertheless, these outbreaks and the possibility that the mild neutrophilia which the infections normally stimulate may be protective against major pathogen infections have increased the interest in these types of infection. Analysis of extensive herd data indicates that the degree of protection does not appear to be of practical significance.

Mixed infections

Surveys of the clinical mastitis in herds and large field experiments have shown that over 10% of infections are 'mixed', that is two or more pathogens are present. The associations are not random; the probability of an *S. aureus* infection being mixed with *Str. dysgalactiae* is twice that with *Str. uberis*, and ten times greater than with *E. coli*. *C. bovis* is rarely found in mixed infections.

The pathology of the diseases caused by the separate pathogens differs, but the variation that occurs in the severity of each type of infection makes it impossible to be certain of the cause of an infection by physical examination of udder quarters and their secretions.

Detection of clinical mastitis and diagnosis of infection

The detection of clinical mastitis by farmers and veterinary surgeons is nearly always by examining foremilk or by palpating the udders. The milk is best examined using a black plastic disc (foremilk cup) or a device called a mastitis detector which is a small gauze filter in the long milk tube of the milking machine (Fig. 8.2). Providing these are always examined as each cow is milked, both methods are effective in detecting clots but much less so for sediment and discoloured milk.

Because most mastitis is subclinical there has been a constant search for the ideal simple test that would detect all levels of mastitis inflammation. The large number of tests that have been devised measure directly or indirectly one or more of the changes in milk composition that occur when quarters are inflamed. Most are laboratory tests on milk samples, but there are simple cow-side tests. Currently, measuring equipment is being developed that can be fitted into the long milk tubes or claws of milking machines for continuously recording the

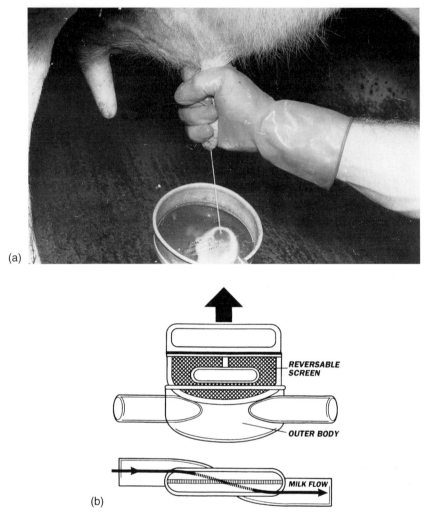

(a)

(b)

Fig. 8.2 Detecting clinical mastitis: (a) by using foremilk cup to detect abnormal milk; (b) by Ambic in-line filter fitted in long milk tube to detect clots in milk.

conductivity and temperature of the milk from each cow, factors that are altered by intramammary infection. The most commonly used laboratory test for mastitis inflammation is the somatic cell count of milk. The milk from a normal uninfected quarter will usually have fewer than 100 000 cells/ml. The rise with the inflammatory reaction due to mastitis varies, but with typical subclinical infections the counts are up to 10^6 cells/ml and with clinical mastitis counts exceeding 10^7 cells/ml are not uncommon. Cell counting was a tedious microscopic routine until 1966 when electronic methods of counting particles in milk were devised which could be standardised and mechanised to enable large numbers of milk samples to be counted in an automated system. The first method used a technique of counting particles of the appropriate size with the Coulter Counter, but this has been superseded by equipment for measuring fluorescing stained somatic cells such as the Fossomatic instrument. The Whiteside Test is a simple indirect method of estimating cell count in the laboratory. It is based on the degree of coagulation when a small amount of milk is mixed with sodium hydroxide. This has been superseded by the California Mastitis Test (CMT) which also gives a measure of the degree of coagulation when mastitis milk is mixed with the reagent and has the advantage that it can be used as a simple cow-side test.

The increase in the sodium and chloride content of milk from inflamed quarters has been the basis of a number of tests measuring the electrical conductivity of milk, either with laboratory or cow-side equipment. Most recently, equipment has been developed for measuring the conductivity of the milk as it enters the milking machine. The records can be made at every milking and with a farm-based microprocessor the deviation from normality can be assessed. For maximum sensitivity the comparisons are made between the quarters of individual cows. This type of equipment will detect small increases in inflammation, but for practical use the problem is to decide on the best threshold value to adopt. The test is so sensitive that even at a low threshold most infections are detected, but at the same time there are many false positive results. Set at a higher threshold the equipment should detect infections with a marked inflammatory response with few false positive results.

Tests measuring the effect of mastitis on the lactose content of milk have been used for over 75 years. Currently, there is interest in measuring the increases in mastitic milk of bovine serum albumin (BSA), and in certain enzymes such as N-acetyl-β-D-glucosaminidase (NAGase) and antitrypsin. There is evidence that the latter tests make it possible to distinguish between changes in milk composition that are the result of tissue damage and those that normally occur with advance in lactation.

The tests for inflammation are made on milks that range from the visually normal to secretions approximating to blood serum. The measurements are continuous variables and there is no absolute dividing line that separates normal and mastitic. Because the tests measure different physiological and chemical changes the results obtained do not correlate perfectly and the correlation coefficients between the results of different tests vary from about 0.5 to 0.9. These tests for inflammation are useful in both research and routine mastitis control, but when investigating the causes of mastitis, microbiological data are essential.

The bacteriological tests to discover the cause of infection are standard procedures that have remained substantially unchanged for many years. For initial investigation small quantities of milk (0.01–0.05 ml) are plated on blood agar which is incubated at 37 °C for 48 hours. The milk samples are either fresh or kept under refrigeration prior to plating. The common mastitis pathogens are identified by colony appearance and if there is doubt the diagnosis is confirmed by biochemical tests. Providing a good aseptic sampling routine is followed, the milk from an uninfected quarter will not show any bacterial growth other than an occasional contaminant. There will be colony growth, with one or more species of bacteria, from about 90% of single samples from subclinically infected quarters and from about 80% of clinical quarters. There are various reasons why bacteria are not detected. Bacterial growth may be prevented by naturally occurring inhibitors or antibiotic residues in milk, but the main reason is that the number of bacteria in the milk of infected quarters is variable and when the numbers are low they are not detected in the small amounts of milk plated. Fortunately, with the common types of mastitis infection the probability that pathogens will not be detected in two consecutive samples is low (<0.01) and diagnostic routines based on confirmed states of infection are accurate. The milk samples from uninfected quarters are contaminated more often when teat ducts are colonised. With a colonised duct the pathogens, usually either *S. aureus*, *Str. dysgalactiae* or *Str. agalactiae*, can be regularly recovered on swabs from the duct even after careful disinfection of the teat-end. However, unlike true intramammary infections the pathogens are not found in milk samples taken from the teat sinus by teat-wall puncture. When iodine- or chlorine-based teat dips are used regularly, teat duct colonisation is rare (<1% of teat ducts).

Accurate diagnosis requires competent laboratory staff, but even the most experienced cannot produce useful information unless *the milk samples are taken aseptically*. This is time consuming and requires each teat orifice to be scrubbed with a disinfectant (e.g. 75% ethanol) for at least 20 seconds before sampling.

Epidemiology

The prevalence of mastitis in herds depends on many factors. These are not fully understood, but the most important appear to be those that influence the degree of exposure of the cows' udders to pathogens. However, the wide differences between herds in the levels and patterns of infection cannot all be due to variation in exposure to pathogens. Additional factors influence the cows' susceptibilities; some are genetic (bovine and bacterial), others physiological (age and stage of lactation). Physical factors affect the penetration of the teat duct by bacteria, and cattle nutrition and levels of stress in the herd may play a part.

Exposure of teats to microorganisms

In all herds, even those using teat disinfection, the teats of cows will be regularly exposed to most of the major pathogens (Fig. 8.1). The degree of exposure by transfer from primary sites is usually relatively small. In herds with over 20% of quarters infected with staphylococci it may not be possible to detect the pathogen on 50% of teat skin swabs unless these are incubated before testing. This is not surprising because the concentration of bacteria in the milk of infected quarters is usually relatively small (<10000 bacteria/ml of milk) and the small quantities of this milk that transferred on teatcups is constantly being washed off with milk from uninfected cows. There will be exceptions when the milk from a clinical quarter contains very large numbers of pathogens (>10^8 bacteria/ml) which occasionally occur, especially with streptococcal infections. A further factor reducing the numbers of bacteria on cows' teats is that the common major pathogens do not persist on *healthy* teat skin and their presence indicates recent contamination.

In addition to exposure by transfer from primary sites the teats are also exposed to bacteria from the secondary sites where mastitis bacteria multiply. This exposure will be many times greater than by transfer at milking and can be maintained at high levels for long periods and is most important in the epidemiology of mastitis. The main sites of multiplication have been mentioned above in the description of the various types of infection; they are colonised teat lesions and ducts and bedding materials. Teat lesions of various types are common in lactating dairy cattle and unless special steps are taken they invariably become colonised by either *S. aureus*, *Str. dysgalactiae* or *Str. agalactiae*. When this happens there will be very high numbers of pathogens at or near the teat orifice until the lesions heal. Usually there are insignificant numbers of mastitis pathogens in clean, dry straw, sawdust and wood shavings. However, in bedding these are moistened and contaminated with dung, urine and milk and the temperature will be raised by composting or the body heat of the cows. When this occurs *E. coli* and *Str. uberis* can rise to astronomic numbers (>10^7 bacteria/g of bedding) within a few days. Cows that lie down with their teats touching this bedding are exposed to very large numbers of pathogens.

The factors that determine both the level of exposure of the teats to bacteria and the predominant types are obviously complex. There will be marked differences between herds and even, from time to time, in individual herds. Some exposure is inevitable and there will always be transfer between teats and from cow to cow at milking time. The level of this transfer from primary sites is relatively small, but it increases considerably when there are other sites of pathogen multiplication near the cows' teats (Fig. 8.3). Clearly, once there are infected lesions on cows' teats or the cows lie on grossly contaminated bedding the *direct* transfer of pathogens from cow to cow ceases to be a significant factor influencing the *total exposure* to pathogens. The recognition of this was necessary before effective hygiene routines could be developed.

Obviously factors other than the level of exposure to pathogens influence the probability of a cow becoming infected, but on current evidence it appears to be the major one. Under experimental conditions, raising the level of exposure increases the rate of infection in both lactating and dry cows and under practical conditions infection rates increase when teat lesions are common and decrease when steps are taken to reduce the exposure.

Teat lesions

Bovine teat skin is devoid of sweat glands and hair, forming a relatively smooth covering interrupted only at the apex where the outer layer invaginates to form the lining of the streak canal (Fig. 8.4a). Teat skin is usually free from lesions until first calving and lesions heal in the dry period, but in lactating cows they are common. The methods of milking and housing cattle are the main factors affecting the condition of teat skin.

Some lesions are caused by physical damage or skin infection. The most common are chaps (Figs. 8.4b,c), which are fissures due to the loss of skin elasticity, and changes in the external structure of the teat duct caused by the action of the milking machine. The latter is known as hyperkeratosis, sometimes called

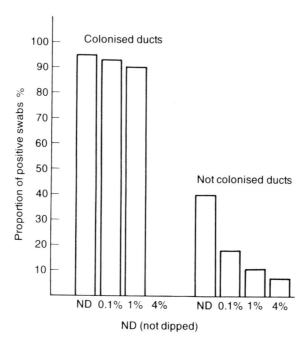

Fig. 8.3 Recovery of *S. aureus* from swabs taken from skin of teats of uninfected cows before milking. At the preceding milking each test cow was milked after a cow with all four quarters infected with *S. aureus* and then teats were dipped in a solution of sodium hypochlorite at concentrations of 0.1, 1 or 4% or were left undipped (*ND*). Note the most important factor determining presence of *S. aureus* was colonisation (i.e. *S. aureus* repeatedly found on teat duct swabs) and there were no colonised teat ducts with the 4% dip. (Neave, 1965, unpublished data.)

teat erosion or eversion (Fig. 8.4d). Infectious lesions can also be caused by infection with the paravaccinia virus (Fig. 8.4e) and much less frequently by bovine herpes mammillitis (Fig. 8.4f) or by staphylococci. Mammillitis can occasionally cause a serious herd outbreak and can be controlled by vaccination.

Blackspot is a lesion of the teat orifice which occludes and sometimes completely blocks the teat duct. It follows the infection of the duct with *Fusobacterium necrophorum* and is associated with hyperkeratosis and poor housing conditions. It can be prevented by eliminating faulty milking machine factors, regular post-milking teat disinfection and improved housing.

All types of lesion except hyperkeratosis occur most often in winter and spring, particularly with cows under dirty conditions exposed to bad weather. In summer flies can increase lesions and prevent them healing. In an ADAS/NIRD survey of 56 herds not using post-milking disinfectant teat dips, teat examinations were made at 3-monthly intervals for 1 year. Excluding teat orifice damage, 6% of teats were chapped and 6% had other lesions. Individual herd readings ranged from nil to 51% with chapped teats and to 40% of teats with other lesions.

Hygiene and good husbandry greatly reduce infectious lesions, particularly using teat dips containing hypochlorite or iodophor. These disinfectants do not damage teat skin, but neither do they reduce the incidence of chapping (Fig. 8.4g).

Chapped teats can be reduced considerably by using an iodophor teat dip or spray containing an emollient such as glycerol. Cream salves are frequently used to attempt to improve skin condition, but they are inconvenient, can reduce the life of rubber teat cup liners and are usually less effective than emollient teat dips.

Milking hygiene

Once it was recognised that bacteria were spread by hands and equipment that touched the udder during milking, various hygiene practices were recommended. These included adding disinfectants to udder wash water and dipping milking machine clusters in disinfectant before each cow was milked. The surfaces of hands, udder cloths and the rubber of milking machines are, in microbiological terms, very rough and in the short time available during milking cannot be adequately disinfected chemically. When the use of chemical disinfectants is employed there is still transfer of pathogens and it does not prevent the colonisation of lesions and ducts (Table 8.3). Routines that include a massage of the udder spread pathogens from foci of infection, such as teat lesions, over the skin surface (Fig. 8.1). These hygiene practices did not control infection and if hygiene was to be effective better methods were required.

The transfer of pathogens from cow to cow on udder cloths can be prevented if a separate boiled cloth or paper towel is used for each cow. With milking machines the transfer is prevented if the clusters are treated with water at a temperature exceeding 85 °C for at least 5 seconds before each cow is milked (Table 8.4). Unfortunately there is no practical way of preventing the transfer on hands even if milkers wear smooth rubber gloves and rinse them in disinfectant when moving from cow to cow. The numbers of pathogens transferred may be small, but they could be sufficient to colonise teat lesions and teat ducts and once this happens the exposure levels will be high.

The problem of colonised ducts and lesions was overcome by the introduction of the use of disinfectant teat dips after milking (Fig. 8.5). This was first proposed in 1916 and from 1945 was recommended by Cornell University, but its value was not realised until a series of experiments were carried out at the National Institute for Research in Dairying, Reading, in the 1960s. With correctly formulated iodophor, hypochlorite and chlorhexidine teat disinfectants the colonisation of teat ducts is almost eliminated and infectious lesions are rare (Table 8.5). When teat skin is damaged and other lesions occur they heal much more rapidly. The degree of success can be judged from the results of tests under commercial conditions. Without teat disinfection up to 70% of the teat ducts in a herd can be colonised by *S. aureus*. After a few weeks' teat dipping with 4% hypochlorite the level is less than 1%. Teat chaps present a special problem, but they can be reduced considerably by keeping cows under clean conditions, not exposing them to adverse weather and by using a teat dip containing an emollient such as glycerol.

Small-scale experiments in a research herd demonstrated that over 80% of infections caused by *S. aureus* and the common streptococci could be prevented by a hygiene routine that included washing udders with separate boiled udder cloths, pasteurising milking equipment before each cow is milked and

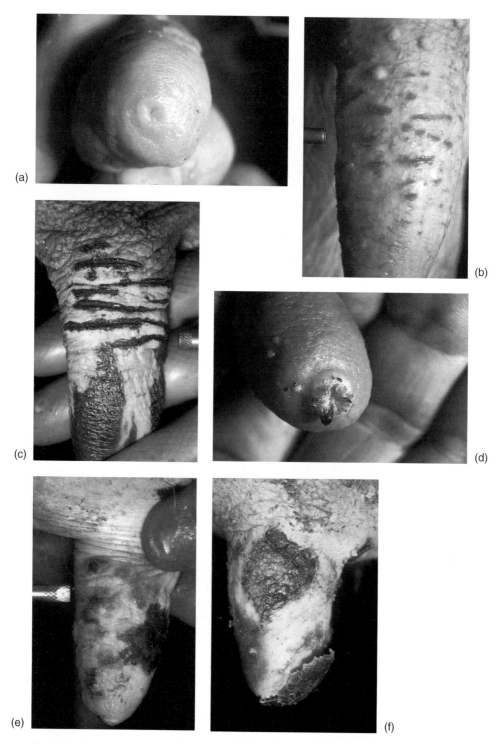

(a)

(b)

(c)

(d)

(e)

(f)

Fig. 8.4 For descriptions see opposite.

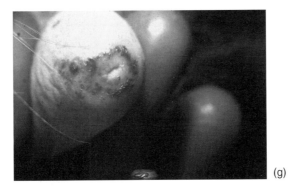
(g)

Fig. 8.4 Examples of lesions at teat duct and on barrel of teat. Photographs by M. F. H. Shearn. (a) Normal teat orifice, (b) small chaps, (c) large chaps, severe lesions, (d) teat orifice with hyperkeratosis, (e) extensive lesions due to exposure to severe weather or dirty housing with no teat disinfection, (f) bovine herpes mamillitis lesions, (g) lesions that occasionally occur with hypochlorite teat dipping – they rapidly heal.

Table 8.3 Efficiency of washing methods in removing *S. aureus* from teats of cows artificially contaminated. The hypochlorite wash contained 0.06% available chlorine and each treatment is the mean of 18 swab tests from teat skin. (From Neave in Dodd and Jackson, 1971.)

Treatment of teats	Geometric mean colony count of *S. aureus*/swab
Foremilk taken, no washing	23 000
Water wash from bucket with cloth	1 630
Chlorine wash from bucket with cloth	128
Chlorine wash from hose using hand	69

Table 8.4 Disinfection of teat cup clusters after removal from cows with mastitis. Each cluster was disinfected by steam before milking and was tested after milking only one cow with mastitis or with artificially contaminated teats. (From Dodd and Neave, 1970, p. 30.)

Treatment of cluster	Time	Number tested	% Swabs positive	Number of *S. aureus* recovered/swabs
Cold water flush	5 sec	19	100	100 000–800 000
Cold hypochlorite circulation (0.03%)	3 min	19	100	50–2000
Circulation of water at 66 °C	3 min	18	22	0–80
Circulation of water at 74 °C	3 min	85	0	0
Circulation of water at 85 °C	5 sec	530	3	0–15

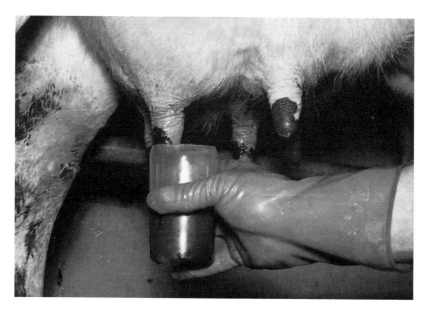

Fig. 8.5 Dipping teats in disinfectant after each milking greatly reduces pathogen contamination and prevents colonisation of lesions and ducts.

Table 8.5 The skin-disinfecting properties of some disinfectant teat dips. (From Dodd and Neave, 1970, p. 32.)

Teat dip	Concentration	Additive	pH	Geometric mean count of *S. aureus*/swab
Hypochlorite	0.1%		8.8	416
Iodophor	0.5%	33% glycerol	4.6	206
Iodophor	0.5%	15% glycerol	4.7	107
Chlorhexidine	1.0%	Pyrollidine	6.2	40
Iodophor	0.5%		4.9	17
Hypochlorite	1.0%		10.3	14
Hypochlorite	4.0%		10.9	6

Each teat dip was tested on 18–24 teats of cows free from infection, teat lesions and residual teat contamination. One hour before milking, teats were dipped in a culture containing 5×10^7 *S. aureus*/ml and tests made 1 hour after dipping.

post-milking disinfectant teat dipping. Such experiments give little indication of the quantitative response to hygiene under normal farm conditions, nor the relative values of its component parts. This was subsequently demonstrated by experiments carried out on commercial dairy farms that were organised by the National Institute for Research in Dairying, Reading. They are known as the Mastitis Field Experiments (MFE) and compared hygiene routines in commercial herds under close supervision, measuring both clinical and subclinical mastitis. The first (MFE 1) used 14 herds for 1 year and the second (MFE 2) 15 herds for 18 months. These experiments demonstrated that a combination of hygiene methods would reduce the rate at which mastitis infection occurs by at least 50% under a wide range of herd conditions (Fig. 8.6). The methods examined were

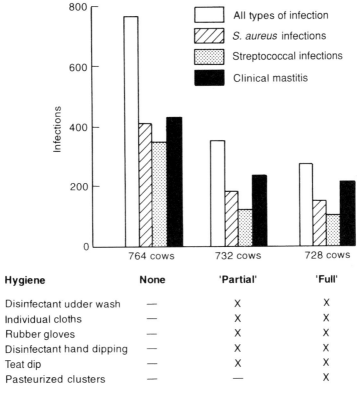

Fig. 8.6 Reduction in udder infection with two routines of milking hygiene. The experiment used 15 herds over a period of 18 months (MFE 2). (From Kingwill *et al.* 1979, p. 255.)

disinfectant udder washing, udder washing with separate sterile towels, use of rubber gloves, dipping gloved hands in disinfectant when moving between cows, dipping cows' teats in disinfectant after milking and heat disinfection of clusters before each cow is milked. Although the maximum benefit was obtained when all methods were used, the omission of cluster pasteurisation, the most costly component, did not materially reduce the effectiveness of the hygiene. As expected the reduction in infection occurred with the bacteria that colonise teat lesions, *S. aureus*, *Str. agalactiae* and *Str. dysgalactiae*.

Post-milking teat disinfection fails against *E. coli* and *Str. uberis* because these organisms do not colonise skin, and the main exposure comes during the milking interval from contaminated bedding. This exposure precedes milking and therefore *pre*milking teat disinfection has been introduced in the USA with evidence that it can reduce infection by environmental pathogens. This type of disinfection must lower the levels of exposure during milking and therefore infection will be reduced. The extent of the reduction will depend on whether pathogens tend to penetrate the teat ducts in the milking interval or during milking itself. Research in the UK has not confirmed the value of this type of disinfection under a range of farm conditions and more research is needed.

Other hygiene factors that occur infrequently at milking can cause outbreaks of clinical mastitis in herds. The concentration of pathogens in the milk of infected quarters is normally not high (i.e. less than 10^3 cfu/ml), but occasionally the numbers are enormous (i.e. more than 10^8 cfu/ml). The latter usually occurs with clinical streptococcal infections and providing these are detected and treated the high numbers persist for only a few days. High levels of exposure for individual teats can also occur if there is an undetected split in the barrel of a teat cup liner. Because the pulsation chamber of the teat cup becomes contaminated with milk and is not included in the routine plant cleaning, it soon becomes grossly contaminated with various pathogens which are spread on the cows' teats during milking. If approved methods of cleaning milking machines are used, preferably those that raise the temperature of the washing water to over 75 °C, the carryover of pathogens on milking equipment from one milking to the next is insignificant.

Housing and bedding

Few if any of the important major mastitis pathogens can be found in clean baled straw, kiln-dried sawdust and shavings, shredded paper and washed sand. However, when these materials are used for bedding cattle they become contaminated with dung, urine and milk and with the exception of sand the counts of certain mastitis pathogens can increase rapidly to very high figures ($>10^8$ bacteria/g of bedding material). This occurs when the bedding temperature is raised either through composting or by the body heat of cattle. With straw the pathogen is usually *Str. uberis* and with wood products coliforms. These very high counts can occur in bedding that appears to be clean (i.e. free from dung) providing it is moist, warm and there is a source of nitrogen. It is not surprising that when this happens outbreaks of clinical coliform and *Str. uberis* mastitis occur.

Mixing bedding materials with lime or disinfectants reduces the growth under laboratory conditions but is ineffective on farms. The counts can be held at much lower levels if *all* the soiled bedding is removed frequently from the rear *half* of cubicles and replaced with fresh bedding. To be really effective this should be a daily routine (Table 8.6). For larger herds the routine should be mechanised, which has been done by mounting a rotating brush on a tractor to remove the soiled bedding from cantilever cubicles. Unfortunately no commercial equipment is available. Rebedding the cubicles with chopped straw or sawdust could also be mechanised. With daily renewing of the bedding material the total use need not exceed that used when rebedding occurs every 7 or 14 days with larger amounts.

Other types of bedding materials have been used, but all the organic materials will have problems similar to straw and sawdust and are likely to be more costly. Using washed sand greatly reduces the clinical mastitis with coliforms and *Str. uberis* because composting does not occur. However, sand is heavy and abrasive and increases the problems of slurry storage and spreading.

Machine milking

From their first introduction, farmers believed that milking machines were an important contributory factor causing mastitis. Their role as a vector was recog-

Table 8.6 Effect of cubicle management on coliform count of sawdust bedding. Sawdust samples were taken from the part of the cubicle that the cow's udder comes in contact with when lying down. Note the much lower coliform counts when sawdust is renewed daily. (From Dodd *et al.*, 1984.)

Day	Mean coliform count g of sawdust ($\times 10^6$)	Routine management
1	59.0	Fresh sawdust added to cubicle every 7 days
15	290.0	
21	4.0	
35	740.0	All bedding removed and cubicles cleaned and disinfected
36	1.5	Bedding removed from back of cubicle and replaced
37	0.5	with fresh sawdust *each* day
38	1.0	
39	0.8	
40	0.4	
41	2.6	
42	1.4	
44	4.0	Fresh sawdust added to cubicle every 7 days
46	14.2	
52	47.4	
58	59.8	

nised and high vacuum level, overmilking and certain designs of teat cup liner were believed to be significant factors. Research demonstrated that these did increase mastitis but less than was generally believed. Work on the relationship between machine milking and mastitis was stimulated by the clear demonstration that somatic cell counts (SCC) were higher in herds milked by machines with inadequate vacuum reserve. Subsequently it was demonstrated that the key adverse factor was the vacuum fluctuation in the teat cup liner.

In milking machines the bore of the teat cup liner is connected via rubber tubes to the clawpiece and pipes regulated at a constant vacuum level of about 50 kilopascals (kPa). However, when high frequency electronic recorders became available it was demonstrated that the vacuum within the liner could fluctuate considerably (i.e. from 35 to 65 kPa) in every pulsation cycle. This occurs because the milk leaving the liner prevents the free flow of air through the tubes. In each pulsation cycle the changes in air pressure in the pulsation chamber of the teat cup, induced by the action of the pulsator, cause the liner to open and close about once each second. When the liner is open milk flows from the teat and when closed the liner compresses the teat end, stopping milk flow. The collapsing liner reduces the volume of the liner and because the short milk tube is full of milk the vacuum in the liner falls rapidly. However, the milk moving rapidly along the short milk tube acts as a piston, creating a marked increase in vacuum behind it, that is, in the collapsed liner. This high vacuum is relieved only when the milk clears the short milk tube and there is again a free flow of air. This air moves rapidly from the claw to relieve the low vacuum in the liner and carries with it milk droplets that impact on the teat. These droplets impact the teat end with sufficient force to penetrate the teat duct and if they are carrying pathogens they are likely to cause infection. From this brief description it is clear that it is not the vacuum fluctuations per se that cause infections but the impacts that they generate. These effects are accentuated if liners slip on the teats during milking, allowing air to enter the clawpiece. This does not increase the impacts on the teat where the slip occurs but on the other teats.

This discovery of milking machine-induced infection led to modifications to the design of milking machines. The vacuum fluctuations are generated by pulsation and liner wall movement, but they are enhanced when there are air leaks into the milk tubes (i.e. 'liner slip'). The fluctuations are reduced by increasing the diameter of the short milk tube, providing an adequate air bleed into the claw to encourage movement of milk from the claw, improving the designs of the liners and to a much lesser extent increasing the volume of the claw bowl (Fig. 8.7).

It is impossible with the standard design of milking machines to prevent all impacts. Therefore another approach to this problem was to fit small deflector plates or shields at the junction of the short milk tube and barrel of the liner to

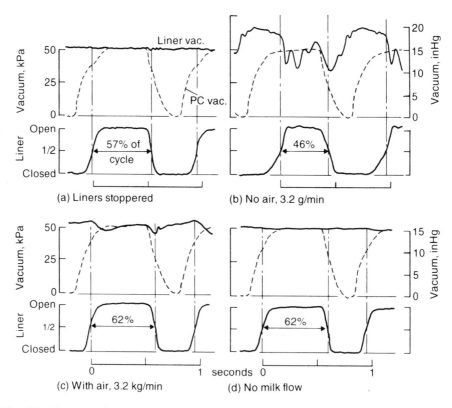

Fig. 8.7 Teat cup liner (*solid line*) and pulsation chamber (PC) (*dashed line*) vacuum changes and consequent liner wall movement: (a) before milking, (b) and (c) during milking without and with an air bleed at the claw and (d) after milk flow has ceased. (From Mein in Bramley *et al.*, 1992.)

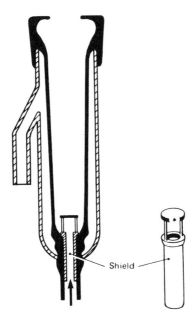

Fig. 8.8 Shields fitted into a teat cup liner to deflect milk particles travelling up the short milk tube when liner opens. These droplets impact the teat end and can penetrate the teat duct causing infection if they carry pathogens. (From Griffin and Grindal in Bramley *et al.*, 1981, p. 170.)

prevent the droplets reaching the teat (Fig. 8.8). These 'shields' do not restrict milk flow and in small experiments using enhanced exposure to pathogens they prevented over 90% of machine-induced infections. In large experiments on commercial farms the total infections were reduced by 10–15%.

A more radical solution was a claw which prevents both impacts and the transfer of milk from teat to teat during milking. This was achieved by fitting 'ball valves' where the short milk tubes connect with the claw. For conventional milking these claws require an airbleed to be fitted in the short milk tubes of the liners and used in this way they appear extremely effective in preventing both impacts and the cross transfer of pathogens between teats during milking. In the course of determining the necessary size of the airbleeds it was discovered that cows could be milked quite effectively if they were omitted, but the action of the liner in removing the milk was completely different. This new principle now named 'hydraulic milking' gives protection against machine-induced infection and faster milking.

Pulsation was incorporated in milking machine action about 100 years ago in order to minimise the adverse effects on the teats of applying a constant vacuum. Subsequently it was discovered that milking was faster if the 'pulsation rate' or frequency was increased and the 'pulsation ratio' (the ratio of the time that the liner is open to closed) was widened. The usual values are now a rate of about 60 cycles per minute and ratios within the range of 1:1 to 2:1. Because pulsation is the prime cause of impacts the effect of milking without pulsation has been re-examined. With some cows this gives problems with milk ejection and also mastitis increases. This appears to be due to the constant vacuum damaging the teat duct. Further investigations indicate that the duration of the rest or closed phase of each pulsation cycle should not be less than 0.3 seconds.

The pressure exerted on the teat by collapsing liners depends on the thickness and hardness of the rubber. Stiff liners increase the pressure and cause more hyperkeratosis. Unless there is effective post-milking teat disinfection this will increase the probability of orifice colonisation by pathogens.

There is no doubt that a poorly designed, incorrectly installed or inadequately maintained milking machine can be an important factor in increasing mastitis. However, there are no good estimates of the relative importance of milking machines and other factors. In some herds a very poor milking machine can be the major factor, but the results of recent experiments and surveys suggest that less than 25% of mastitis can be attributed directly to machine factors. It appears that, providing a milking machine conforms to the basic BSI or ISO standards (see below), it will not be a major factor influencing mastitis infections.

In order to improve the standards of milking machines used on farms the British Standards Institute (BSI) and the International Standards Organisation (ISO) have drawn up standards for design, installation, mechanical properties and cleaning which are updated regularly. Contracts for new parlours or for upgrading equipment should require compliance to these Standards. To help ensure that milking machines on farms are maintained correctly portable equipment has been devised to measure the mechanical properties of vacuum pumps, pulsators, regulators, etc. Various agencies (e.g. Genus and ADAS) provide services to test farm milking machines and to give advice on the steps necessary to correct any faults found.

For a much fuller account of the design, properties, use and testing of milking equipment refer to the chapters by Dr G. A. Mein in *Machine Milking and Lactation* (Bramley *et al.*, 1992).

Feeding and management

There are reports attributing mastitis to many aspects of general cattle management, feeding and 'stress'. They are often subjective and associations that could have other explanations. Many attribute mastitis to excess protein feeding and high levels of feeding in the dry period. Recently, higher levels of mastitis have been found in areas deficient in selenium. The role of general management and feeding in mastitis is interesting and potentially important, but current evidence does not indicate that individual items are crucial in mastitis aetiology.

The dynamics of infection in herds

In addition to general factors that influence all the cows in a herd there are others that influence the probability of individual cows becoming infected in a common environment. Some of these are genetic and others physiological.

Age

Calves can become infected from birth and there are occasional reports of mastitis when group-fed calves are fed milk from cows with mastitis. Summer mastitis can cause serious problems with calves on some farms, but intramammary infection with major pathogens is uncommon up to first parturition, and normally less than 2% of quarters are infected at first calving. Subsequently levels of subclinical infection and clinical mastitis increase with age. This is due to an accumulation of persistent infections and also a higher new infection rate in older cows (Fig. 8.9).

Stage of lactation and the dry period

Although mastitis is usually associated with lactating cattle, infection can occur at any time. Prior to the introduction of drying off therapy the highest rates of infection were immediately after drying off and at calving; thus levels of infection were higher at calving than at the start of the dry period i.e. at drying off (Fig. 8.10). Infection in the dry period reduces the yields of the quarters in the subsequent lactation.

Structure of the udder

The anatomy of the udder and teats influences infection in a number of ways. There is more infection in cows with udders that are pendulous. About 60% of infections occur in hind quarters. Because infection follows bacterial penetration

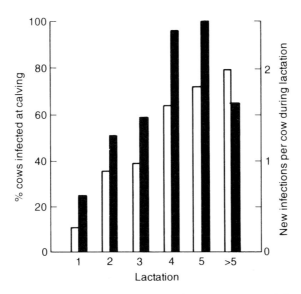

Fig. 8.9 Both level of infection (*open bars*) and frequency of new infection (*solid bars*) increase with age of cow. (From Kingwill *et al.*, 1979, p. 234.)

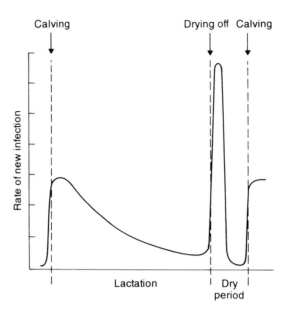

Fig. 8.10   Relative frequencies of new infections during lactation and the dry period. (From Kingwill *et al.*, 1979, p. 239.)

of the teat duct it is not surprising that fast milking cows which have more patent teats are more prone to infection.

Prevalence or level of infection in herds

The level of infection in a herd is a function of the *new infection rate* and the *duration of the infections*; both are equally important. Under farm conditions the way in which these factors operate is complex. The herd population changes, infections of different types have different durations, a quarter can be infected with more than one pathogen and cows do not lactate continuously. Nevertheless, over a period of time (e.g. 12 months), the principles apply and can be expressed by a simple relationship:

> Average level of infection in a herd (% quarters infected) (A) = Proportion of quarters infected during the period (B) × Average duration of the infections (% of period) (C) × 0.01.

For example, if in the course of a year 30% of the quarters in a herd are infected (B) and the average duration of the infections is 50% of the year (C), the average level of infection in the herd, as measured at herd tests, will be 15% of quarters (A).

From this relationship it follows that the level of infection can be reduced either by preventing quarters becoming infected or by reducing the duration of infections; both are equally effective. A 50% reduction in either rate of infection or duration of infection will reduce level of infection by half, but if both are reduced by 50% the level will fall by 75%. Thus a marked reduction in level can be obtained by modest reductions in both new infection and duration of infection. This is the basis of effective control.

The success of a control programme is usually assessed by the extent of the reduction in mastitis and the time it takes for this to be achieved. A control that gives no reduction for a year will be regarded by farmers as a failure even if it ultimately gave good results. The main factor controlling the *rate* of decline is the duration of infection – the longer the durations of the infections the slower the decline. If most infection is staphylococcal it always takes several years for the full benefit of a control to be achieved, but for coliforms it is almost immediate.

An understanding of the dynamics of infection in herds is necessary not only in devising control schemes but also to interpret mastitis data. Measuring levels of infection at a 'herd test' either by bacteriological tests or indirectly by the SCC or other test on herd bulk milk will overestimate the importance of infections of long duration, e.g. *S. aureus*, and underestimate the short duration infections such as *E. coli*. The latter are rarely found at herd tests but may cause 20% or more of the clinical mastitis. The difference in duration of infections is also the main reason for the poor correlation between herd incidences of clinical mastitis and their levels of infection and cell count.

Elimination of infections

Once infections are established they will persist unless eliminated by the host's defence mechanisms, cured by therapy or the cow is culled. Because it is impossible to prevent all infections it is important to examine the potential value of these methods of elimination.

Spontaneous recovery

In large-scale farm experiments it is usually found that over a period of a year 20–25% of infections by major pathogens are eliminated spontaneously by the host's defence mechanisms. This is probably an underestimate and does not include some infections of short duration that recover before detection and coliform infections that appear to be cured by therapy but are very probably eliminated by the host's defences. Nevertheless, most infections persist for weeks or months unless they receive therapy. For example, extensive farm data show that 90% of untreated *S. aureus* infections persist for at least 3 months and 80% of infections present at drying off persist beyond calving. The exceptions are coliform infections and also *Str. uberis* infections starting in the dry period, many of which are eliminated at or about the time of calving. Most *E. coli* infections last only a few days, but in this short time there is often considerable damage to secretory tissue.

For spontaneous recovery to be really useful in mastitis control ways have to be found of increasing its frequency. There are possibilities of achieving this by immunisation and much research has been in this field, so far without much success.

Culling

The sale of cows for any reason eliminates infections from herds. The number of infections is reduced with a policy of culling cows that repeatedly have clinical mastitis and there is an involuntary culling for mastitis when culling is based on milk yield. In one large field trial the cows culled for any reason had twice the level of intramammary infection compared to those of the same age that were retained even though the farmers did not have access to the laboratory infection or somatic cell count information. On first inspection culling appears to be a powerful tool in mastitis control. Extensive data collected over 20 years ago showed that over 50% of clinical mastitis occurred in 10% of the cows. Today the level of clinical mastitis is much lower and the concentration of infection in the most susceptible cows may not be so clearcut. Furthermore, in a self-contained herd culling for all reasons is limited to about 25% of cows each year and usually more than half of these will be barren cows and casualties. This means that selective culling on the basis of milk yield, milk quality, temperament, mastitis, etc. will be restricted to 10%, or less, of the herd each year and the cows with most clinical mastitis will tend to be the older, higher yielding animals. There is evidence that, at least in the short term, it is likely to be more economic to cull on the basis of milk yield rather than *increasing* the culling for mastitis.

Antibiotic therapy

The first improved therapy for clinical mastitis was oral dosing with sulphonamide, but this was superseded in 1945 by the intramammary infusion of penicillin. For the first time a high proportion of infections could be eliminated with a simple treatment. Soon several other antibiotics formulated singly or in mixtures were available. There is an extensive literature on antibiotic therapy for mastitis dealing with the pharmacokinetics, pathogen sensitivities, and cure rates when subclinical infections are treated. To succeed a drug must be maintained at the minimum inhibitory concentration (MIC) at the site of infection for an adequate period. There is a need for a broad spectrum of activity to cover both Gram-positive and Gram-negative bacteria and no single antibiotic meets all the criteria.

The introduction of antibiotic therapy was the most important single development in mastitis control. It is by no means fully effective, but it is unlikely that effective mastitis control could have been developed without it. In spite of the massive amount of literature, there is a dearth of information on the real value of the many products available *when used under practical farm conditions* and on the best way to use them in control schemes.

The most extensive data on the results of antibiotic therapy when used on farms in the normal way to treat clinical infections are for the semi-synthetic penicillin cloxacillin. They were collected in a series of experiments on commercial farms in 1960–1970 (Fig. 8.11). The products tested are still in general use

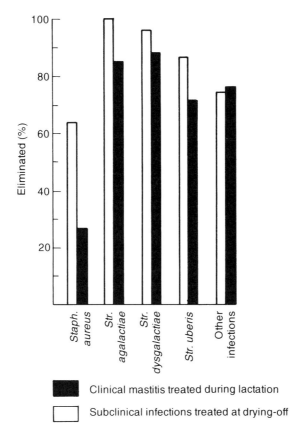

Fig. 8.11 Proportions of treated infections eliminated by cloxacillin therapy given to about 3000 clinical lactating quarters and about 3000 subclinical infected quarters at drying off. (From Dodd and Neave, 1970, p. 50.)

and it is unlikely that the results that are currently obtained with other products are materially different.

Most therapy is by intramammary infusion given to cows with clinical mastitis without any knowledge of the pathogen causing the infection. Under these conditions there is usually a clinical recovery with over 95% of treated quarters. More than 80% of infections caused by *Str. dysgalactiae* and *Str. agalactiae* are eliminated. The success rate for *Str. uberis* infections is less, only 70% are eliminated, and for *S. aureus* infections it is only 25%. Clinical mastitis may result in a spontaneous cure of infections, but this is probably uncommon except for coliform infections. The cure rates are higher for all pathogens when the treatment is for subclinical infections, though the highest rates of all are obtained when subclinical infections are treated after the last milking of lactation with preparations formulated to persist in the non-lactating udder (see Fig. 8.12).

Antibiotic therapy is ineffective against some of the less common types of infection such as pseudomonas, mycoplasma and *C. ulcerans* whereas virtually all *C. bovis* infections are eliminated by drying-off therapy.

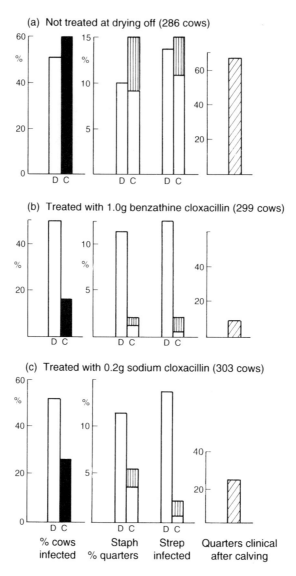

Fig. 8.12 Effect of drying-off therapy on levels of infection at calving. Note that if cows are not treated, levels increase during the dry period. D = At drying off; C = at calving. (From Dodd and Neave, 1970, p. 42.)

The major limitation of antibiotic therapy either in lactation or at drying off is the poor cure rate against *S. aureus*. This failure is *not primarily associated with antibiotic resistance or tolerance* but may reflect either the intracellular survival of the bacteria or the pathological changes induced by some infections. *S. aureus* can survive within neutrophils and be protected against the antibiotic in the surrounding fluid. The efforts to overcome this weakness have not yet been successful.

Because most streptococcal infections have a high cure rate the variation in response between infections in different cows and herds is small. With staphylococci, and to a lesser extent *Str. uberis*, the variation is large and potentially important in mastitis control. Even in herds treated with a synthetic penicillin to which all the strains of *S. aureus* are sensitive, the average *herd* rates of cure can vary between 10% and 65% for treatments given for clinical mastitis. This variation is not understood; it does not appear to be due to the different strains of staphylococci in the herds but to some aspect of the management of the cows.

Even within herds there are marked differences in the response to therapy of individual staphylococcal infections (Fig. 8.13). For example, field experiments show that 46% of clinical quarters infected with staphylococci were cured when treated for the first time. The cure rate for the next treatment for those that had failed was 21% and if further treatments were given to persisting infections the responses were less than 10%. This selection process will account to some extent for the between-herd difference in cure rates and for the observed lower cure rates of infections in older cows and cows with more than one infected quarter. The rates of elimination are also lower for cows treated in early lactation and with quarters with more severe mastitis.

Although the elimination of infection plays an important role in mastitis control, very few studies examine the relative importance of culling, spontaneous recovery and therapy. Care is needed in interpreting the data because they are not independent of each other. For example, if therapy is discontinued all infections are eliminated by spontaneous recovery or culling. Also the proportions eliminated depend on the duration of the study. Normally in a period of 6 months more than half of the infections present at the start are still present at the end, whereas they will virtually all have disappeared in 3 years.

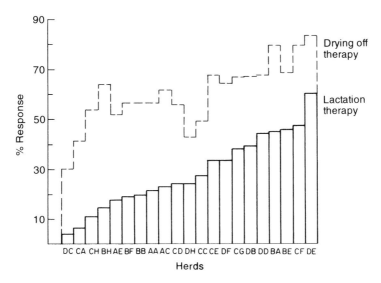

Fig. 8.13 Elimination of *S. aureus* infections from treated quarters in 21 herds over a period of 3 years; 1140 quarters were treated in lactation when clinical and 1327 as subclinical infections at drying off. In laboratory tests none of the *S. aureus* isolates were resistant to cloxacillin. (From Dodd and Neave, 1970, p. 52.)

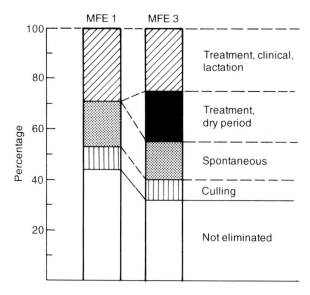

Fig. 8.14   Relative importance of the various ways in which infections are eliminated. Data from the first year of two large field experiments; in one cows were treated at drying off (MFE3) and in the other they were not (MFE1). (Dodd, 1992.)

In spite of this complexity the patterns of elimination are important in deciding on a strategy of control. Figure 8.14 shows data from studies in commercial herds in which measurements were made over a 1-year period. In herds not using drying-off therapy, treating all clinical infections eliminates only 31% of infections, approximately the same as the total by culling and spontaneous recovery; 41% of infections persist until the end of the year. When drying-off therapy is introduced it eliminates 22% of infections and the total for therapy rises to 48%, reducing the proportion persisting to the end of the year to 29%. The benefit of drying-off therapy is greatest for *S. aureus* infections. It appears that antibiotic therapy given when cows are detected with clinical mastitis, though necessary to reduce the damage to udder quarters, is, on its own, relatively ineffective in a control scheme as a means of eliminating infections. This is not because most treatments fail – the average elimination rate for all infections is 70% – but because only about 40% of the infections are discovered by the stockman and receive therapy. This detection rate limits the success that can be achieved with this type of therapy.

Control

It is impossible to eradicate most mastitis pathogens from a herd environment, and even when it is possible (e.g. *Str. agalactiae*) it is impractical on a national scale. Immunisation may give a degree of resistance against specific pathogens or reduce the severity of the infections, but on current evidence its efficiency is not sufficient for it to be the basis of a control scheme. Therapy is essential to reduce the damage caused by infection, but the rates of eliminating infections are poor with some important pathogens and, because therapy is given mainly to clinically infected cows, either many infections do not receive it or it is long delayed. Culling cows with repeated clinical mastitis is useful, but most herds have limited scope for voluntary culling. Many of the factors affecting susceptibility are genetic but, using conventional methods of cattle breeding, the reduction in infection will inevitably be slow.

In examining the options for controlling mastitis most workers came to the conclusion that the only practical scheme was to prevent infection by improved cattle management. However, dairy farming is a business and so many management factors were associated with infection that it was impractical for farmers to adopt all the recommendations. The problem was to discover a few simple methods that together prevent most infection by the major pathogens.

There was no mastitis survey using modern methods of diagnosis before 1945 and levels of subclinical mastitis in UK herds can only be estimated from published experiments in commercial herds. It would appear that more than half the cows had at least one quarter infected and the predominant infection was *Str. agalactiae*. The proportion of quarters infected exceeded 35%. There was no effective therapy and infections persisted and were repeatedly clinical. The number of clinical cases exceeded 150 per 100 cows per year and the somatic cell count of the bulk milk of many, possibly most, herds would have exceeded 1×10^6 cells/ml. Cows with blind quarters were commonplace.

With the introduction of penicillin therapy in 1945 eradication of *Str. agalactiae* became practical and many believed that this would solve the mastitis problem. National and regional schemes for eradicating *Str. agalactiae* were started in several countries, detecting infected cows using laboratory tests, treating them with antibiotics and giving advice on hygiene and management. These schemes were not widely adopted, laboratory costs were high, infection with other pathogens persisted and it became clear that a more effective cheaper method of control was required.

Research on the many management factors that were believed to affect mastitis was carried out in many countries. This did not discover any single all-important factor, but the most promising line of research was milking hygiene even though previous advice in this field had not been successful. The development of this research, described above, led to the clear demonstration under a wide range of farm conditions that a simple hygiene routine based on disinfectant teat dipping after milking could reduce the rate that quarters became infected with the pathogens then causing most infection by at least 50%. However, because of the persistence of infections, particularly those caused by *S. aureus*, and the high rates of new infection in the dry period, a control based solely on reducing new infection in lactating cows had little effect on levels of infection in the first year of use. In fact, reducing new lactating infection by 50% reduced the proportion of quarters infected by less than 10% in a year. A practical way of overcoming this problem was to give antibiotic therapy to all cows at drying off. With this, all persisting infections were treated and, because it gave a much higher cure rate for *S. aureus* infections, it greatly reduced the average duration of infections. The drying-off therapy also prevented most new infection in the dry period and partially controlled summer mastitis. New antibiotic formulations were devised for infusion at drying off and field experiments demonstrated that these eliminated over 70% of infections present at drying off and prevented about 80% of new infections in the dry period (Fig. 8.12).

A mastitis control routine consisting of partial hygiene, which was essentially disinfectant teat dipping after milking coupled with antibiotic therapy for clinical mastitis and for all cows at drying off, was tested in the UK and USA with over 5000 cows in 60 herds for 3 years. The experiments were organised in the UK by the NIRD, Reading, and the Central Veterinary Laboratory, Weybridge, and in the US by Cornell University. The results of the experiments were almost the same in the two countries. Levels of infection fell by over 75% and clinical mastitis by over 50% (Fig. 8.15). It was also clear from the results of the experiments that the levels of infection would ultimately decline by more than 90% if the routine was used over a longer period. However, the experiments also demonstrated the limitations of the routines, principally that the system was not very effective against environmental pathogens, where the main exposure to cows comes from a non-bovine source such as bedding materials. The routine gave no reduction in coliform mastitis and only a partial control for *Str. uberis*. It was also clear that although all herds benefited there was considerable herd variation in the responses. The scheme had the advantage that it did not require routine laboratory testing of cows but was a simple procedure that could be incorporated in day-to-day management. Subsequent research has aimed at reducing the infection directly attributable to milking machine action and at ways of reducing the

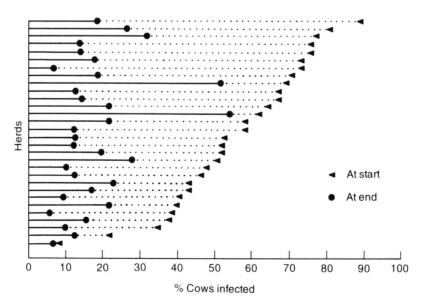

Fig. 8.15   Reduction in levels of infection in 3 years in 30 UK herds after introduction of the NIRD/CVL 'Five Point Plan' mastitis control routine (MFE3).

mastitis caused by environmental pathogens. As the results became available milking machines were modified, farm testing and maintenance were improved and advice on bedding cattle included in the routine.

The current advice based on hygiene, therapy, improved machine milking and housing is outlined below. The full routine applied conscientiously will reduce infection by both major and minor pathogens to low levels. Most farmers have adopted at least the main components of the method, but some will do so inefficiently or intermittently. Nevertheless, the levels of infection and clinical mastitis in the UK have declined considerably and the somatic cell count of herd milk has fallen from a level in the order of 900 000 cells/ml in 1960 to 180 000 cells/ml in 1996. Surveys of farmers with herds with a continuing clinical mastitis problem and high cell count in herd milk usually show that they do not follow the routine.

A routine for controlling mastitis

The NIRD/CVL routine was introduced in 1970 and became known as 'The Five Point Plan'. These are the first five in the following list; the others were added later as more information became available.

(1) Use a milking machine designed and installed to the standards laid down by ISO 5707 (1996). Give regular routine maintenance and have its mechanical performance tested at least annually *and correct the faults found.*
(2) Adopt a simple hygiene system during milking to reduce infection. The main component of this is post-milking teat disinfection of all teats with a disinfectant proved effective for this purpose.
(3) At each milking examine all cows for clinical mastitis using a foremilk cup or mastitis detector. Treat all clinical quarters according to veterinary advice.
(4) Keep records of treatments and cull cows with three or more cases of mastitis in a lactation.
(5) After the last milking of lactation treat all quarters of all cows with an appropriate long-lasting antibiotic product.
(6) Follow good general husbandry practices; avoid sudden major changes in management and feeding that impose stress on cows.
(7) House and manage cows in ways that maintain teat skin clean and free from lesions so that udders and teats do not require routine udder washing.
(8) With cattle housed in cubicles avoid accumulations of organic bedding materials (e.g. straw, sawdust and shavings). Remove bedding from the rear half of the cubicles frequently and renew. Alternatively, use washed sand as bedding.
(9) It is best not to house milking cows on straw yards because of the risk of clinical outbreaks of *Str. uberis* mastitis. If they are used, re-straw daily with dry straw and do not move cows through bedded passageways or feed and water from the straw bed. Do not use calving boxes that have accumulations of soiled bedding. (See page 286 onwards.)

(10)   In herds where summer mastitis is a problem in July and August avoid grazing dry cattle in fields with a history of this problem. Adopt fly control measures and if necessary repeat the dry cow therapy in mid dry period.

In the 20 years since the main parts of this routine were recommended other items have been suggested. Pre-milking teat disinfection has been recommended as an additional item to control infection by environmental pathogens. The evidence for this is not conclusive, but it could be a useful option in herds where this type of infection is a problem and does not respond to improving the housing methods.

Some advisers have recommended selective dry cow therapy. Various methods of selection have been suggested. These included cows with a record of clinical mastitis, old cows and cows that indirect tests (i.e. cell count or California Mastitis Test) indicate are probably infected. The aim was to reduce farm costs and to avoid problems that were anticipated with routine antibiotic treatments for all cows. In fact, in 25 years of widespread use problems have not developed. These types of selective treatment would probably result in treating the majority of infected quarters, but the untreated cows would not be protected against high levels of infection that occur in the dry period or from summer mastitis. The effect of selective therapy will inevitably reduce the benefit of the control method. In this respect it is most important to recognise the synergism of methods of reducing new infection (e.g. teat disinfection) and reducing duration of infections (e.g. drying-off therapy). The effect of the two together has a much greater effect than either alone (Fig. 8.16).

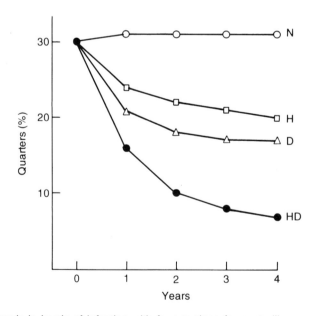

Fig. 8.16   Trends in levels of infection with four routines for controlling mastitis. Data are calculated from results of large experiments in commercial herds. All cows were treated when clinical mastitis was detected. N = No specific hygiene or drying-off therapy; H = disinfectant teat dipping only; D = drying-off therapy only; HD = teat disinfection and drying-off therapy.

Udder washing has not been included in the mastitis control method. This is because its effect is either neutral or detrimental because it is a vector of pathogens, even when disinfectants are used. Some authorities have recommended it should be omitted, but mastitis is not the sole factor in planning a milking routine. Some udder cleaning is necessary as part of the hygiene for producing milk with a low bacterial count.

Monitoring progress in controlling mastitis

There are a number of ways that progress in controlling mastitis can be measured.

Clinical mastitis

Recording trends in the incidence of clinical mastitis appears to be the easiest way to monitor mastitis, but it has limitations and unfortunately many dairy farmers do not keep adequate records. The minimum information on each case that should be recorded is: date, cow identity, quarter(s) affected and treatment given. Additional information on severity, date of calving and date when the cow's milk was included in the bulk tank is also useful, as is the bacterial cause of mastitis if this is identified at a later stage. A case of mastitis is normally defined as an incident affecting one or more quarters at any one time, and a new case is recorded if a period of more than 7 days has elapsed from the end of the last treatment. The incidence is usually reported as the annual number of cases per 100 cows, although the simple total is sufficient for examining within-herd trends.

Because mastitis in most herds follows a seasonal pattern of incidence, which in part is related to housing methods and seasonal patterns of calving, it is preferable to use the annual rolling total, or average, to monitor mastitis. The present UK national average is estimated to be about 40 cases per 100 cows per annum. The target is to keep the annual incidence below 20 cases per 100 cows with not more than 15% of cows in the herd affected.

Subclinical mastitis

Direct measurement of subclinical infection is impractical for most herds because it requires the bacteriological examination of quarter milk samples from all cows on a regular basis, at the very least twice a year. When these data are available the target should be to have less than 10% of the cows and less than 4% of the quarters infected at any one time.

Bulk milk cell count

Bulk milk cell counts measure the average effect of the mastitis infection on herd milk. All UK herds have a cell count on their bulk milk at least once a week for payment purposes. The 3-month geometric (logarithmic) average of these counts is used to determine the payment class of the milk each month. Under EU Directive 92/46 all herd bulk milk must have a cell count below 400000 cells/ml. Currently, bonus payments are paid by some dairy companies for herd milks with cell counts of 150000 cells/ml or less. These cell counts can be used as a herd monitor of mastitis. However, because of the normal variations due to calving patterns and season, they should be averaged over a rolling 12-month period before any significance is attached to the overall average or to trends.

It is important to remember the limitations of bulk milk cell count as a measure of mastitis in a herd. It does not have a good correlation with the incidence of clinical mastitis and occasionally will be markedly increased by undetected clinical mastitis in only one cow, even in a herd of 100 cows. When interpreting bulk cell counts the proportion of milk that has been withheld from the bulk tank either because cows are under treatment or specifically because they have high cell counts must be taken into account. The milk withheld should not exceed 0.6% of total milk production, excluding the milk produced and withheld for the first 4 days after calving. These considerations are increasingly important with the current price penalties based on cell count.

Individual cow cell counts

Almost 40% of UK herds now receive monthly cell counts on the milks from individual cows. This information can be used to monitor the mastitis situation, whilst recognising that not all low cell count cows are uninfected and transient high cell counts may not represent infection.

It is generally accepted that cows producing milk with a cell count exceeding 200000 cells/ml are likely to be infected. The target is to maintain the proportion above this limit at less than 20% of the herd and less than 10% of first lactation cows. In herds of more than 70 cows it is possible to use the monthly results for monitoring provided they are not block calving. Smaller herds and those block calving herds should use the annual averages.

Cow-side testing

The results obtained from regular testing of a herd using an indirect cow-side test such as the California Mastitis Test (CMT) provide a good monitor of infection within a herd. It is a time consuming exercise to test and record the result on every quarter of every cow in milk, but it should be carried out at least twice a year and preferably more frequently. As with subclinical mastitis, the target is to maintain the proportion of positive reactions at less than 10% of cows and less than 4% of quarters.

Conclusions

In practice, the most regular monitor is likely to be the bulk milk cell count and records of clinical mastitis, supplemented by individual cow cell counts if available. Although the bulk milk cell count supplied by dairies to farmers is a rolling geometric mean a simple arithmetic average of these figures can be used as a guide to progress. Thus, the annual average is the average of the last 12 figures and the rolling average is calculated after adding the current month's figure and deleting the data from the equivalent month 1 year ago. The target should be to keep the annual average below 200 000 cells/ml, and many herds are now successfully keeping below 100 000 cells/ml. Provided the count is below 200 000 cells/ml no further action should be necessary. However, if the trend is significantly upwards over a period, for example if the annual average has increased by more than 10 000 cells/ml each month for 3 months or longer, the cause should be investigated. Individual cow cell count data or the CMT can be useful in this situation.

It is now a legal requirement that records of all treatments are kept, and this is particularly important with mastitis in order to prevent the contamination of milk with antibiotic residues. These records can provide an excellent monitor of mastitis in the herd and they should be checked monthly and analysed regularly for maximum value. It is essential to have both measures, the clinical mastitis incidence and the bulk milk cell count, in order to monitor accurately the mastitis status of a herd.

Investigating the causes of high levels of mastitis in herds

Herds with levels of mastitis that require investigation will have either a bulk milk cell count that is higher than average or rising, or a high incidence of clinical mastitis or both. The causes can be complex, but many can be discovered by observation of the herd management and examining records that are, or should be, available on the farm. Some problems cannot be solved without the additional information that can be provided by a diagnostic laboratory to determine the types of infection in the herd.

The first step is to examine the records of clinical mastitis, the bulk milk cell count data and if available the individual cow cell counts. The investigator must make a judgement on the reliability of the clinical records in relation to information on antibiotic usage. From these data tentative conclusions can be drawn. If the cell count is consistently high it can be assumed that the average level of subclinical infection is high and that the most likely cause is infection with *S. aureus* and/or the common streptococci. This conclusion will apply with or without high levels of clinical mastitis in the herd. If the herd cell count levels are below average with occasional high values but clinical mastitis is frequent the most likely cause is infection with the environmental pathogens *E. coli* and/or *Str. uberis*. This conclusion is strengthened if the clinical mastitis occurs mainly in cattle that are housed and in early lactation. It is important to recognise that if both cell counts and clinical mastitis are high it is possible that both types of infection are causing the problem. The other records to examine are the most recent milking machine test reports, evidence that any machine faults detected have been corrected, information on the types of antibiotics used for treating clinical mastitis and cows at drying off, and the monthly records of the hygienic quality of the milk (i.e. Bactoscan/TBC). If the Bactoscan counts are mostly below 50000 cells/ml of milk (TBC below 10000 cells/ml) but there are frequent high values it suggests that clinical mastitis caused by *Str. uberis* is a likely cause of the infections.

The next step is to observe the milking and the associated management. It is better not to precede this by asking if the milker adopts 'The Five Point Plan'; this will become obvious during the observation. The important points to observe are:

- Examine the most recent test results of the mechanical efficiency of the milking equipment. Have the faults been corrected?
- Is post-milking teat disinfection effectively carried out *on all cows?*
- What chemical is used, and at what dilution? How much is purchased?
- Is the general hygiene at milking satisfactory?
- Are the cows' udders grossly soiled before milking?
- Does the milker use a foremilk cup or detector to look for clinical mastitis *on all cows?*
- Are there gross faults in the use of the milking machines (e.g. excessive over-milking, frequent fall-off of units, removal of units under vacuum)?
- Are teat lesions common (i.e. on more than 15% of teats)?
- Do many teat orifices show marked hyperkeratosis (i.e. erosion)?
- Is the general hygiene of the milking parlour/cowshed satisfactory?

The final step is to examine the management of the cows between milkings:

- If the cows are outdoors or at pasture are the udders grossly soiled?
- Are the cows troubled by flies?
- If the cows are indoors is the bedding satisfactory and are the cows clean?
- If the bedding is with sawdust/shavings how frequently is fresh material added?
- If straw is used how deep is the bed and is it likely to compost?

With this information it is usually possible to determine the likely cause of a herd mastitis problem without recourse to a diagnostic laboratory. Herds that follow the recommended routine fully and consistently rarely have a mastitis problem. If the cell counts are high it will usually be due to a failure to disinfect the teats with the correct disinfectants, not using dry-cow therapy or gross faults in the milking machine. If teat lesions are common a teat disinfectant containing an emollient should be used. When the incidence of clinical mastitis is high with acute mastitis in freshly calved cows and the teat disinfection and machine milking are correct the cause is probably related to the method of housing or the bedding material. It is best not to use sawdust/shavings or deep straw beds. If possible use washed sand in cubicles or renew organic bedding materials very frequently. Particular care should be taken with bedding materials over the calving period and in early lactation because most clinical mastitis occurs at these times.

In a few herds a problem cannot be resolved by a routine investigation of the type described and in some cases it can be difficult to discover the causes even with the assistance of a diagnostic laboratory. The cause may be infections with atypical pathogens, or with strains of common bacteria that are more invasive or pathogenic, or with bacterial infections that cannot be eliminated by routine therapy. These factors may be associated with an abnormal management or milking machine factors, but they can be fortuitous.

In this brief review it is impractical to detail the various strategies for solving the more difficult problems, but the following notes indicate a systematic approach:

- Make special checks to make certain that the correct mastitis control routine is actually being followed. Some stockmen when questioned on their routine work are 'economical with the truth'.
- Determine the pathogen causing most of the infections. If the herd has high cell counts this information can be obtained by bacteriological tests on a sample of the older cows. If the herd has a clinical problem with low cell counts the bacteriological tests have to be from the affected cows. *Bacteriological data are useless unless samples are taken aseptically.*
- Poor cure rates with standard antibiotics for infections caused by the common mastitis pathogens are rare except for *S. aureus* and occasionally *Str. uberis* infections. This situation can be detected by tests on recently treated quarters (but not within 21 days of the last infusion). There is little correlation between cure rates and antibiotic sensitivity tests on the pathogens. Some of the less common mastitis pathogens, e.g. *C. ulcerans* and pseudomonas, have extremely low cure rates.
- Laboratory tests of any type rarely indicate the underlying causes of a mastitis problem, but they can be invaluable in indicating where a solution may be found. For example, if *Str. agalactiae* infection is common poor teat disinfection is the likely cause, if *E. coli* predominates then bedding is the likely source of the infections, etc.
- If the problem is found to be *E. coli* mastitis, an infection with a short duration, and the underlying cause is removed the problem is immediately resolved, but with long duration infections such as *S. aureus* the reduction in infections will be gradual, taking months and even years.
- If after investigation the levels of infection are reduced by treating infected quarters or culling infected cows, the benefit will last only a few months unless action is taken to eliminate the factors causing new infections.

When investigating the more difficult problems assistance can be obtained from the services of ADAS or Genus or the veterinary practices that specialise in this type of work.

Postscript

Of the cattle diseases of major economic importance to dairy farmers, mastitis has been the most refractory, in spite of it being the most researched. The slow progress was partly due to the complexity of mastitis which is several diseases caused by different pathogens, each with a different epidemiology and requiring a different approach for control. It was not until 1970 that a practical economic and effective control for the most common types of mastitis was developed and proved. One of the two key components of this control, post-milking teat disinfection, was first proposed in 1916, and the other, drying-off therapy, in 1950. These passed unnoticed in the multitude of unproven proposals that were put forward to solve the mastitis problem. The key to progress came when it was possible to assemble a team of workers from veterinary science, microbiology, engineering, and animal science who were able to concentrate on developing and testing a method of control based on the epidemiologies of the various types of infection. The first proposals were based on the results of their own research and the accumulated published work of many other scientists. They cooperated with the chemical and pharmaceutical industries and had the good fortune to have the resources to be able to test their hypotheses in large experiments on commercial farms, the only place that a control can be proven. In this way the major weaknesses in the first attempts at control were discovered and corrected through detailed investigation. Subsequently in further farm experiments an effective control scheme was proved.

The main weakness of the mastitis control that was developed, the poor control of environmental mastitis, was revealed in the field experiments 30 years ago. Subsequent research has increased the understanding of these infections, but there is not yet a proven practical method of control of them. It is difficult to believe that this will be achieved unless it is possible to mount a multidisciplinary team approach similar to the one that was successful against the most common types of infection.

References

Bramley, A. J., Dodd, F. H. & Griffin, T. K. (1981) *Mastitis Control and Herd Management.* Technical Bulletin no. 4 National Institute for Research in Dairying, Reading.

Bramley, A. J., Dodd, F. H., Mein, G. A. & Bramley, J. A. (1992) *Machine Milking and Lactation*, p. 113. Insight Books, Newbury.

Dodd, F. R. (1992) In: *Large Dairy Herd Management* (M. H. van Horn & C. J. Wilcox, eds), p. 450. American Dairy Science Association, Champagne, IL.

Dodd, F. H. & Jackson, E. R. (1971) *The Control of Bovine Mastitis.* National Institute for Research in Dairying, Reading.

Dodd, F. H., Higgs, T. M. & Bramley, A. J. (1984) Cubicle management and coliform mastitis. *Veterinary Record*, **114**, 522–3.

Dodd, F. H. & Neave, F. K. (1970) *Mastitis Control*, pp. 21–60. Biennial Reviews. National Institute for Research in Dairying, Reading.

Kingwill, R. G., Dodd, F. H. & Neave, F. K. (1979) *Machine Milking.* Technical Bulletin no. 1. National Institute for Research in Dairying, Reading.

Kitchen, B. J. (1981) Bovine mastitis: milk compositional changes and related diagnostic tests. *Journal of Dairy Research*, **48**, 167–88

Munch-Petersen, E. (1938) *Bovine Mastitis: Survey of the Literature to the End of 1935.* Imperial Bureau of Animal Health, Weybridge.

Further reading

Booth, J. M. (1988) Update on mastitis. 1. Control measures in England and Wales. How have they influenced incidence and aetiology? *British Veterinary Journal* **144**, 316–22.

Bramley, A. J. & Dodd, F. H. (1984) Mastitis control – progress and prospects. *Journal of Dairying Research*, **51**, 481–512.

British Standards Institution (1988) *Milking Machine Installations. Part 2. Specifications for Construction and Performance. Part 3. Methods for Mechanical Testing. BS 5445.* BSI, London.

International Dairy Federation (1975) *Proceedings of Seminar on Mastitis Control,* Reading, 7–11 April. Document no. 85. IDF, Brussels.

International Dairy Federation (1981) *Laboratory Methods for Use in Mastitis Work.* Document no. 132. IDF, Brussels.

International Dairy Federation (1985) *Progress in the Control of Bovine Mastitis.* IDF Seminar, Kiel, Germany, 21–24 May. Verlag Th. Mann, Gelsenkirchen-Buer, Germany.

International Dairy Federation (1987) *Machine Milking and Mastitis.* Document no. 215. IDF, Brussels.

Sandholm, M. & Mattila, T. (1986) *Mechanisms of Infection and Inflammation of the Mammary Gland – An Overview*, pp. 7–13. Proceedings of a Symposium on Mastitis Control, Espoo, Finland, 1986. College of Veterinary Medicine, Helsinki 55, Finland.

Saran, A. & Soback, S. (eds) (1995) *Proceedings of the Third International Mastitis Seminar,* Tel Aviv, Israel, 28 May–1 June. National Mastitis Reference Center, Kimron Veterinary Institute, PO Box 12, Biet Dagan 50250, Israel.

Schalm, O. W., Carroll, E. J. & Jain, N. C. (1971) *Bovine Mastitis.* Lea and Febiger, Philadelphia.

Wilson, C. D. & Richards, M. S. (1980) A survey of mastitis in the British dairy herd. *Veterinary Record*, **106**, 431–5.

Chapter 9
Genetics of Disease Resistance

Roger Spooner

Introduction

Farmers have been breeding animals and selecting types suited to particular uses or environments for millenia. However, genetic variation in resistance to disease is only now becoming a topic of serious consideration in animal production. Domestic animals have been attacked by viruses, bacteria and parasites since domestication started and there must have been very active selection for resistance to disease. Today this natural resistance can be clearly seen in the tropics where disease challenge is more intense and local breeds can survive whilst imported stock, particularly European, cannot unless very considerable management input is expended to keep them alive.

History

The concept of genetics is relatively recent, starting with the work on peas by Mendel in the 1860s. Soon after this, around the turn of the century, there was a massive development in bacteriology and parasitology which, coupled with advances in therapy, largely pushed the concept of genetic resistance in animal populations into the background. Pasteur developed his vaccine against anthrax, and vaccines were then developed against a wide range of organisms. Many diseases in addition to anthrax, including clostridial infections, tetanus and smallpox, were controlled by vaccines. There were major steps forward in treatment, drugs such as penicillin and subsequent antibiotics, and the many parasiticidal drugs that were developed to combat malaria and trypanosomiasis to name just two. DDT was developed and it was widely believed that it would be only a matter of time before mosquitoes would be exterminated and malaria with them. However, resistance to DDT developed, side effects to DDT usage were realised and the programme was stopped. Anthelminthics, acaricides and antibiotics are constantly having to be replaced as resistance develops and the new drugs are normally more expensive than the ones they replace. This resistance to drugs not only had relevance to the control of the disease and the target organism, but also is being increasingly seen as a problem in human nutrition because when antibiotics are being used as food additives for pigs and poultry to increase growth

Table 9.1 Tropical theileriosis in Morocco.

	Holstein	Crossbreed	Local breed
% Farms using acaricide	100	60	6
% Carriers	22	40	52
% Clinical cases	23	34	—
% Of clinically ill that died	24	—	—

rate, there is the danger of introducing antibiotic-resistant bacteria into the population. Thus, the cost of treatment and prevention increases and becomes less efficient whilst at the same time multidrug-resistant organisms are becoming common. The only way to avoid this is to develop genetically resistant stock which do not need treatment.

Even within Europe there was evidence in the 1960s of variations in resistance between European breeds and it was shown that Red Danish cattle had a higher incidence of most infections than Danish Friesians and Jerseys and that these differences markedly affected the herd life of cows in these breeds. Little note was taken of this type of data at the time and selection for milk yield continued in the absence of any thought about disease.

In the tropics where disease challenge is greater, genetic solutions have only very recently been considered. The International Laboratory for Research into Animal Diseases was set up in Kenya in the 1970s, but in the first decade of its existence it did no work on genetic resistance and it is really only in the 1990s that a serious effort to study the genetics of resistance to trypanosomiasis has been instituted. In India, European dairy breeds particularly Holsteins and Jerseys have been widely disseminated throughout the country, but they have to be crossed with local breeds to have a reasonable level of survival. Although there has been suggestive evidence for many years that there are breed differences in disease resistance in cattle, there has been too little use of this fact in the improvement of animals for the tropics. Although the Belgians were using trypanosomiasis-resistant N'Damas in commercial cattle production in the Congo, many animal breeders were advising Africa to import European breeds as the best way of improving their cattle productivity. Tropical theileriosis has become more important as European cattle breeds have been exported to the tropics and exposed to the disease. Similarly, *Theileria sergenti* infection was not a problem in local cattle breeds in China but is now reported to be killing cattle in pure Holstein farms. With *Theileria annulata*, the cause of tropical theileriosis, there is a highly effective vaccine; with *T. sergenti* there is not, but it would be of great value if it were possible to identify resistant genes to both these organisms. With tropical theileriosis in Morocco there is clear evidence that the disease is most pathogenic in pure Holsteins, less in crossbreds and does not cause clinical disease in local cattle. Results from an experiment in Morocco are shown in Table 9.1.

Whilst vaccines and therapy were leading the way in the control of disease in both domestic animals and humans, there were, however, quite a lot of experiments studying genetic resistance in laboratory animals to a range of diseases such as tuberculosis, salmonellosis, scrapie and many others. In every case where attempts had been made to select animals for resistance to a disease, resistant and susceptible populations had been developed. Often, selection took place in very few generations suggesting that only a few genes are involved. However, it was not uncommon for an animal resistant to one disease to became susceptible to another and so a general resistance to disease was not common in these experiments.

In human beings there is a rapidly expanding list of diseases and predispositions, from schizophrenia to renal failure, where genetic components have been identified. There are many single gene diseases, some of which are recessive, such as cystic fibrosis and others that are dominant such as neurofibromatosis. Diabetes, particularly the early onset insulin-dependent diabetes, shows marked genetic effects and the relevant genes are being identified. Infectious diseases are more difficult to study, but amongst the parasitic diseases there is evidence of major genetic effects. Malaria is a good example and was also one of the first where a marker for resistance was identified. It was many years ago that it was shown that the highly disadvantageous mutation causing sickle cell haemoglobin is common in malarial areas. It was found that although the homozygous sickle cell individuals were at a severe disadvantage, those with only one copy of the sickle gene were more resistant to malaria and survived better.

Modes of inheritance

The genes that control a particular trait are situated at a particular site on one of the chromosomes. In most animals one copy of the gene is inherited from the mother and one copy from the father. These genes are composed of nucleic acid (DNA) and the sequence of the nucleotides in this DNA determines the protein produced and hence the function of that particular gene. By early in the next century the nucleotide sequence of the entire human genome will have been determined. Many genes occur in different versions, caused by slight differences in the nucleotide sequence, and these versions are called alleles. Often different alleles show no effect on the animal, but some alleles cause disease or other variation in phenotype.

Dominant genes

Where an allele of a gene is expressed and fully functional, even if there is a different allele at the other copy of the gene, it is said to be dominant. The white face in the Hereford is an example of a dominant allele. Dominant alleles producing severe disease effects are likely to be lethal and so will not be perpetuated, and therefore dominance that persists in the population tends to produce fairly minor effects, or none at all, as with alleles of genes controlling colour.

Penetrance

Dominance may be irregular, in other words fully expressed in some animals but not in others, e.g. the environmental stress may vary and modify the effect of the gene and this is commonly known as incomplete penetrance. In other words, several animals may have the same alleles for a particular trait, but it is partially visible and expressed in some and not in others. Hereditary ataxia in Aberdeen Angus illustrates this type of inheritance; transmitting bulls mated to non-carriers leave around 25–40% of the calves affected instead of the expected 50%, so penetrance is from 50 to 80%. If there was complete penetrance then 50% would be affected.

Semi-dominant genes

With semi-dominant genes the allele is expressed partially in the heterozygote when there is only one dose of the allele but more strongly when there are two doses. The Dexter mentioned later is a good example of this. One dose of the 'Dexter' allele converts the Kerry into the small achondroplastic Dexter, but a double dose produces monsters.

Recessive genes

With recessive genes the normal allele is dominant and the abnormal one does not show when it is present in a single dose. However, when there are two doses of the gene then the effect is seen, i.e. neither parent is affected but the defect has in fact come from both parents.

In matings of carriers, one in four of the offspring are normal (RR), two are carriers (Rr) and one in four will be affected (rr). Examples of this type of inheritance are mentioned later. Bovine leukocyte adhesion deficience (BLAD) and Weaver are two examples and, as will be noted, it is not uncommon for the heterozygotes, the animals with one dose of the gene, to be better in some way than the normals. Although not proven, this may well be the case with BLAD and Weaver. New recessive mutations where the heterozygote has some advantage can very rapidly spread in the dairy population. When one considers that a bull may well have 100000 daughters, such spread can happen rapidly. BLAD, which rose to 12% frequency in the American cattle population by the time it was recognised, is a good example.

Polygenic inheritance

In some traits such as polled, BLAD, Weaver, etc. there is one gene at one locus causing the trait. However, with many traits such as milk yield, growth rate, disease resistance and susceptibility many genes are involved, some playing a large part, others a small. Quantitative genetics has developed to create the mathematical tools to analyse such traits whilst only being able to measure the phenotype. However, in spite of not knowing any of the specific genes, it has been possible to select for increased milk production. Very considerable progress has been made in selecting bulls whose daughters produce more milk. However, as the mapping of the bovine genome continues and the genes contributing to the control of yield are identified, it may turn out that even traits such as milk yield, which have been assumed to be controlled by many genes, are controlled by only a few.

Identifying genetic differences in susceptibility

There are many traits, such as growth rate and milk yield, where no single gene has been identified and it has been assumed that many genes are involved. Population geneticists were then able to develop statistical methods for studying the effects of all of these genes at the same time and they coined the term 'heritability'. The main area where genetic traits have been measured and applied is production traits. In the dairy industry, before new bulls are used widely in the AI system, they produce 200–400 daughters, with a few daughters on each farm so that on any one farm there are daughters of several bulls. The milk yield and other traits of these daughters can then be measured and compared within the same environment. From this, the breeding value or PIN number of the bull and the heritability of the trait are calculated. The next generation of bulls will be chosen from matings between the best bulls of the previous generation and high-producing cows.

Heritability is a term used to describe the proportion of the genetic variation in a trait due to additive genetic effects after statistically allowing for differences in other attributable effects such as sex, year, date of birth, type of birth, farm, and management regime. With heritability one can then predict the likely response to selection. The heritability of milk yield which is between 0.3 and 0.4 has enabled steady improvement in milk yield in the dairy population over the past 30 years. Heritability estimates for susceptibility to diseases are now being made.

At the same time as these quantitative traits were being studied statistically and before there was any definition of genes controlling specific diseases, it was nevertheless known that a number of conditions were genetically controlled and controlled by single genes. However, as knowledge of the genome has developed, not only have genes controlling these single gene diseases been mapped to particular parts of the genome or in some cases actually identified and cloned, but also it has been found that there are often only a few major genes contributing to some of the traits formerly thought to be controlled by many genes.

The dissection of these effects has been extended very considerably in recent years and in some cases single genes have been identified which have major effects on disease resistance. In the mid 1970s it was shown that a group of inbred strains of mice could be divided into two populations when challenged with *Salmonella typhimurium*. They were either highly resistant or highly susceptible. It was then found that there was a single gene controlling this resistance on chromosome 1 in the mouse. Later it was found that this same gene was involved in resistance to relatively low virulence tubercle infection of mice by BCG and *Leishmania* infection. As a result, the gene was variously called Ity/Bcg/Lsh. Another instance where genetic variation was found was in the incubation time of mouse strains to scrapie; this has become of much more relevant and interest recently as a result of BSE. It was found that some mouse strains had a very long incubation period to a particular strain of scrapie, whereas others had a short incubation period for that same strain. However, the complexity of the interaction was underlined when it was found that with a different strain of scrapie the long-incubation-period strain of mice with the first strain had a short incubation period with this second strain and vice versa.

Arguments against selection for disease resistance

There have been many attacks on the concept of the usefulness of genetic variation in disease resistance in animal populations. It has been commonly assumed and claimed that bacteria and viruses mutate very much more rapidly than animals or plants and therefore there is no point in attempting to develop resistance because the organism will rapidly evade that resistance. Although the development of strains of viruses, bacteria and parasites resistant to drugs is the norm, this is not the case with infectious disease and, once developed, resistance is normally maintained.

Moreover, the concept of a pathogen continually evolving new strains in response to the evolution of resistance in the host may be misleading since a virulent strain would tend to eliminate its host, its major resource, either by killing it directly or by reducing its reproductive capacity and, thus eliminating itself, a stable host–pathogen relationship is more likely to evolve. A classic example of this is the prickly pear cactus which became a major weed in Australia. The moth *Cactoblastus cactorum* Berg, introduced to control it in 1925, rapidly reduced its density and both populations initially showed a series of damped oscillations, since when they have coexisted in stable equilibrium at low density. It appears that each species has influenced the genetic composition of the other. Another example also demonstrated in Australia is myxomatosis in rabbits which was introduced to control the rabbit population. The disease spread rapidly and for a time did control the rabbit population, but then resistant animals gradually bred and replaced the susceptible population and the virus has not mutated to produce more virulent forms. Now myxomatosis is of little relevance to rabbit control. There are some examples of virulence increasing. With Marek's disease virulent strains have developed which cause vaccine breakdown before slaughter age.

In addition to the objections about organisms mutating more rapidly than animals, other objections are often raised regarding the feasibility of selecting disease-resistant stock and undue weight is given to them. Some examples are:

- Only a relative resistance to any specific disease is obtainable (but this may be better than no resistance).
- Selection emphasis on production characters is reduced (this is true: the more

characters that one includes in the selection index the smaller the effect of any single character). However, diseases like mastitis may have sufficient genetic variation and be sufficiently economically important to justify selection against them. The Milk Marketing Board and now the Milk Development Council and Meat and Livestock Commission do not collect disease information in this country, nor is such information collected in most other EU countries. The major exception is that information on mastitis, ketosis and a number of the economically important diseases is collected in Norway and now Finland and Sweden and the information is then included in a selection index of animals in those countries.

- There is automatic selection against diseased animals. Another way of putting this is that we are already selecting against disease, so why bother? This would be true under natural conditions, but now we are keeping alive, through our therapeutic efforts, animals that should have been discarded. In fact, there may well be virtual selection for disease susceptibility by selection in the absence of challenge.

Genetics of disease resistance and susceptibility

The evidence for genetic variation in disease can be considered under three headings: (1) longevity, (2) single gene defects and (3) quantitative multigene traits. The single gene defects may be defects in a metabolic pathway or in some cases of unknown aetiology but known to be a single gene. The multigene traits are the more quantitative traits, such as susceptibility to mastitis, ketosis, metabolic diseases and reproductive problems.

Genetic variation in survival

Selection for viability or longevity could be practised. Groups of bulls whose offspring showed similar first lactation yields could by selected and then only those daughters with the longest working lives chosen. Moreover, if the genes that are controlling longevity could be identified then this would not have to be repeated for each generation and the genes could be utilised in selection of young males.

Longevity is an important parameter because the survival of a cow in the dairy herd represents the farmers' positive assessment of her economic worth. Studies on the survival of daughters of various bulls indicate that longevity has a large genetic component which is independent of yield. Figure 9.1 indicates the variation in survival of daughters of bulls of similar breeding value. The breeding value is a prediction of the increase in yield that the use of the bull would produce. As can be seen, there are bulls with the same breeding value but with greatly differing proportions of their daughters surviving to third lactation. There are two bulls with a breeding value of 114, but one has 75% of his daughters surviving, the other 53%. There are five bulls with around 54% of their daughters

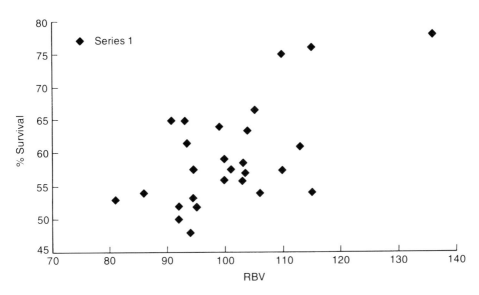

Fig. 9.1 Survival of daughters of bulls correlated with breeding value.

surviving but with breeding values ranging from 80 to 115. These results were obtained from an average of 400 daughters per bull and thus the sampling error is unlikely to have produced much variation. This implies that bulls are transmitting other factors besides yield that determine whether farmers cull females, and a heritability for survival is obtainable from variation in progeny survival. This varies with breed and the point at which survival is measured. In Ayrshires it has been estimated at 20% to sixth lactation, but since longevity is an all or none trait the precision of this estimate is low. In a crude measure such as survival, yield and disease cannot be separated, and hence it provides no guidance on what specific disease factors would justify selection. The trend (Fig. 9.1) is mainly due to heavy culling of low yielders in early lactation but also to the preferential treatment of high yielders which may produce a longer life. While the trend indicates that selection for yield is not increasing disease incidence markedly, otherwise the slope would be negative, it does not imply that it is inadvisable or unnecessary to select for viability. The relationship between yield and survival may also have altered under current conditions.

Longevity is something that can be deduced from data collected in our current milk recording schemes. The importance of doing this is now being recognised and the Animal Data Centre is introducing a breeding value for lifespan.

Specific diseases

Although this chapter is about cattle, one cannot discuss genetics without considering evidence from other species as well and in this section a number of diseases will be considered some of which are common to several species. Others are seen only in one species. Poultry provide an example of a species where genetic resistance has and is being used commercially. The poultry industry is now in the hands of a very few large commercial firms worldwide. They provide the majority of the layer and broiler stocks in use in the world and they are now becoming, or have become, seriously interested in genetic resistance to disease. The pig industry is moving in the same direction. There is also work in sheep.

Diseases caused by single genes

BLAD

Starting with single gene diseases, one that has had recent and very widespread publicity in the dairy population is BLAD, bovine leukocyte adhesion deficiency. In many ways this is a quite remarkable story because it was only identified a very few years ago when a veterinarian, Marcus Kerhli, working in Ames in Iowa found some calves that were dying before a year of age from various bacterial inflammatory conditions. Because of some similarities with a human condition he suspected some fault in leukocyte adhesion. He found that the animals he was looking at had a particularly popular bull on both sides of their pedigree. From there he identified a defect in an adhesion molecule which prevented leukocytes adhering to the walls of blood vessels. Because they could not adhere they could not get out to sites of infection so that animals died of whichever infection they were exposed to. He identified the mutation in the gene, developed a test for it and set up testing of American AI bulls. Before the disease was barely known in this country it had already been identified and removed from the USA. The disease is caused by a recessive mutation in the CD18 gene and it is only the homozygote recessives that are affected. This mutation, however, had reached 12% frequency in the USA before it was identified and it is not impossible that the heterozygotes may have been more productive than normal cattle and that this was why it had been selected for in these elite bulls.

Weaver

Weaver is another single gene defect where the homozygote recessives are affected but the heterozygotes are not. Weaver is almost entirely confined to Brown Swiss cattle. It is first seen at around 5–8 months of age and is characterised by progressive signs of pelvic limb paresis, ataxia and proprioceptive placing deficits. Affected animals are mentally alert and reveal normal motor and sensory reflexes, gonadal atrophy in both males and females and Wallerian degeneration in the white matter. Affected animals are homozygous for a recessive gene and a microsatellite has been identified which can be used to identify carriers of the gene. It seems that, as with BLAD, weaver may have been inadvertently selected for as the heterozygotes are reported to produce more milk than normal cattle. However, with the microsatellite it is possible to screen out carriers and in time the gene should disappear.

Mannosidosis

Another condition that has caused considerable problems particularly in the Aberdeen Angus and Murray Grey cattle in New Zealand is mannosidosis, a deficiency of a specific lysozomal hydrolase enzyme mannosidase. This causes the accumulation of mannose and glucosamine in secondary lysozomes. The signs develop from 1 to 15 months of age and most animals die by 1 year. There is at first slight hind leg ataxia and then a fine lateral head tremor, slow vertical head nodding, aggression and loss of condition. Diagnosis is based on reduced tissue and plasma levels of mannosidase. Histologically the accumulations of mannose and glucosamine are seen in the nerve cells, fixed macrophages and epithelial cells of the viscera. Tissue and plasma levels of mannosidase are around half the normal levels in the heterozygous animals and so these can be detected. A genetic screening programme was instituted in New Zealand in the late 1970s and this has largely removed the problem.

Now the gene controlling the enzyme has been identified and mapped and a screening programme is underway to remove the faulty mutation from the Salers breed.

Dwarfism

Genes for dwarfism were also intentionally bred for in the early part of the century. This was not confined to dogs, with monsters like the Boston Terrier and the Bulldog, but also took place in cattle. An extreme example of this is the Dexter breed where the dwarf gene produces the small Dexter in the heterozygous state whilst the homozygous is lethal. This is a single gene defect and when Dexters are mated together 25% of the offspring are Bulldog, 50% are Dexters and 25% are normal long leg Kerrys. There seems to be no particular value in this mutation other than that the offspring are unusual. A similar gene, called the Spider syndrome, has developed in Suffolk and Hampshire sheep in North America since the 1980s.

Diseases where several genes are involved

Some of the best examples of disease genetics are not in cattle but in faster growing and reproducing species such as poultry. They do, however, give an example of what might be expected in cattle.

Marek's disease

Marek's disease which is confined to poultry is an interesting example in that this was one of the first diseases where genetic variation in resistance was sought. Animals were selected by exposure to the virus and resistant strains were bred. It was also noted by people working with chicken blood groups that in years when there was an outbreak of Marek's disease, animals with a particular B blood group survived better than those without. Subsequently it has been shown that other B blood groups, notably the B[21] blood group, bestow significant resistance. It is now known that the B blood group system is part of the major histocompatibility complex, the region of the genome which controls many aspects of the immune response; thus presumably the resistance to Marek's disease is a function of the ability to develop immunity. However, as this information was being produced, a vaccine was developed for Marek's disease and many people forgot about genetics. Now, however, with the development of more virulent strains of the virus it is being found that the vaccine does not protect fully until commercial slaughter age and that one needs both genetic-resistant stock and the vaccine.

Coccidiosis

There are some seven species of *Eimeria* which can cause coccidiosis in chickens. Ingestion of oocysts leads to intracellular infection of the gut wall, in which the parasites undergo several cycles of asexual replication before entering a sexual phase which is followed by the release of oocytes into the gut lumen. The oocytes are then excreted with the faeces and become infective for other chickens. Infection appears to be self limiting if ingestion of further oocysts is prevented and in most species a strong protective immune response is developed which prevents the establishment of subsequent reinfections. Bumstead (1996) has challenged various inbred chicken lines with these seven *Eimeria* spp. and found that resistance to some of the strains is highly correlated whereas others it is not. Basically, animals that are resistant to *Eimeria tenella* are susceptible to most of the other species. However, there is genetic resistance to *E. tenella* which is economically the most important species.

Infectious bronchitis virus (IBV)

Infectious bronchitis virus (IBV) is a highly contagious respiratory disease of chickens due to a corona virus, causing respiratory infection in young birds and reduced egg production and poor egg quality in older animals. Other bacteria such as *E. coli* exacerbate the morbidity caused by infection and, as with salmonellosis and coccidia, there is variation in resistance between different inbred lines. However, a very important finding from the research is that lines resistant to one organism are not necessarily resistant to another and in fact the line most resistant to one pathogen is in some cases the most susceptible to another.

Pink eye (see also p. 38 onwards)

Pink eye or infectious bovine keretoconjunctivitis is a serious problem in some tropical and temperate regions. Much work has been undertaken on the causal organism or organisms, but work in Australia (see Table 9.2), has shown big differences between zebu and European breeds in their susceptibility to pink eye. It was shown that zebu could be totally resistant whereas European

Table 9.2 Incidence of pink eye in cattle in Australia exposed to natural infection.

Breed	% Affected at 15 months
Hereford and Shorthorn	72.5
Afrikander cross	22.1
Brahmin cross	8.4
Afrikander	6.1
Brahmin	0

breeds were highly susceptible. Thus the apparent complexity of the microbiology of pink eye may in part arise from variation in susceptibility between individual cattle.

Intestinal parasites

Little is known about the variation in resistance to intestinal parasites in cattle. Although there has been much work on intestinal nematodes in sheep, there has been little work on lungworm or fasciola. Using the number of eggs per gram of faeces as a reasonable measure of the level of infection, variation in susceptibility to internal nematodes has been demonstrated, particularly in Australia. Although with some parasites, such as *Ostertagia*, correlation between faecal egg counts and worm number is not always high, there has been clear evidence of genetic variation in *Haemonchus contortus*. In Australia there was the 'golden ram' whose offspring had a significantly lower faecal egg count than those of other rams. However, in spite of this the offspring of this particular ram have not repopulated Australian sheep.

Stear *et al.* (1997) working in this country have been studying resistance to *Ostertagia circumcincta*. They have shown that there is very considerable variation between sheep in the resistance to infection as assessed by both how many and how long each worm is, together with the production of eggs or infected larvae. One of the interesting things about this work is that there are no genetic differences between animals in response to the parasite before 3 months of age; in other words, the resistance develops as animals get older and by 6 months of age the heritability of resistance is similar to that for milk yield in cattle. Thus it is possible to consider breeding for resistance. Moreover, as it has been shown that there is a strong correlation between resistance and growth rate, and as growth rate is the major economic criterion, it could be well worthwhile selecting for more resistant sheep.

Escherichia coli resistance

The main aetiological agent for piglet diarrhoea is *E. coli* possessing the K88 antigen. The strains can adhere to the intestinal mucosa which makes it much easier for them to colonise the gut and cause diarrhoea. Some pigs lack the intestinal receptor for K88; thus the organisms cannot bind to the gut and the animals are much more resistant to diarrhoea. Selecting for this resistance gene is quite difficult because one has to identify the phenotype in the gut which either means killing the animal or taking a biopsy, not an easy test for routine use. However, it does indicate that there is genetic variation in susceptibility to *E. coli* and that it is likely that similar variation occurs in other species.

E. coli is also very important in calves from the point of view of diarrhoea and in adult cattle with regard to human nutrition. A gene has now been identified affecting resistance to *E. coli*. Not surprisingly perhaps it has been patented.

Salmonellosis

As noted in the introduction, a single gene affecting resistance to *Salmonella* spp. was identified in mice many years ago. Experiments have also been carried out by Bumstead in poultry to show that resistance to salmonella is strongly correlated with different serotypes and again you can select resistant and susceptible animals. This work, however, has been looking at resistance of the bird to *Salmonella* spp.; another aspect that has been less studied is the ability of animals to carry *Salmonella* spp. even though unaffected and this is becoming increasingly important with the problems of salmonellosis in the human population resulting from eating poultry meat and eggs.

Variation in suceptibility to salmonellosis is also being studied in pigs. There has been little work on the genetics of salmonellosis in cattle, although it is likely that genetic variation exists both in susceptibility to illness and in development of the carrier status and infection of the human population.

Brucellosis

Brucella abortus is another intramacrophage parasite like *Salmonella*. It appears that not all animals are susceptible to brucellosis, the disease it causes. Moreover, of those that are susceptible to the disease only a proportion are protected by S19 vaccination. Workers in Texas A&M university have studied this disease and have bred resistant and susceptible animals and shown that in the resistant animals the macrophages are much more efficient at destroying the organism than in the susceptible (Templeton, personal communication). They have not as yet identified the particular genes involved in this resistance, but clearly the *Nramp* gene which controls resistance to salmonellosis in mice, and to a lesser degree in chickens, is a strong candidate and is one of the genes that they are investigating.

Lameness (see also Chapter 6)

Lameness in cattle is a major constraint to dairy production and there has been much work on causes of lameness. There is little hard data on whether any of these are subject to genetic variation.

Mastitis (see also Chapter 8)

In this country, at least, there has been no collection of mastitis data. I was interested, in the 1970s, in asking whether bulls with a high breeding value for milk production produced daughters that were more or less susceptible to mastitis. I approached the Milk Marketing Board and asked for their assistance in providing data to answer this question. They were unable to do so because no disease data had been collected. However, they subsequently provided me with funds to study the genetics of culling for mastitis in dairy herds in East Anglia and this study showed us that there were in fact very large differences between bulls in the percentage of their daughters that were culled for mastitis; furthermore, if one looked at a list of the bulls that were in use in the areas we were working in, and listed them in order of the proportion of their daughters that were culled for mastitis then there were very popular bulls with high genetic merit for milk production at the top and bottom of the list. Putting it another way, there were bulls with high genetic merit whose daughters were not culled much for mastitis and others where many of their daughters were. Overall, in this survey there was no genetic correlation between yield and mastitis, and we found little difference between bulls in the reproductive problems of their daughters.

There have been numerous estimates of the heritability of mastitis. Some have approached that of milk yield, but most have been very low. Selection against mastitis is relatively recent and is confined so far to Scandinavia. Although the heritability of mastitis may be less than that of milk yield, that of somatic cell count, which is very highly correlated with clinical mastitis, is higher. In Norway they started a country-wide programme for compulsory recording of veterinary treatments of disease in cattle, and this applied to all veterinary surgeons. They recorded treatments for common diseases such as mastitis, ketosis, milk fever, etc. The scheme has been running in Norway since the early 1980s and they have now been joined by Sweden and Finland.

Data are being collected by the Scottish Livestock Service from farmers in southern Scotland and in the DAISY scheme, which has now been taken over by the National Milk Records, and some mastitis data have been collected. Compared with Scandinavia, however, this is minimal.

Economics

The cost effectiveness of selection against disease and for viability depends upon (1) the economic importance of the disease and (2) whether there is a sufficient genetic variation in the population of AI bulls to make rapid progress. Little is known about the economic importance of many diseases because very little work has been done on them; mastitis may be an exception. National recording schemes do not record disease. However, disease data are being obtained in other countries and, as noted earlier, Norway and the other Scandinavian countries collect disease data from the dairy population on a routine basis. This information is then included in a selection index: bulls are selected in part on the disease resistance of their daughters.

Markers of resistance

Much work over the years has looked for associations between markers of resistance that one could measure and traits of importance; an early association was polymorphism in transferrin, the serum protein that carries iron. There are several discrete transferrin alleles in cattle and the question was asked, 'Do animals with one allele produce more milk than those with another?'. Effects were found but they were very weak and often not reproducible. However, there is no great rational reason why transferrin polymorphism should have any relationship with milk production. In humans, associations were sought between blood groups and gastric cancer or ulcers. These associations too were very weak; perhaps the first really strong association seen was with the sickle cell haemoglobin gene when, in the homozygote form, the red cell actually sickles as haemoglobin crystallises out, particularly under oxygen stress. This gene is therefore, if not lethal, very disadvantageous, but in areas where malaria is endemic it is maintained at high frequency because the heterozygotes of normal and sickle haemoglobin are more resistant to malaria. Similarly, there are two species causing malaria – *Plasmodium falciparum* and the less pathogenic *P. vivax*. It has been found that the Duffy blood group is essential for *P. vivax* to enter red cells. Individuals that have no Duffy on their red cell surfaces are totally refractory to infection. Duffy negatives are almost unknown in Caucasians and are confined to people of African origin. If one is resistant to *P. vivax* one is better able to survive *P. falciparum*.

Identifying disease genes

The identification of genes for disease is now becoming feasible. Genome maps are now available for the major agriculturally important species and it is possible to start searching for genes for disease resistance. There are now well over 1000 markers on the bovine genome, distributed fairly evenly over the chromosomes, so that it is possible to search for the area of the genome controlling resistance if you have a suitable population in which to do that. One can also paint animal chromosomes with coloured probes specific for individual human chromosomes and find which human chromosome each part of the animal chromosome corresponds to. By this means animal geneticists can benefit from the massive investment in research in the human genome and it means that the model for animal genome research is no longer the mouse but man.

Double muscling

There has been very intense selection for leanness particularly in pigs and cattle and a number of genes have been identified. One has been selected for in cattle double muscling, a trait seen in Charolais, Belgian Blue, South Devon and the Welsh Black. It causes massive muscular hypertrophy and in the Belgian Blue most affected calves are delivered by Caesarean section. The trait is maintained by the higher value of the meat in spite of the increased management costs.

The speed at which information can be obtained on traits today has recently been shown very vividly with this disease. In May 1997 a paper was published on a knockout of a myostatin gene in mice, i.e. mice that did not have this particular gene. It was found that these animals all had extremely large muscles and that this muscle hypertrophy started *in utero* very like the situation in double-muscled cattle. Michel George and Ruedi Fries in Germany both immediately recognised that this might well be the gene involved in double muscling. They knew where and on which bovine chromosome the double muscle gene was but did not know what it was and had not been able to clone it. They therefore went immediately to libraries of bovine genes and to a particular fragment of that library which they knew contained the double muscle gene and attempted to clone out the gene that had been inactivated in these rapidly growing mice. They cloned the bovine equivalent, then looked at the same gene from double-muscled and non-double-muscled animals, and were able to identify a mutation in the double muscle gene which is almost certainly the cause of double muscling. What this has shown is that this gene is a suppressor of muscle growth and the mutation in fact inactivates the gene and makes it unable to control and modulate muscle growth and so muscles grow very fast (some would say too fast). The initial paper on the mouse knockout came out in May 1997 and the description of the mutation in this myostatin gene in double-muscled cattle was submitted to *Nature* in early July and published in *Nature Genetics* in September of the same year. A group in the USA followed exactly the same route and their paper was published in *Genomics* just days after the *Nature* paper.

Similarly in pigs, the very active selection for growth rate has become linked with malignant hyperthermia. Animals selected for high growth rate occasionally dropped dead particularly following sudden stress and had pale soft exudative (PSE) pork. Three characteristics of the disease – sudden death, PSE and halothane-induced malignant hyperthermia – were found to be controlled by a single gene which was generally more frequent in breeds that had been selected for rapid growth rate. The gene is recessive and it is the homozygous recessives that are particularly at risk. Initially halothane was used for diagnosing the presence of the gene, but more recently the actual gene, a ryanodin receptor, which is a Ca^{2+}-release channel protein, was identified. It is not the same as the double muscling gene. A diagnostic test based on the mutation in the gene was set up and now this disadvantageous mutation has been largely removed from the pig population. With double muscling in the Belgian Blue it is exactly the reverse and in Belgium, particularly, breeders have selected for the gene. The killing-out percentage of the animals is significantly increased from 65% of the carcass being lean meat for the conventional animal to 80% for the double-muscled animal. Consumers are also prepared to pay more per kilogram for the meat even though that meat bears similarities to the pale soft exudative pork seen in stress-susceptible pigs. This increase in economic value occurs in spite of the fact that the milk yield of affected animals is around one-third lower than in normal animals and there are other detrimental effects on fertility and age at first calving.

Trypanosomiasis

As mentioned above, the taurine cattle of West Africa, the N'Dama and Baoulé cattle are tolerant to trypanosomiasis and dermatophilosis. They can survive and produce in areas where European breeds cannot. This resistance was recognised many years ago by Belgium ranchers in what was formerly Zaire who imported N'Damas from West Africa and ran highly successful farming operations in tsetse-infested areas in Africa. Serious efforts are now underway in the International Livestock Research Institute in Kenya to search for the genes that might be controlling this resistance in N'Dama cattle. To do this they have set up populations of N'Dama and susceptible Boran cattle and have crossed these to produce F1 and then subsequent F2 populations. When they look at these animals they find that they are segregating for many of the colour traits present in the parent populations and when they challenge them with trypanosomiasis they find that they are also segregating for resistance to trypanosomiasis. They are thus at the stage when they can identify which genes are segregating in individual animals with resistance or susceptibility. Setting up crosses of this nature and challenging with disease is a very expensive operation. However, the payoff would be if one could identify genes associated with resistance and could then use these for selecting animals to live in high challenge environments.

Enzootic bovine leukosis

Bovine leukaemia virus is a C-type retrovirus that causes lymphosarcoma and persistent lymphocytosis (PL) in about 1% and 30% of infected cattle respectively. Lymphosarcoma and PL cause at least a US $86 million loss to the dairy industry in the USA each year. An association has been found between a BoLA class I antigen A14 and resistance to PL and delay in seroconversion in several herds. Moreover, animals with the A14 allele had longer lifespans in two Holstein herds with a high prevalence of BLV. Resistance to PL has now been mapped, not to the class I region but to the class II region and a particular MHC class II allele DR 3 11 is dominant and has been shown to be closely linked to the A14 class I allele. Thus, if one was to increase the frequency of the A14 DR 3 11 allele so that animals in herds with a high level of BLV all had one copy of the gene, this would have a controlling effect on the disease. Moreover, it has been shown that animals with A14 have significantly increased yields of fat, milk, fat percentage and income over feed costs and decreased scores on the California mastitis tests, also suggesting that having a high frequency of A14 in these affected herds would be beneficial from a number of scores.

Dermatophilosis

Dermatophilosis is another disease that is particularly a disease of European breeds imported into the tropics. Like pink eye, the aetiology is complicated because one needs both the organism and *Amblyomma* ticks; thus it is only present where *Amblyomma variegatum* exists. It has now been shown that a particular MHC class II DRB3 allele is associated with susceptibility; thus, reducing the incidence of this allele would significantly reduce the incidence of the disease.

Ticks

Similar experiments are underway in Australia to study tick resistance in both taurus and zebu cattle. Australian agriculture has to some degree already carried out its selection in that in the more tropical areas of the north, there is a high percentage of zebu blood. Further south there are zebu/taurus crosses and then in the extreme south pure taurus predominates. However, the genes for resistance are being sought and in the zebu it appears that there are several genes whereas in taurus, where there is also genetic variation, resistance seems to be controlled by a single gene.

Tropical theileriosis

Another disease, tropical theileriosis, kills imported European breeds from Morocco to China. It is of major economic importance in the tropics and occurs in southern Spain and Italy. There is a wealth of evidence, much of it at the level of clinical impressions, indicating that local breeds (which in North Africa are taurus not zebu) are more resistant to the disease than imported black and whites and that the crossbreds are somewhat intermediate between the two. However, if you look in Morocco at the black and white population being exposed to the disease, one finds that in each tick season about 40% of the animals that have not seen the disease become exposed to ticks and are infected, but only about 40% of those infected animals become clinically ill. One might ask what relevance this has to British agriculture and at the moment it has none – because of BSE we cannot export cattle. However, if we could export we could identify the genes that determine whether cattle become clinically ill or not. This would be of great economic importance and one could sell animals at a premium.

Relevance to Europe

Some of the diseases mentioned above may not appear at first sight to be of great relevance to British agriculture, but they will and do demonstrate that it is possible to identify genes that play an important role in specific diseases if one is prepared to set up the resources to do so. A collaborative programme between Holland Genetics and the New Zealand Dairy Board is looking for genes controlling milk production in the national herds of the two countries. Although this is clearly a feasible operation for milk yield, it is not for disease as disease traits are not measured.

Challenging animals with disease is not something that can be carried out on the normal commercial population. It may be possible with a large commercial poultry organisation to challenge animals with Marek's disease or salmonellosis and to use these results in selecting elite stock. In the field, however, one hopes to identify markers or preferably the actual genes controlling the disease which can be used in marker-assisted selection (MAS). As mentioned earlier in relation to Marek' disease, this is being used to help the poultry industry by selecting for the B^{21} allele. However, further work is taking place to identify other genes, hopefully with larger effects, and once identified these too can be used.

There has been much work on the major histcompatability complex (MHC), a group of genes controlling a range of immunological functions, and whether there is a rational reason why particular genes within the MHC might be associated with resistance. As mentioned above, the blood group that was found to be associated with Marek's disease has subsequently been shown to be an MHC gene. However, going into particular parts of the genome, even when there is a very rational reason why that region of the genome might be associated with the disease, has largely been superseded by the approach of genome mapping. Genes or DNA sequences have now been identified throughout the genomes of domestic animals. The experiment of studying trypanosomiasis resistance in Kenya is an example of addressing the question of whether particular genes are segregating with resistance or susceptibility. The aim will be to find for one of these loci a large discrepancy from the normal random 50:50 split in the frequency of the two alleles being inherited from the parents in the susceptible and resistant offspring. By this means it is possible to deduce that a particular locus is close to the locus controlling resistance to trypanosomiasis. This leads on to further detailed investigation around the area where the gene is located, hopefully to find the actual gene controlling resistance.

One or many genes?

In salmonellosis in mice a single gene (*Nramp*) has been identified as controlling resistance. This has now been cloned and shown to play a role in macrophage function. However, although this gene is of major importance in a particular *Salmonella typhymurium* challenge in mice it is not the only or even major gene controlling resistance to *Salmonella* in poultry. Other genes have now been found with greater effects than *Nramp*. Thus, the candidate gene approach to identifying genes controlling resistance has value but may involve a lot of work and produce no results.

Development of resistance

In a number of cases you may well find that naive animals from different breeds are equally susceptible but one breed develops resistance very much more quickly than another. This is seen well with infection with *Boophilus microplus* in cattle. The Australians have developed a test where they put 20000 larvae in a band around a cow and then measure the number engorging. As shown in Table 9.3, when they compared naive zebus and Shorthorns there was no differ-

Table 9.3 Development of immunity to *Boophilus microplus* as measured by number of ticks engorging following application of 20 000 larvae.

Application	Brahmin	Shorthorn
1st	4932	4845
2nd	2026	4996
3rd	1428	4685
4th	1514	5062

ence in susceptibility to ticks. However, with successive infestations there was no development of immunity in the Shorthorns whereas there was in the zebu, strongly suggesting that the immune response is in some way involved.

A similar situation occurs with *Eimeria tenella* in chickens. Bumstead selected a number of lines of chickens for resistance to various *Eimeria* spp. and on first challenge at an early age there is no difference between them in resistance to *Eimeria tenella*. However, as time progresses resistance develops. A similar situation occurs with *Ostertagia* in sheep. This late development of resistance strongly suggests differences in the ability to develop an effective immune response.

Efficiency of production

It is commonly thought that big is beautiful, and animal breeders have been advised in places such as West Africa that they should replace the small Boulé, Lagune and N'Dama cattle with large fast-growing European breeds. If this is done European breeds die either from susceptibility to diseases or because they are unable to walk far enough to obtain water. However, it has been shown that if a comparison is made between British breeds of their efficiency of food conversion then there is more variation in food conversion efficiency within breeds than between breeds. In other words, the large breeds, such as the South Devon, are no more efficient as converters of food into meat than the small Dexter, the difference lying in the fact that they eat more and therefore grow faster. Large appetites are a distinct disadvantage where food supplies are limited.

If in the absence of disease and climatic stress there is no difference in efficiency, it is likely that under stress the large non-adapted animals will be less efficient than the small adapted breed. This is borne out by the experience in Australia where under temperate conditions a Shorthorn or Hereford grows faster than the zebu or zebu crosses whilst in tropical areas the zebu grows fastest.

Selection for resistance

How do you select against disease? As mentioned earlier, in the early parts of the century many experiments challenged animals with diseases such as tuberculosis and then selected survivors. However, for many diseases this is impossible – one could not conceive setting up a challenge experiment with foot-and-mouth disease, for example. It is also difficult if not impossible for the farmer or veterinarian in the field to carry out selection as they only see a very small snapshot of the population. With cattle, in particular, a farmer will only have one or very few offspring of a particular bull on his farm. If there is some increase in susceptibility to a particular disease in the offspring of that bull, he will never see it. Nor will he be able to identify the bull as the cause of a problem that he may have in only one offspring. If he has four daughters of a bull and two have mastitis sufficiently seriously to require culling he is unlikely to associate it with the bull. If, however, it was known that 50% of that bull's daughters across all farms were being culled for mastitis he would not use that bull again.

At the moment our milking industry operates with very high management inputs and animals are shielded from disease. However, in the future one can foresee that pressure for low input systems will increase. It is already happening with the pressure to put pigs and poultry into extensive management systems. It is likely that there will be pressure to reduce the use of antibiotics in feed and generally to reduce the use of drugs in any animal products destined for human consumption. Thus, the need for genetic resistance will increase and it would be hoped that individuals in the field will be observant, as was the case with BLAD, and that pressure will be put on the funding agencies to support work on disease genetics. For example Bumstead has lines of chickens that differ in susceptibility to coccidia and *Salmonella* spp. However, it is very much easier to produce lines of chickens that differ in disease susceptibility and to carry out experimental challenges to produce those lines than it is with cattle, and the costs and time involved in asking genetic questions in cattle are great. However, as in the case in the dairy industry, 100 000 offspring from a particular bull is not uncommon and if it were possible to know that disease resistance genes were being transmitted, this would have great economic value. Increasingly such knowledge will become essential for successful cattle breeding. The potential of genome mapping and the identification of disease-resistance genes will be helped by the massive work in man and in the smaller mammals and birds. It may well be possible to foreshorten the effort in cattle by making use of the information in other species.

Where do we go from here?

As mentioned earlier, from the beginning of the progeny testing schemes it was shown that there were differences in the survival of the offspring of bulls with the same breeding value. This still occurs and animals with the same PIN value will produce daughters with differing survival rates. Attempts to utilise this information are already being made. There are some indicator type traits that are known to be correlated with daughter survival and these traits are included in ITEM (index for total economic merit), which together with PIN value gives an estimate of the sire's worth. However, there are plans to expand this because data are collected within the national system on daughter survival and new statistical techniques are being developed which will enable this information to be directly included in bull proofs. The Animal Data Centre is including a breeding value for longevity in those proofs. Moreover, Scottish Livestock Services and the management system formerly known as DAISY, now managed by the National Milk Records, are collecting some information on survival and culling for mastitis which can be included in future.

Bull selection

There is no general proposal at the moment to include or to introduce a system such as the one that occurs in Scandinavia, where all veterinarians record their treatments for mastitis, ketosis and other diseases, and these are then included in the PIN value for the bull. As was mentioned earlier in this chapter, a single gene affects susceptibility to *E. coli* in pigs. There is also another single gene affecting *E. coli* resistance in cattle which has been patented and is soon to be released. There may be variation in the ability of cattle to carry and pass on to the human population pathogenic *E. coli* and *Salmonella* spp.

It is only 10 years ago that a scientist researching calf diarrhoea commented in a talk that it 'runs in their jeans'! One can no longer make fun of genetic resistance. Until there is strong enough pressure to collect data on disease and set up specific experiments to study susceptibility and resistance to pathogenic organisms in our cattle this data will not be collected. Over the past 30 years it has been shown conclusively that it is to the financial advantage of the farmer to select for traits giving higher production. In the future the cattle and beef industries need to become convinced that selecting against disease susceptibility or for disease resistance is economically beneficial and environmentally and socially advisable. It may well be that consumer pressure will force movement in this direction, but it would seem sensible that the industry itself should take the initiative. The poultry and pig industries are already doing so.

Further reading

Axford, R. F. E., Bishop, S. C., Owen, J. B. & Nicolas, F. W. (Eds) (1999) *Breeding for Disease Resistance in Farm Animals*, 2nd edn. CAB International, Wallingford.

Bumstead, N. (1996) Breeding for disease resistance. In *Poultry Immunology* (T. F. Davison, T. R. Morris & L. N. Payne, eds), pp. 405–11. Carfax Publishing Company, Abingdon.

Gray, G. D., Wollaston, R. R. & Eaton B. T. (1995) *Breeding for Resistance to Infectious Diseases in Small Ruminants*. Australian Centre for International Agricultural Research (ACIAR) Monograph 34, Canberra.

Office International des Epizooties (1998) *Genetic Resistance to Animal Diseases*. Revues Scientifique et Technique, Vol 7.

Stear, M. J., Bairden, K., Bishop, S. C. *et al.* (1997) The genetic basis of resistance to *Osteragia circumcincta* in lambs. *Veterinary Journal* **154**, 111–19.

Chapter 10
Internal Cattle Building Design and Cow Tracks

John Hughes

The influence of cubicle design on cow lameness and cow comfort (see also Chapter 6)

Lying requirements

The natural enviroment for the cow is the field. When she lies down she is cushioned by a carpet of grass. She needs this because she supports 80% of her body weight on her two knees and her hock joint. If you look at the 'form' made by a cow where she has lain overnight, it gives a good indication of her space requirements in terms of what she needs for a bed. The average Holstein/Friesian measures 1.8 m (6 ft) from tail to brisket and 60 cm (2 ft) from brisket to nose. This means that when the cow is lying in her normal position with her head outstretched for cudding she takes up an overall length of 2.4 m (8 ft) (Fig. 10.1). In this position her jaw will be 38 cm (15 inches) above the pasture. The indentation in the grass will show that the overall width taken up by stomach and hip is 1.2 m (4 ft).

Cows like to lie uphill as this helps to take away the pressure exerted by the rumen on the diaphragm and consequently the heart and lungs. If a field has a slope they will always take advantage of it and very rarely will you see a cow lying facing downhill. Close examination of the indentations in the ground made by the two knees and the hock indicates the pressure exerted at these points.

Video recordings have shown that when a cow gets up she makes an average of 30 separate movements (Fig. 10.2). Because the back leg and hock joint are used for support in the lying position, when rising the cow has to draw the other leg in and position the foot as close to the body as possible so that she can use it to lift up the hindquarters. The force exerted on this foot is indicated by the fact that a hole about 5 cm (2 inches) deep is often left in the ground. As the hindquarters rise, the head slides forward over the grass approximately 60 cm (2 ft) which makes the overall length taken up by the cow when lying and rising in the field 3 m (10 ft). With the hindquarters raised and on her knees the cow extends one foot 45.7 cm (18 inches) and again using only one leg lifts her

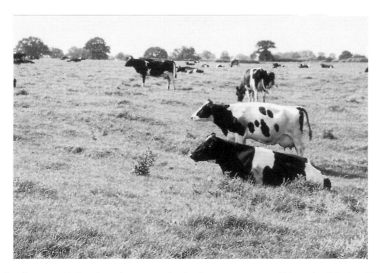

Fig. 10.1   A cow with her head outstretched takes up an overall length of 2.4 m (8 ft).

forequarters, but because the forequarters are significantly heavier than the hindquarters she assists the lifting process by throwing up her head.

Common cubicle design (see also p. 39)

When cows come in for winter housing, the cubicle bed should allow them the freedom to perform all their natural and essential movements without difficulty. Unfortunately a comprehensive study of conventional cubicles revealed this was not so, and that certain major design faults existed which were likely to cause lameness, discomfort and injury. Cows were restricted in the stalls and the natural 30 movements made in the field when rising were reduced by half. The average length of cubicle is 2.13–2.28 m (7–7 ft 6 inches) and since the modern cow is at least 2.4 m (8 ft) long and each generation of heifers appears to be getting larger she is forced to lie either tight against the front wall of the stall or with her hindquarters hanging over the kerb. If she lies forward her head is at a right angle which restricts rumination (Fig. 10.3) and if she lies back she experiences extreme difficulty rising (Fig. 10.4) and often has to resort to a dog-sitting position (Fig. 10.5).

   The solid lower rail of the stall divisions causes pressure on the hip bones which frequently results in lesions. The restricted length of the cubicle means that when the cow gets up she has to lunge sideways between the top and bottom rails of the stall division. The top rail is often set only 91 cm (3 ft) high and when a head rail is attached it means that the cow has no head movement and is virtually trapped (Fig. 10.6).

Lameness due to cubicle design

The majority of cubicles have been concreted and the popular bedding materials are chopped straw and sawdust. When spread over concrete the bedding

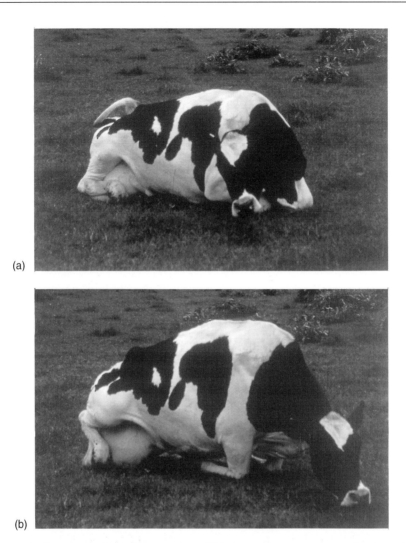

Fig. 10.2 A cow goes through an average of 30 separate movements as she rises. (a) This is an early movement; (b) another early movement in rising, soon after that shown in (a).

disperses as the cow lies down and knees and hock are exposed to bare concrete. Since the two knees and the hock, as previously mentioned, form a tripod supporting most of the body weight, the result is that she attempts to form protective pads over vulnerable areas, such as joints, which would otherwise be damaged and this leads to swellings, which can become quite gross and often develop infection (Fig. 10.7). When large cows lie in conventional cubicles with solid lower rails the pressure against the protruding hip bone results in lesions (Figs. 10.8 and 10.9).

Constriction, discomfort and the inability to ruminate force cows to stand, and, because the cubicles are frequently too short and/or where a head rail is fitted, they are compelled to stand half in and half out of the beds. Since the average

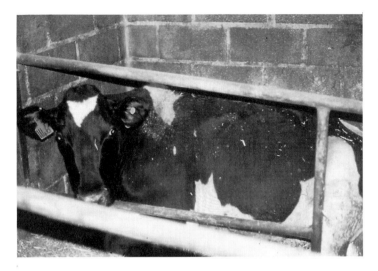

Fig. 10.3 A modern cow in a traditional cubicle. The head is at an angle that restricts rumination.

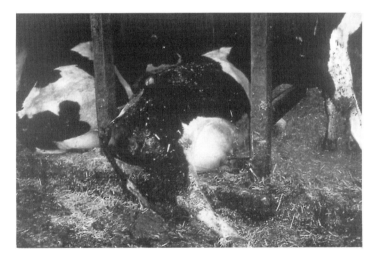

Fig. 10.4 A cow lying back in too small a cubicle, which leads to extreme difficulty in rising.

height of the kerb to the cubicles is 25 cm (10 inches) (railway sleepers were the convenient means of shuttering the concrete to form the beds), standing with her back feet in the channel imposes undue stress on the flexor tendon which eventually weakens, causing her to put pressure on the heel and this results in the overgrowth of detached horn and erosion (Fig. 10.10). When a cow stands normally she has 60% of weight on her front feet and 40% on her back feet. Standing half in the cubicle reverses this. In addition to the stress on the back feet, slipping on the kerb when rising and when attempting to back out causes haemorrhaging which predisposes the hind feet to sole ulcers.

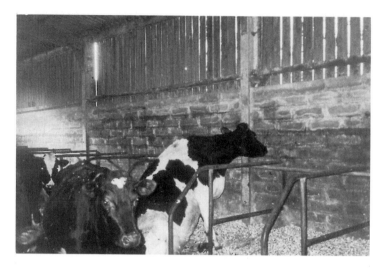

Fig. 10.5 A cow in a dog-sitting position as the cubicle is too small.

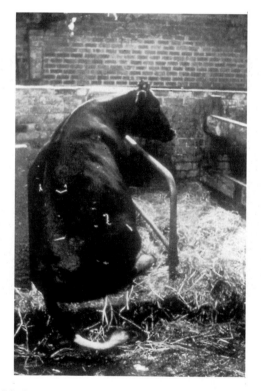

Fig. 10.6 This cubicle has almost no room for head movement, leaving the cow virtually trapped.

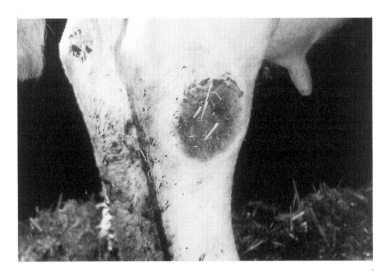

Fig. 10.7 Damage to the hock and skin of the leg from too narrow and too short a cubicle.

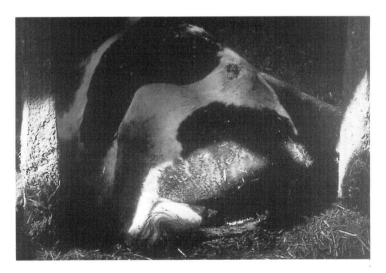

Fig. 10.8 Damage to hip bones.

Cows gradually come to terms and adapt to the constriction and discomfort of cubicles, but the autumn calving heifers take several weeks to adapt and during this time they may have an average lying time of only 2 hours in 24. The effect of this often manifests itself in stiffness, lameness, loss of condition and infertility.

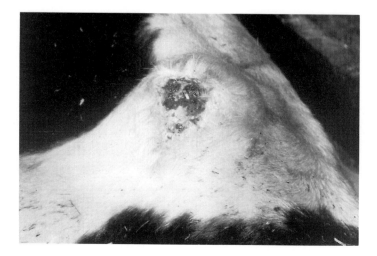

Fig. 10.9   Damage to hook bones (tuber ischii) caused by a too small cubicle.

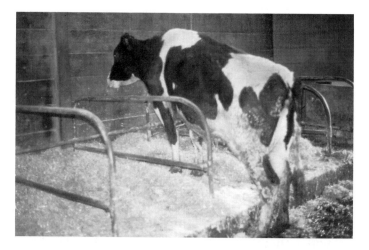

Fig. 10.10   Cow standing with her feet in the dung passage, thereby placing undue stress on the flexor tendons.

The ideal cubicle (Figs. 10.11 and 10.12)

The problem with many of the current cubicle sheds is that they were constructed and designed 20–25 years ago when the main aim was to fit as many cubicles into a building as possible. The plans were frequently drawn up by people who had little contact with or understanding of cows. The issue has been complicated further in recent years by the introduction of the Holstein cow which is a, significantly larger animal. By careful study of the cow's behaviour at pasture and observing all her movements it is possible to design a cubicle that gives her virtually every comfort and freedom that she enjoys in the field.

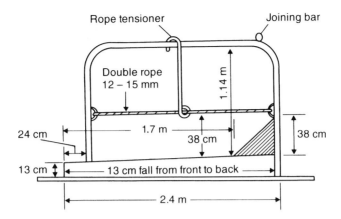

Fig. 10.11 A single cubicle.

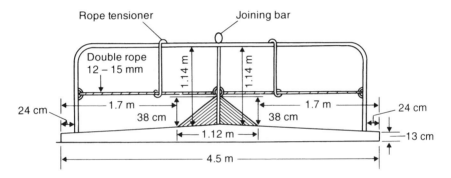

Fig. 10.12 A double fronted cubicle.

The ideal cubicle should be 2.4 m (8 ft) long and 1.14 m (3 ft 9 inches) wide with a fall from front to back of 13 cm (5 inches). There should be no head rails. Cows should be positioned in the cubicles by means of a concrete fillet, the base of which should start 1.7 m (5 ft 8 inches) forward from the edge of the kerb, and the apex of the fillet should be 38 cm (15 inches) high (Fig. 10.13). It is very important that the cubicle kerb height should not be more than 13 cm (5 inches). For the base of the cubicle beds you have the option of rammed clay, bitumenised stone or concrete. If concrete is used, mats are required to provide an adequate cushion to prevent injury; long straw is a possible alternative but it needs a considerable quantity applied daily (Fig. 10.14). The front end of the cubicle stall divisions should be 1.14 m (3 ft 9 inches) high and the lower rail flexible (Fig. 10.15). For head-to-head cubicles the fronts should be open and the cows positioned on the beds by means of a concrete pyramid. The base of the pyramid should start 1.7 m (5 ft 8 inches) forward from the kerb and the apex should be 38 cm (15 inches) high. Because the cows have maximum forward lungeing space the length of the open-fronted cubicles can be reduced to 2.28 m (7 ft 6 inches). To divide the two rows of cubicles, a tubular rail should be fitted 76 cm (2 ft 6 inches) above the apex of the pyramid.

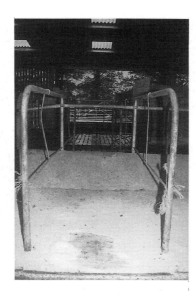

Fig. 10.13   Concrete fillet 1.7 m (5 ft 8 inches) from the edge of the kerb.

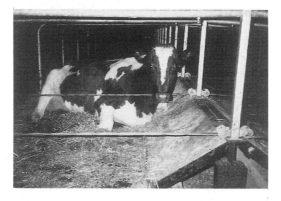

Fig. 10.14   Well-bedded cubicles of a suitable design.

Where this modified design has been introduced the indications are that there is virtually 100% acceptance by heifers, lying time is close to that recorded at pasture, enlarged knees and hocks rarely occur and the incidence of lameness is significantly reduced.

Management and design of straw yards

Cow behaviour

To discover what cows need in terms of comfort and welfare you just have to watch them when turned out to spring pasture. Entering the field after morning

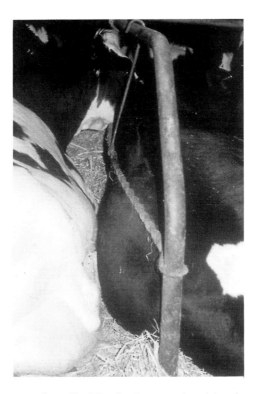

Fig. 10.15 Use of a rope allows flexibility for the cow when lying down.

milking they will graze avidly and then lie down to cud for about 2 hours on a comfortable cushion of grass. Cows at pasture will lie for approximately 12 hours out of 24 and of this time they spend 7 hours ruminating. Of the ruminating time, 5.5 hours is spent lying down and 1.5 hours standing. Straw yards equate very favourably to this pattern.

Winter housed in a well-designed straw yard, cows will lie down on average 13 hours out of 24 and cud for 8 hours. Of the ruminating time, 6 hours is spent lying down and 2 hours standing. The extended ruminating and lying times on straw can probably be accounted for by the fact that food is conveniently near and straw that is eaten excites rumen activity. All the movements made when lying and rising are the same as in the field. The shortcomings of conventional cubicles for winter housing compared to straw yards can be assessed when we contrast a lying time of 13 hours on straw compared with 8 hours in cubicles and a lying cudding time of 6 hours on straw compared with only 1.5 hours in cubicles (see Table 10.1). Also in cubicles, the 30 normal movements made when rising is often reduced to 15.

Advantages of straw yards

It is for these reasons that most farmers changing from a conventional cubicle shed to loose housing on straw comment on a substantial increase in milk

Table 10.1 Time spent by cows in various activities per 24 hours.

	Lying	Ruminating	Ruminating lying	Ruminating standing
At pasture	12	7	5.5	1.5
On straw	13	8	6	2
In cubicles	8	7	1.5	5.5

Table 10.2 Mastitis records for farm T during winter housing before and after entering straw yards.

Year	New clinical cases	Cell counts (×10³ cells/ml)	TBC (band)
1993/1994*	14	84	A
1994/1995**	19	69	A
1995/1996**	10	111	A

* In cubicles.
** In straw yards.

Table 10.3 Mastitis records for farm LH during winter housing before and after entering straw yards.

Year	New clinical cases	Cell counts (×10³ cells/ml)	TBC (band)
1991/1992*	19	152	A
1995/1996**	14	82	A

* In cubicles.
** In straw yards.

production of up to 500 litres per cow and dramatic decline in lameness where lameness has been a problem. A recent study has been completed in which the prevalence and incidence of lameness and mastitis were measured when cows were originally housed in cubicles and later when the same animals were changed to loose housing on straw (Tables 10.2 and 10.3; Figs. 10.16–10.19). Unfortunately this comparison was made between conventional cubicles constructed about 20 years ago and newly designed straw yards. What is required now is a straight comparison between a new well-designed cubicle shed and a new well-designed straw yard.

One of the undoubted advantages of the straw yard is seen in respect of the autumn-calving heifer. She is spared nearly all the stress resulting from confrontations with bully cows. Furthermore, she has a much better chance because of lying time to overcome the tenderness in the feet which nearly always manifests itself in the post-calving period. These two factors can have an important influence on fertility.

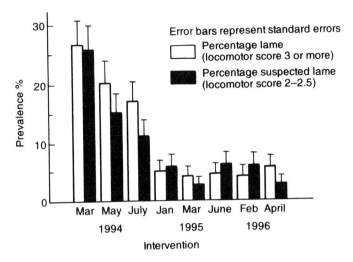

Fig. 10.16 Prevalence of lameness on farm T before and after intervention.

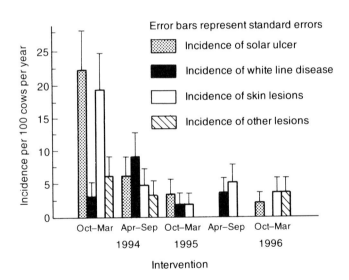

Fig. 10.17 Incidence of lameness of farm T before and after intervention.

Disadvantages of straw yards

Whilst extolling the virtues of the straw yard we also have to be aware of the problems that can be encountered. The cost of straw is often a deciding factor; in the arable areas of the eastern counties it can cost as little as £10 per tonne whilst in the western regions of Devon, Cornwall and Wales it can be up to £70 per tonne. The quality of the straw is also of vital importance. It should not exceed 15% moisture content. All too often the bales are left uncovered and the beds are littered with damp material. This provides an open invitation to mastitis

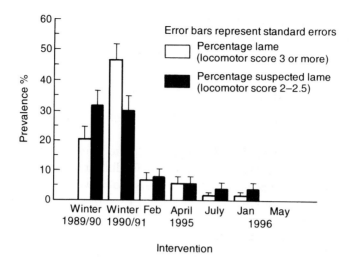

Fig. 10.18 Prevalence of lameness of farm LH before and after intervention.

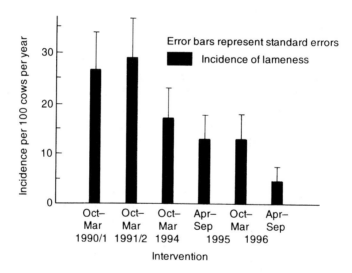

Fig. 10.19 Incidence of lameness on Farm LH before and after intervention.

pathogens, particularly *Streptococcus uberis* (see p. 247). Good ventilation is also an essential ingredient for a straw yard. This means adequate height to the eaves and a well pitched roof. To avoid trodden teats and excessive poaching of the litter the bedded area should never exceed 10 m (30 ft) in width and there should be open access to the feed area along the whole length of the shed.

The incidence of environmental mastitis so feared by farmers who contemplate adopting a straw yard system is above all the result of humidity in the building and the heating up of the bed as a result of fermentation. Once the substrata of litter reaches 37 °C multiplication of pathogens is so rapid that the challenge to the teats becomes too great and cows start to breakdown with infection. Experience has shown that, with careful design of the building and regular cleaning out, the risk of mastitis can be reduced to insignificance.

A successful straw yard

My guidelines for the design of a successful straw yard are as follows:

- The building should be divided longitudinally to allow 7.3 m (24 ft) for the bedded area and 3.7 m (12 ft) for the loafing/feeding area (see Fig. 10.20). This gives the flexibility that, should the need arise to convert to cubicles at some future date, the 7.3-m (24-ft) bed allows for two rows of 2.75-m (9-ft) cubicles with a 24-m (8-ft) slurry passage, with the feeding arrangements remaining unchanged. The allocation of space for the bedded section should be based on 6.5 m² (70 ft²) for the freshly calved, 5.57 m² (60 ft²) for mid lactation cows, and 4.6 m² (50 ft²) for dry cows. Additionally, 2.3 m² (25 ft²) per cow is required for the loafing/feeding area. It should be divided by means of railway crossing sleepers set into right-angled steel joist (RSJ) sections. The RSJs should be firmly set in concrete and allowed to protrude 30 cm (1 ft) above floor level. When the sleepers are slotted in the RSJ sections, allowance should be made for a 2.5-cm (1-inch) gap between the sleepers and the floor to allow for seepage from the bedded area onto the concrete loafing area.
- The bedded area should have a slope of 1:60 towards the loafing area. If the water table is high or if the land is not free draining, this section should be concreted; otherwise well-consolidated hardcore can be used.
- The water trough should be of large capacity and set into the bedded area,

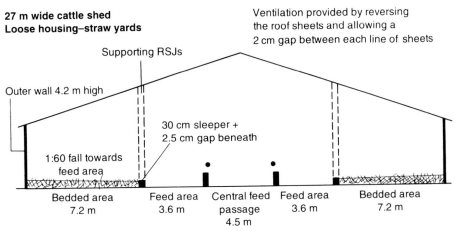

NB: The base of the feed manger should be made 62.5 cm high and the top rail fitted 65 cm above and inset 5 cm towards the forage

Fig. 10.20   A 27.5-m (90-ft)-wide cattle shed with loose housing.

with the front of the trough in line with the sleeper division to assist scraping. The water trough should be built around on the bedded side up to approx. 135 cm (4 ft 6 inches) above the level of the bedding to force cows onto the loafing area to drink; otherwise poaching of the bedding will occur (see Fig. 10.21).

- The feeding passage/loafing area should be constructed of flat concrete with convenient doorways to facilitate daily scraping. The feeding passage should never be less than 3.66 m (12 ft) wide.

- The bed should be formed by a 10-cm (4-inch) layer of sand topped with straw. The sand acts as a soakaway and, as it is inert, helps to prevent heating up of the bedding which can lead to the incubation of coliforms. If the straw is removed every month the use of sand is not so essential. The usage of straw should be based on 2.5 tonnes per cow for a 180-day housing period.

- Good ventilation is essential to the success of a straw yard. To ensure this I recommend that the roof sheets are reversed when put on and that a 2-cm (¾-inch) gap is left between each sheet. As an alternative, spacers can be fitted in the horizontal line of the sheets or, where there is an existing roof, slots can be cut to let the roof breathe (see Fig. 10.22). The ridge should be open or preferably fitted with upswept ventilators. Traditional roof cowls should be avoided as they tend only to produce a downdraught. The building should have a height to the eaves of 4 m (14 ft), with a solid wall up to 3 m (10 ft) high. The gap between the wall and the eaves should be fitted with space

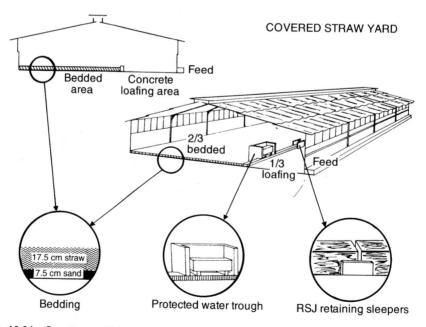

Fig. 10.21   Structures within a covered straw yard.

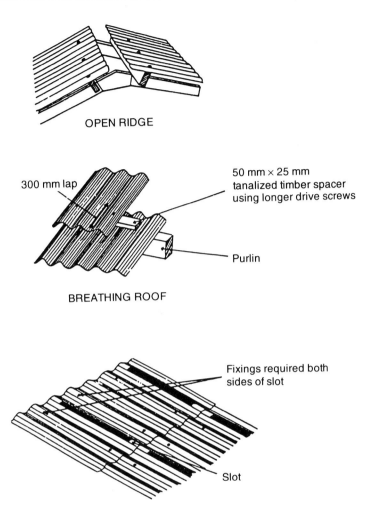

OPEN RIDGE

300 mm lap

50 mm × 25 mm
tanalized timber spacer
using longer drive screws

Purlin

BREATHING ROOF

Fixings required both
sides of slot

Slot

CUT SLOTS

Fig. 10.22 Ventilation for a covered straw yard.

boarding with 3.8 cm ($1\frac{1}{2}$ inch) gaps. Space boarding should also be fitted in the gable ends. Alternatively, if it is not subject to prevailing harsh weather conditions it can be left open.

For methods of ventilation.

• Cows are best divided into groups in a straw yard and the optimum number for a group is 40. The maximum number is 60. When cows are in groups of 40 they quickly establish their social order and this reduces stress and bullying, especially when heifers are introduced to the herd. It also means that the yards can be cleaned out and rebedded in about 2 hours.

- When cleaning out, if necessary an electric fencing wire can be set up along the line of the dividing wooden sleepers and by this means cows can be confined to the feeding/loafing passage where food and water is available to them, thus causing no privation.
- To overcome the manual task of spreading the straw over the bedded area, machines are now available that will rip (not chop) the bales and blow the straw evenly over the beds, reducing the time spent in littering to a matter of minutes.

Conclusion

There is no doubt that cows enjoy greater comfort in a straw yard, there is rarely any problem with lameness, pollution is diminished and farmers adopting the system often comment that milk yields improve. It is my opinion that a straw yard is the best place for first-calved heifers and any infirm cows. The only problem is the cost of the straw for bedding. In practical terms it means you need an acre of arable land for every cow or alternatively a local supply of straw at a reasonable cost.

Cow tracks

Historical perspective

The modern cow is very different from her indigenous predecessors the Short-horns, Ayrshires and conventional British Friesians. The swing towards the pure Holstein and the fact that we currently source 80% of the semen from abroad, where many cows are permanently yarded, has resulted in a much larger, angular and often more fragile animal. Milk yields have increased significantly and the types of animals now giving 9000 litres are having to carry between their hind legs the equivalent of 50 kg (1 cwt) in milk and udder tissue on their journey from pasture to farmstead.

For centuries the gateways and the lanes from farm to field were designed primarily for the horse and cart. The gateways were drained where necessary, and made up with cobblestones to prevent a heavy-ladened cart pulled by two horses from sinking. The lanes were built up with large cobblestones set deep to expose only the rounded tips. A ditch usually ran alongside to prevent the roadway flooding. The cows shared these facilities in the summer and such surfaces were well suited to their needs.

The coming of tractors, drawing ever larger tankers and trailers, resulted in the collapse of the gateways and the disintegration of the cobbled lanes. The drains and ditches disappeared. To provide the necessary access for the tractors and large vehicles the sunken damaged roadways were either levelled off with large quantities of shale or concreted. Neither surface was suited to cows. The shards of stone pierced the white line and often resulted in infection and abscess formation, whilst small stones on unforgiving concrete punctured the soles and heels. If there were grass verges alongside these roads cows took advantage of them and walked in single file abandoning the stone and concrete surfaces for the kinder grass and soil.

Cow track design

It was this observation that cows showed a preference to walk in single file that led to the development of purpose-built cow tracks. The preferment for moving in single file is demonstrated not only where they walk alongside roadways but also when they cross large pasture fields. It was also reasoned that if horses required all-weather gallops then surely a herd of cows needing only a comparatively narrow track deserved a similar surface. Consequently discussion with Terram Ltd., the suppliers of the geotextile used in the making of horse gallops and schooling rings, led to the development of cow tracks. Figures 10.23 and 10.24 demonstrate the methods of building a cow track.

Essentially, it involved cutting out a trench 1 m (3 ft 3 inches) wide and 30 cm (12 inches) deep. The trench was lined with a white permeable geotextile membrane, the purpose of which is to prevent sinkage of the track occurring. (A similar material is used to support motorways.) With ordinary farm roadways, sinkage is often one of the main problems since it leads to water-filled potholes and the eventual disintegration of the surface.

Having lined the sides and bottom of the trench with white membrane, angular 35-cm (1.5-inch) stone aggregate is then introduced to a depth of approx 20 cm (8 inches). If the land over which the track passes is particularly wet then a perforated plastic drainage pipe is incorporated in the layer of aggregate and allowed to discharge into a convenient ditch or soakaway. The crushed stone is then covered with a black geotextile membrane which permits water and mud to permeate downwards through it but prevents any return to the surface of mud and stones. The track is given a final topping with 'Cundy' peelings to a maximum depth of 10 cm (4 inches). 'Cundy' peelings are the by-product of stripping pine fencing posts. Many different materials were tried for topping the tracks, such as woodchips, wood bark and quarry dust. None of them really stood up to heavy storm conditions except for the peelings, which in all aspects, including durability and cleanliness, proved excellent.

The concept was extended to gateways and the surrounds to water troughs. Excavating an area about 15 m (49 ft) wide at the approach to gateways from the fields and building up as described for the tracks will provide a firm clean approach to the gateways rather than the churned up mud which so often results in spring and autumn. A separate gateway formed with white Terram as a base (to prevent sinkage and flooding) and topped with stone should be created for tractors and farm vehicles alongside the field access for the cows.

The tracks need to be topped up with peelings twice during the grazing period and where they run along a hedge bank the hedge needs to be regularly cut back,

(1) Excavate a trench one metre wide (3'3") by 30 cm (12") deep and to the required length. Unwrap the Terram membrane and note it comprises two contrasting fabrics—the WHITE material to line the track and the BLACK material to lay above the aggregate.

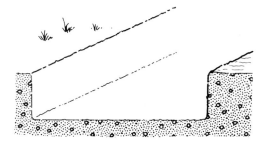

(2) Roll out Terram membrane to full length required. Lay the WHITE material across the trench to within 10 cm (4") of the opposite side and keep the BLACK material unfolded on the adjacent track or bank. If you wish, weigh it down with stones. The joint between both materials should now be positioned around 10 cm (4") from the trench side.

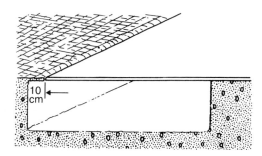

(3) Push the WHITE material into the trench to line both sides and bottom. Make sure the material joint lies on one side of the trench, 10 cm (4") down from the top. The BLACK material should remain in position at one side of the trench and the WHITE material fold out on the opposite side by around 0.5 metres (20") prior to trimming.

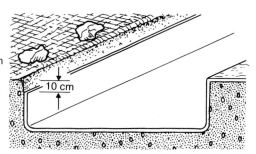

(4) Pour in the aggregate on top of the WHITE material to a depth of around 20 cm (8"). Trim the open edge of the WHITE material which is protruding so when you fold it back on top of the stones, it is no longer than 15 cm (6"). You can cut the material with scissors or a sharp knife.

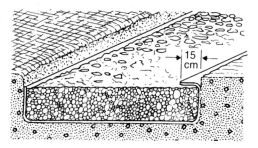

Fig. 10.23   Six easy steps to building a track.

(5) Compact the drainage aggregate to give it stability. Fold back the BLACK material over the stone and push the edge down the back of the WHITE material on the opposite side to secure it. Take out any slack in the BLACK material before moving onto the next stage.

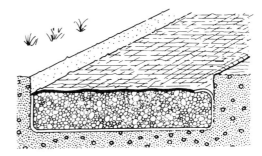

(6) To complete the track, cover the top of the BLACK material with cundy peelings to a maximum depth of 10 cm (4").

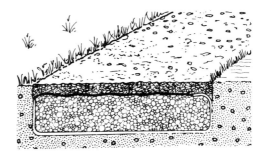

NB: The track is made for cows and will not be strong enough for tractors and trailers.

Fig. 10.23 *Contd.*

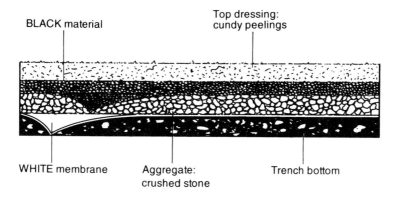

BLACK material

Top dressing: cundy peelings

WHITE membrane   Aggregate: crushed stone   Trench bottom

Fig. 10.24 Building method for a cow track.

otherwise growth along the base of the hedge will force cows off the track. Even nettles and thistles can do this.

The cost of the laying down of the cow track is about £15 per running metre (1.2 yds). This can be reduced to £8 if farm labour is used.

The advantages of the cow tracks and improved gateways are:

- Grazing can be extended at either end of the summer period.
- Lame cows show minimal distress or restriction in movement.
- Bruising and puncturing of the feet is virtually eliminated.
- Unnecessary soiling of teats, udders and feet is prevented.
- They provide a significant contribution to the welfare and comfort of the dairy herd.

Acknowledgements: This chapter was partly originally published as articles in *UK Vet* (Hughes, 1996, 1997) and these are printed here with the permission of the editor.

References

Hughes, J. W. (1996) The influence of cubicle design on lameness and cow comfort. *UK Vet*, **1** (7), 70–4.
Hughes, J. W. (1997) The management and design of straw yards. *UK Vet*, **2** (3), 17–21.

Chapter 11

Dairy Farming Systems: Husbandry, Economics and Recording

Dick Esslemont and Mohamed A. Kossaibati

The dairy cow's life cycle

The life cycle of the dairy cow can be split into two: (1) the rearing phase and (2) the milking phase.

The rearing phase

A dairy cow lives for an average of only six-and-a-half years, milking for about four lactations. A similar culling rate (23.8%) has been reported in a recent UK study (Kossaibati and Esslemont, 1995). As the cost of keeping an animal for the rearing phase is high (about £1100), and usually the cost of replacing a cow in the herd is more than the money received for selling the cull animal, farmers should try to get the young animal into the herd quickly, and keep her in the herd for as many fit and productive years as possible. The target for any herd should be an average of six lactations; hence a 16% replacement rate should be sought (Kossaibati and Esslemont, 1995).

As cows age, so they become more susceptible to disease. Provided a sensible breeding programme has been followed, as time passes the replacements available to the farmer are also generally of a higher genetic potential. Thus, the farmer has a decision to make as to when to cull a cow, incurring a replacement cost, and when to carry on with her in the herd. Sadly he often does not have the luxury of making such a decision, as most cows are culled for failing to become pregnant.

Cows give more milk as they grow older (Table 11.1), so replacing a cow with a heifer generally means that the herd yield will be reduced. Broadly speaking, the balance is achieved between genetic gain and yield reduction with an 18% replacement rate (Gartner, 1980).

Assuming sufficient quota is available, in a 100-cow herd, reducing the age at first calving from 3 to 2 years increases the typical farm profits by £12915 (Table 11.2), as the hectarage for the heifers required is cut back significantly (see also Table 11.3). The gross margin per hectare from youngstock rearing is very

Table 11.1 Effect of lactation number on milk yield (305 days).

Lactation number	Yield (%) of a mature cow
1	75
2	87
3	95
4+	100

Table 11.2 Benefits of earlier calving in a 100-cow herd.

Physical benefits	Calving at	
	3 Years	2 Years
Area available (ha)	70	70
Area available for cows (ha)	45	54
No. of cows (0.45 ha/cow)	100	120
Area available for youngstock (ha)	25	16
No. of heifers calving per year	25	30
Financial benefits	£	£
Gross margin from cows (£2131/ha)	95 895	115 074
Gross margin from youngstock (£696/ha)	17 400	11 136
Total gross margin	113 295	126 210
Gross margin per ha	1 619	1 803

Table 11.3 Effect of age at first calving on hectarage required.

Age at first calving (years)	Replacement rate (%)	Number of heifers reared each year	Hectarage required
2	20	40	10
3	20	60	18

low, especially when carried out extensively. If alternative enterprises to dairying have to be sought, it is important to choose those with as high a gross margin as possible.

A heifer takes a minimum of around 2 years to reach the size and weight suitable for calving, and to produce a worthwhile lactation. Even so, this lactation is a 'loss leader', as the gross margin is only just about matched by the total costs of producing the heifer (about £1100). Any delay beyond the 2 years increases rearing costs more than the small amount of extra income gained from the higher yield from older calving heifers. An extra day of rearing costs about £1.50 (£1100 divided by 730 days) more than the benefits.

A Holstein heifer should calve at no younger than 22 months old, but at a weight (pre-calving) of around 630 kg (ADAS, 1996; Drew, 1998). The age at calving should be, on average, 24–25 months. The younger calved animals have a longer productive life, and produce more milk per day of life (Table 11.4). There are more difficulties with calving at an older age (over 3 years) than with animals calving at 2 years (Table 11.5). In fact, it is body weight and condition, more than age, that have a key influence on animal performance. Research results published by ADAS (1996) have shown that body condition at first calving has a profound effect on milk yield from first lactation heifers (see Table 11.6).

The heifer herself should be put in calf by dairy semen using a bull with low dystocia rating, so that some replacements can be reared out of heifers. Certainly,

Table 11.4 Effect of age at first calving on lifetime performance. (From data supplied by MMB, 1972.)

Age at first calving (years)	Herd life (lactations)	Lifetime milk production (kg)	Milk yield per day of life (kg)
2	4.00	18 708	8.8
2.5	3.84	17 927	7.8
3	3.78	17 621	7.3

Table 11.5 Effect of age at first calving on calf mortality.

Age (years)	No. of cows calving	% Difficult	% Calf mortality
Under 2	277	16	12
2–2.5	768	10	11
2.5–3	345	13	12
Over 3	60	22	28

Table 11.6 Effect of body weight, condition score and height of Friesian heifers at calving on first lactation performance (305-day mean herd milk yield 5000–6000 kg). (From ADAS, 1996.)

	305-day milk yield (kg)
Body weight (kg) of heifer at calving	
<480 (small)	4172
480–520 (average)	4388
>520 (large)	4549
Body condition score at calving	
Poor (<2.0)	4058
Fair (2.0–2.5)	4327
Good (3.0)	4437
Very good (>3.0)	4571
Withers height (cm) at calving	
<126 (small)	4261
126–130 (average)	4334
>130 (large)	4476

Table 11.7   Effect of age of dam of heifer on yield and performance. (From Furniss *et al.*, 1986.)

	Heifer born to	
	Heifer	Cow
Weight at first service (kg)	370	360
Weight at calving (kg)	496	503
Age at first calving (years)	2.48	2.48
First lactation (305-day) milk yield (kg)	4977	4742
Proportion re-bred	0.80	0.80
Proportion reaching fourth lactation	0.49	0.43
Fourth lactation milk yield (kg)	6308	6153

one round of inseminations can be carried out in heifer groups where heat detection is good (at a rate of at least 60%), before the beef bull is turned in. At 80%
heat detection and 60% pregnancy rate, this means that 48% (according to the
'Fertility Factor') will get in calf in one cycle. Half will be heifer calves, so in a
herd where 25 heifers are introduced each year, an extra 12 or so will be in calf
to the dairy semen, and will produce about six dairy replacement heifers.

While the genetic development will be faster because of this tactic, the milk
yield of heifers out of heifers (Table 11.7) is more than might be imagined
(Furniss *et al.*, 1986). The older cows in the herd can be put in calf to beef semen.
Provided the sires are carefully chosen and the calving is well managed, there
should be little danger of difficult calving. If the recording dates of the AI are
accurate, the heifer can be induced to calve at the appropriate time.

The heifer calves that arrive in the herd early in the season will be much easier
to rear for 2-year calving themselves. This can mean that six more heifers
are reared for calving at 2 years, saving some 8 months in each case. A saving
of 48 calf months at about £1.50 per day is worth £2190 off the costs of heifer
rearing in a 100 cow herd.

Having produced six or so heifer replacements from the dairy heifers
themselves, if we assume the pregnancy rate to a service is 50%, then we
need to produce a crop of 19 or so remaining heifers out of the cows (to make
up the 25 needed). This requires about 80 inseminations with black-and-white
semen in 38 cows. If the herd pregnancy rate is lower than this, say 40%,
then 100 inseminations will be needed in the same number of cows. Usually a
farmer will stop serving his stock with dairy semen after this number is reached.
In well-run farms, this can be finished within 6–9 weeks of the start of the serving
season.

In autumn calving herds, the heifer calves should be born before 1 November.
This allows them to be large enough at turnout to grass next summer (with a
body weight of 150 kg) and at service (380 kg at 15 months) for the animal to
calve successfully at 2 years of age (630 kg body weight prior to calving and
140 cm in height at the withers). These standards are for Holstein heifers
(Drew, 1998; ADAS Bridgets; personal communication). So long as they are at

least 325 kg, it is probably more important to have the heifers at the correct height at service (126 cm) and growing at the correct rate (0.85 kg per day) than be solely concerned about weight; the weight gain post service will compensate (Table 11.7).

Not all heifer calves survive to calve themselves. Losses as high as 22–28% have been recorded owing to a range of causes (Hocking, 1984), including those at birth, through accidents, infertility and abortions. These losses are very expensive, as the animals are sold for about half the costs of rearing them to that stage. According to a survey, 22% of replacement heifers born are lost before their first calving (Kossaibati and Esslemont, 1997). Once calved, too many animals (10% on average) are culled at the end of their first lactation for failing to conceive (Kossaibati and Esslemont, 1995). Better fertility management should allow the farmer to cull low yielding heifers on the basis of yield, and to put the remainder in calf. The most effective strategy is to cull the 10% worst yielding heifers post-partum in their first lactation. It is possible to decide the yield potential before 60–90 days post-partum, and hence have the animals set barren at this stage, saving on the costs of semen (Van Arendonk, 1985). In subsequent lactations, the culling rate increases as a percentage of cows calved (Kossaibati and Esslemont, 1995), with a total of 54% culled by the fourth lactation, 75% by the sixth, and 84% by the seventh. There are, of course, generally very few animals left in their ninth or older lactations. The effect of lactation number on culling is illustrated in Fig. 11.1.

The milking phase

Once calved, the cow should be left for a 6- or 7-week rest period before the 'open season' commences for service. The aim is to have animals in calf between

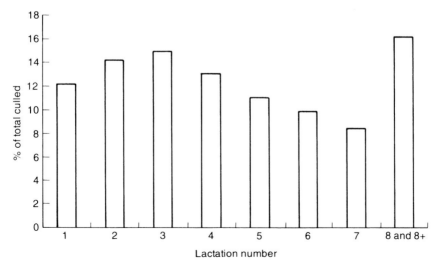

Fig. 11.1   Effect of parity on culling. (From Kossaibati and Esslemont, 1995.)

42 and 100 days after calving. This will produce calving intervals of 322–380 days. Generally, the same profitability per year is obtained for any of these calving intervals. The losses in income per year begin to occur at longer calving intervals (over 380 days).

As the season of calving affects the value of the milk produced in that lactation, and also the margin over all fixed costs per cow, it is as important to consider the date at which the cow will calve next year as it is to consider the interval between calvings. With different dairy companies paying varying incentives for month of production there are no hard and fast rules about which is the most profitable month. It is still commonly true that the best month of calving will produce a margin of some £60 more than the worst.

Cows that are 'late' conceiving lose the farmer about £3 per cow per day (see Table 11.8) off the annual profit (Kossaibati and Esslemont, 1995). Providing the farmer remains under his quota for milk production, the extra milk from the shorter intervals is valuable. If the shortening of the calving interval leads to over-quota production, then the farmer has to make changes in his policy, either

Table 11.8 Total costs of extending the calving interval by one day (for cows yielding 5000–6000 litres). (From Kossaibati and Esslemont, 1995.)

	Unit	Cost (£)	Total (£)
First lactation yield (litre/305 days)	5000		
Milk quality for both lactations			
Butterfat %	4.20		
Protein %	3.30		
Price of milk (£/litre)		0.24	
Drop in yield (per month)	10%		
Extra no. of days in lactation	0.7		
Milk yield at end of lactation (litre/day)	9.22		
Milk quality at end of lactation			
Butterfat %	4.80		
Protein %	3.70		
Extra milk yield (litre)	6.5		
Special milk price for that yield (£/litre) (additional value of £0.04/litre)		0.28	
Return from extra milk			1.81
Second lactation yield (litre/305 days)	6000		
Milk loss for a delay of 1 day (litre)	19.7		
Value of lost milk			4.73
Saving in concentrate			
Quantity (kg/litre)	0.27		
Price (£/kg)		0.147	0.78
Net loss in milk return (*A*)			2.14
Value of calf loss (*B*)			
Price of a calf (£)		120.00	0.33
Cost of extra dry period (*C*)			
Extra period (day)	0.3		
Cost of 1 day (£)		1.78	0.53
Total cost per cow per day of 1 day extra on calving interval (*A* + *B* + *C*)			£3.00

leasing quota at a fee, cutting down on cow numbers, or cutting feeding to reduce yield per cow. He may release forage areas as the stocking rate declines, and these may be used by an alternative enterprise. He may use the released land to grow more forage for the remaining dairy cows. In the calculation of the benefit of shortening the interval, it is assumed that extra quota is leased. There are not many profitable alternative enterprises to dairying, but some intensive cropping methods are worth considering.

The aim is to have an average heat detection rate of 65% and pregnancy rates at 52% or above, but these are standards achieved only by the top 5% (on the FERTEX Score, which is a fertility economics score that takes into account the cost of calving interval and higher culling rates) of farms (Kossaibati and Esslemont, 1995). The effect of the combination of these two indices is the 'Fertility Factor', and this has an important effect on calving intervals and culling rates (see Table 11.9). The Fertility Factor is the multiple of the heat detection rate and pregnancy rate to any one service. Heat (or oestrus) detection rate is the proportion of cows fit to serve seen in heat in 24 days. Fertility Factors, on average, are 26 (Kossaibati and Esslemont, 1995) based on a 56% heat detection rate and 46% pregnancy rate. The effect of Fertility Factor and number of oestrous cycles allowed is illustrated in Fig. 11.2, and these factors determine calving to conception intervals and culling rates.

Most farmers that serve their cows over a 9-month season will stop inseminating cows not in calf when they reach 6 months post-partum, giving most of their cows seven oestrous cycles to be seen, served and got in calf. The target level of culling for failure to conceive is 6% of the herd, leaving 12% (making 18% in total) available for culling for other reasons (Kossaibati and Esslemont, 1995).

The practical target level of this 'Fertility Factor' is 30 (say 50% pregnancy rate and 60% heat detection rates), provided the average interval to first service is below 70 days. In this way, the calving to conception interval is kept below 93 days (373 days calving interval) and the 'infertility culling' is 7% or under.

Table 11.9 Effect of fertility in cows on calving to conception interval and culling rate.

| No. of oestrus cycles allowed | Fertility Factor* | | | | | | | | | | | |
| | 20 | | 25 | | 30 | | 35 | | 40 | | 45 | | 50 | |
	CCI	CR	CCI	CR	CCI	CR	CCI	CR	CCI	CR	CCI	CR	CCI	CR
7	92	21	93	13	92	8	90	5	87	3	84	2	81	1
8	99	17	99	10	96	6	93	3	89	2	85	1	81	0
9	106	13	104	8	100	4	95	2	90	1	86	0	82	0
10+	145	0	124	0	110	0	100	0	93	0	87	0	82	0

CCI, Calving to conception interval (days); CR, Culling rate (%) for failure to conceive in the number of oestrus cycles allowed.

* Fertility Factor is the multiple of the herd pregnancy rate (say 46%) and heat (or oestrus) detection rate (say 56%). UK average Fertility Factor is 26; the top 10% (in terms of FERTEX Score – cost of fertility) of DAISY-recorded farms achieve, on average, 31. See DAISY Report no. 4 (Kossaibati and Esslemont, 1995).

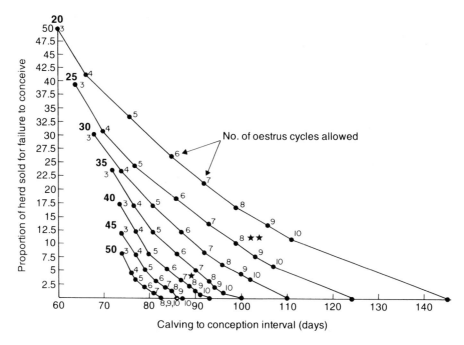

Fig. 11.2 Effect of Fertility Factor and number of oestrous cycles allowed on calving to conception interval and on percentage of herd culled for failing to conceive. ★ Top 10%; ★★ UK average. Fertility Factor (numbers in black circles) = pregnancy rate × heat detection rate, e.g. 50 × 50 = 25. (From Esslemont, 1995.)

Fertility management will have a major effect on the culling levels in dairy herds. In fertile herds the farmer has many more options as far as culling is concerned. Low fertility may be a sign of other husbandry problems, and if the indices are not up to standard, the whole farming system needs examining.

Cows at risk of poor fertility are those that have had calving difficulties, twins, abortions, dead calves, retained afterbirth, endometritis, vulval discharge and lameness. Unless management takes considerable extra care, these cows will have a longer calving interval, lower pregnancy rates, more services per conception, and hence a higher culling rate for failure to conceive. Also, because of the potential risk of disease association (Peeler, 1992), it becomes very important to tackle every single health problem, and keep the levels of production diseases under control to avoid losses in profitability and to maintain the standard of animal welfare (Kossaibati and Esslemont, 1995). An example of the effect of disease on herd fertility is given in Table 11.10. Cows with mastitis are also in a high cull risk category, although not because of lowered fertility.

Normally, the factors that affect fertility are within the control of management. Preventive medicine routines should be installed for each of the potential hazards, helping to keep them to the absolute minimum. If problems do occur, then proper treatment, husbandry and aftercare should return the cow (and herd) to acceptable fertility levels. One of the most important features of this husbandry is good recording and a 'flagging' system for cows at risk.

Table 11.10 Effect of vulval discharge (VLD) on fertility, and its disease association. (From Peeler, 1992.)

	Cows without VLD	Cows with VLD
Fertility parameters		
Calving to first observed oestrus (days)	53.7	56.5
Calving to first service interval (days)	71.3	76.9
Calving to conception (days)	98.8	116.8
Days open*	124.7	150.8
Services per conception	1.8	2.1
Total culling rate (%)	23.2	27.1
Per cent not in calf by day 150	31.1	38.7
Per cent conceived of those originally calved	80.6	77.5
Disease association		
Cows treated for		
oestrus not observed (%)	37.1	43.0
Risk factors		
Cows calving with:		
Aid at calving (%)	10.6	19.3
Calf mortality (%)	4.1	12.0
Twins (%)	1.8	8.3
Retained afterbirth (%)	1.6	12.8

* Average calving to conception for those conceiving plus average calving to culling for those that do not.

Most culling is an involuntary reaction to the results of an earlier slip in management. The fertile sector of the herd, all the cows that do not suffer trauma or disease at calving and are not lame, is generally highly fertile. The culling rate of these animals is often only 3 or 5%. One category that does have a higher culling rate is cows with mastitis (p. 24), and the best policy here, apart from doing all the sensible things to prevent it, is to cull cows with chronic cases of mastitis in that lactation. With good records it should be possible to select out cows that have had mastitis three times in the same quarter, or five cases in all quarters, in the same lactation, also giving the other stock more of a chance to avoid being infected (see Chapter 8).

As far as genetic selection is concerned, the best strategy, provided other culling is at a low rate, is to cull the worst 10% in terms of yield. In UK terms, cows giving an average of less than 12 litres or so per day of lactation are likely to be making a loss. Milk yield and quality are sufficiently heritable to make culling for both factors worthwhile. It is possible to use the first 3-monthly milk recordings to decide the fate of the first lactation heifer (McGuirk, 1992). As far as diseases are concerned, only ketosis and mastitis have sufficient heritabilities to make the selection of the bull to use on this basis worthwhile (Solbu, 1978). Fertility is not a significantly heritable factor to justify selection although in Norway they have incorporated this in their testing programmes.

Cows giving more than 42 litres per day and heifers giving more than 33 litres per day are likely to be more difficult to either seen in heat or get to conceive to services. Most are likely to be in negative energy balance at the time of first service (see Chapter 3).

Growth in dairy herd size

Where quota is not a limiting factor, many farmers are keen to make the herd increase in size. Even those bound by quota often achieve their aim by buying or leasing more. Physical herd growth can be achieved through efficient health and fertility management, so that culling rates are kept down. The effect of a small difference in factors like heat detection and pregnancy rates is considerable over 6 or so years, with a 'fertile' herd increasing in size by 70%, instead of being only 30% larger (see Fig. 11.3). In the better herd, the replacement rate is 7 points lower and the calving interval is 8 days less. These improvements are brought about by only a 10% points improvement in heat detection rate and an 8% better pregnancy rate (Esslemont and Marsh, 1987).

Growth in herd size also comes from reducing the age of first serving of maiden heifers (and hence the age at calving) and by the use of dairy semen on all stock (p. 40 on). Attention to details with calf (see Chapter 1) and youngstock (see Chapter 2) losses is also vital. Attaining a low age at first calving also leads to a longer life for the cow. There is a beneficial effect of the younger age on dystocia (see Table 11.5).

At the expense of producer numbers, which have reduced considerably, herd size has gradually increased, despite a cut in total cow numbers (17%) since the onset of quota in 1984 (see Fig. 11.4). Over the period 1984 to 1994 the average herd size in the UK increased from 58 to 68, and the proportion of dairy cows in herds of 100 cows or more rose from 40.6% to 45.3% (Anon, 1995).

Dairy farms have become more specialised, using more capital intensive

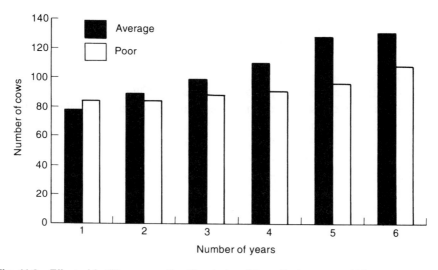

Fig. 11.3 Effect of fertility on growth of herd size. (From Esslemont and Marsh, 1987.)

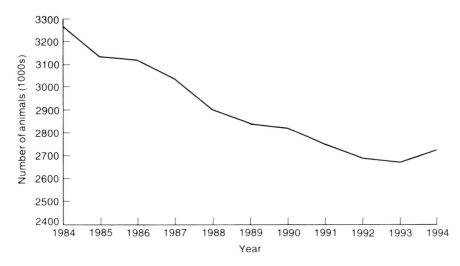

Fig. 11.4 Number of cows and heifers in milk in the UK, 1984–1994. (From Anon, 1995.)

technology and continuing to switch to silage from hay. Maize silage has been increasingly used, along with total mixed rations (see Chapter 3, p. 74). Before the introduction of quotas, product prices were not keeping up with costs, and farm profits fell. Since quotas, farmers have used less purchased feeds, more homegrown forage, spent less on capital equipment, and, with a rise in product prices, the surviving farmers have seen their profits rise too (in real terms) to the highest on record. These are now under pressure because of lower milk, calf and cull prices. Cull and calf prices have been affected by scares over BSE, and milk prices are falling in a response to a decline in demand.

Factors affecting herd size

Generally, quite apart from quota implications, herd size is determined by farm size, as each cow needs about 0.45 ha of forage a year, plus the bought-in concentrates that one still requires. This allows the farmer to maximise the margin from each hectare and litre. Herd size is affected by the time it takes for cows to walk to and from the milking parlour and grazing. Where zero grazing is practised, then other factors, such as machinery costs and slurry handling systems, limit the size of the operation.

Dairy farming is usually a family business, and its size may be affected by the size of the working family and their willingness to milk cows regularly. The herd size is also affected by capital limitations, as the farmer needs to invest considerable amounts of capital in quota, stock and buildings, as well as land, to take in extra cows. In a well-mechanised milking parlour, it takes about 30–40 man hours of labour to look after each cow each year. This excludes any consideration of the time it takes to cope with forage production. If a stockman, or his relief, works 53 hours per week, then he has 2756 hours available in a year. At 35 hours per cow in a year, this allows him to look after about 80 cows 'on his own'.

If there is more investment in equipment, a 'man' may be able to cope with 90 cows or, at the other end of the scale, he may manage 70. In farms where no outside labour is employed, then a common unit size is 60–80 cows. In areas where part-time farming is common, then herd sizes will be lower, at 30–50 cows in a herd. This makes a practical routine possible, involving one member of the family doing the morning milking before leaving for paid employment elsewhere, and a shared responsibility being taken with another family member for other duties. The 30 or so cows will need at least 1050 hours of effort in the year.

Small full-time herds are usually uneconomic because so much of the capital equipment and, indeed, paid labour comes in such large 'units'. A parlour costs £5000 per milking point to install, plus another £10000 for the building. A bulk tank costs £5.00 per litre (£100 per cow in the average herd). Tractors, forage, machinery and concrete yards are all expensive and 'lumpy' in nature, making them expensive for small herds. Herds tend to be found grouped in the sizes that whole units of labour can cope with. Thus, two full-time employees can look after about 160 cows (if 35 hours are required per cow per year). If only 30 hours are needed, then 180 cows can be managed.

If one hard-working farmer or stockman has some help for 1 day a week, then there are 3150 hours available in total, which means, at 35 hours per cow, that almost 120 cows can be kept. Popular herd sizes in the UK reflect this position, with 60, 90, 120, 180 and 240 cow herd sizes being common. Larger herds than this are found, though generally they have not been a success.

The problems of management in herds above 180 cows or so lie more with selecting and keeping staff. Men who excel as stockmen in smaller herds may not have the characteristics needed to organise a team of men in larger ones. Promotion of such stockmen is not likely to be a success, and herd managers who can understand the details of individual animal control, as well as the needs of their staff, have to be found elsewhere. There is a limit to management in the end, and certainly herds of over 240 cows need an extra level of staffing to cope with the volume of work, allow for shift patterns, and yet give the same attention to details. The fact that cow keeping is a work of 7 days a week adds considerably to the difficulties.

In such large herds, there is only a small amount of family labour. There is often a manager who may do some relief milking, and the staff often take their full entitlement of holidays, which may be up to 5 weeks per year. They certainly seek a shift system that includes breaks, to include weekends whenever possible. In a working year of 47 weeks, with a 5.5 day and 50-hour week, one man works 2350 hours. The 240 cows need about 30 hours per cow per year, hence they need 3.1 men to look after them. There may be three herdsmen or stockmen, and the extra cow work needed comes from the owner or manager. The manager may have other enterprises under his direction as well as the cows.

In examples drawn from the USA, there are large economies of scale up to a herd size of 240 cows, but these tail off after that, though they do continue all the way through to the 1400 cow size at the top. The bend in the curve occurs at about 240 cows because of the need at about this size for more investment costs of capital equipment, and more use of professional management. Many of these units do, in any case, keep their cows in sub-groups of about 250 cows. Even in the USA, the economies are gained in the large herds in the warmer west through the use of more automation, zero grazing and simpler housing systems compared with the expensive tie stalls found in the much smaller herds in the eastern half of the country, and in many parts of Europe.

In the UK, despite quotas, herd size is gradually increasing as farmers invest in extra capacity and attempt to benefit from economies of scale. The top 25% of farmers (in terms of margin) are spending an average of £6000 per year on buying quota at around 40p per litre. In depreciation and interest charges, this is equivalent to 15–18p per litre per year and is hard to justify if the money used is borrowed.

Quota leasing costs about 6–8p per litre per year, and again is often hard to justify in terms of return on capital invested. There are often opportunities to improve margins by cutting costs, particularly purchased feed costs, and not simply expanding the output of milk.

Quotas

The rules governing quota are lengthy and complex. A dairy farmer must have either a wholesale quota or a direct sales quota. The quota period is a year lasting from 1 April to 31 March. The quota is issued as litres of milk, and originally was based on 90% of the farmer's milk production in the calendar year of 1983. If an individual's milk delivery to the dairy exceeds his quota, a levy is invoked. At present this levy, based on the 'Target Price', is about 30p per litre, or about 10p more than the farmer will have been paid for that milk already.

The way a farmer's liability to levy payments is worked out is that at the end of the year the net amount of litres that are over quota is calculated. Only if there are more litres produced by over-quota producers than those under quota is a levy liable. Initially, all producers are listed in descending order, according to their percentage over quota. The calculations are done, step by step, with the threshold tested and lowered at each step to the next band of over-quota producers. The total quota and output of all those producing above this threshold is accumulated, and their total levy liability at each threshold percentage is calculated. If this total is less than the 'net amount' over quota nationally, on which the levy is payable, then the threshold is lowered another step and the calculation repeated. The process continues until the net amount is reached. Only those producers over the final threshold percentage pay the levy to meet the total amount due.

There is also a national quota for butterfat (based on a quality of 3.98%). Each producer has a butterfat quota based on the percentage of fat in the milk he produced either in 1984/1985 or 1985/1986 (his choice). If the nation goes over the butterfat quota, each producer has the volume of his quota adjusted for that year, based on the difference between his base butterfat percentage and the percentage in the year in question.

The conversion factor is 18 of volume to 1 of quality. Hence, an increase from 3.77% to 3.97% in a farm's annual butterfat level leads to 18 times the 0.20%

rise. This is a penalty of 3.6% off the volume of quota allocated to that farm. The penalty is calculated on the basis of about 30 p per litre, which is about 10 p more than the sum received in the first place.

Financial performance

In dairying, farm performance can be assessed better than most enterprises. It is a well-recorded industry, with GENUS, ADAS, NMR, feed and fertiliser companies all offering monitoring schemes that, at least, cover the milk sales and feed costs. The typical herd performance is the production of 5300 litres per cow per year, using 1.5 tonnes of concentrates, £18 of other purchased feed, and 0.45 ha of forage for summer grazing and winter supplies of hay and silage (see Table 11.11). Apart from these costs, a farmer has to spend about £52 on other variable or allocatable costs, and from £915 to £1325 per ha (depending on the hectarage over which he can spread them) on fixed or non-allocatable costs (Table 11.12).

At a stocking rate of 2.2 cows per ha, the fixed costs carried by each cow are different for the three size categories (55, 165 and 275 cows). At a gross margin of £853, the profit per cow (before interest) is £257, £351 and £441 respectively (see Table 11.13). If the 'farms' are paying interest on borrowings (say 15% on

Table 11.11   Gross output and gross margin of a typical UK dairy farm. (*Note*: Milk prices are now about 19 p per litre.)

	£/cow	p/litre
Milk (5300 litres @ 24p/litre)	1272	24.00
Calf (allowing for losses)	90	1.70
Less depreciation		
0.25 cull sold @ £400 per head (100)		
0.25 heifer bought @ £700 per head (175)		
Difference £300 per head (75)	−75	−1.41
Total gross output	1287	24.29
Variable costs:		
Concentrates		
0.28 kg/litre, 1.48 tonnes		
@ £146 per tonne	216	4.08
Bulk feed purchased	18	0.34
Forage		
0.45 ha; fertilisers, sprays and		
seeds @ £175/ha	79	1.49
Veterinary medicine	35	0.66
AI recording	30	0.57
Bedding		
0.5–0.7 tonnes of straw	21	0.40
Variable sundries	35	0.66
Total variable costs	434	8.19
Gross margin	853	16.10
Gross margin/ha	1896	

Table 11.12   Fixed costs and profit per hectare of dairy farms, sorted by size (assuming milk yield of 5300 litres per cow, with 0.45 ha per cow).

| | Size of farm (ha) | | | | | |
| | 1–50 | | 50–100 | | >100 | |
	£/ha	p/litre	£/ha	p/litre	£/ha	p/litre
Labour (inc. farmer)	610	5.18	470	3.99	365	3.10
Machinery depreciation	155	1.32	145	1.23	120	1.02
Repairs/tax/insurance	95	0.81	85	0.72	75	0.64
Fuel/electric	70	0.59	60	0.51	50	0.42
General/contract	40	0.34	30	0.25	25	0.21
Total for machinery and power	360	3.06	320	2.72	270	2.29
Rent and rates	185	1.57	180	1.53	170	1.44
Land maintenance	55	0.47	50	0.42	40	0.34
Fixed costs sundries	115	0.98	95	0.81	70	0.59
Total fixed costs	1325	11.25	1115	9.47	915	7.77
Gross margin	1896	16.10	1896	16.10	1896	16.10
Profit	571	4.85	781	6.63	981	8.33

Table 11.13   Effect of herd size on farm profitability.

| | Size of farm (ha) | | | | | |
	1–50 (av. 25)		50–100 (av. 75)		>100 (av. 125)	
No. of cows (0.45 ha/cow)	55		165		275	
			Perfomance			
	£/cow	p/litre	£/cow	p/litre	£/cow	p/litre
Gross margin	853	16.10	853	16.10	853	16.10
Fixed costs	596	11.25	502	9.47	412	7.77
Profit (before interest)	257	4.85	351	6.63	441	8.33
Interest	190	3.58	64	1.20	38	0.72
Profit (after interest)	67	1.27	287	5.43	403	7.61
Profit (£/ha)	149		638		896	
Total profit (£)	3725		47850		112000	

£70000 on average), the fixed costs will be greater by £10500. If the three typical farms are 25, 75 and 125 ha, the interest charge per cow will be £190, £64 and £38 respectively.

This set of illustrative figures shows the effect of scale on profits and the great difficulty that small herds have in surviving financially. In figures drawn from a real sample of dairy herds (GENUS Management, 1993), the factor that is found to determine most how a herd reaches the top 25% in terms of profit is stocking rate, where the better herds achieve 2.06 cows per ha and the worst 25% only 1.79. This factor leads to the better dairy units having a gross margin for the year ending 1993 of £48700 higher than the worst units (see Table 11.14). In addition,

Table 11.14 Profit and disposal of funds (£) in the top and bottom 25% of dairy units. (From GENUS Management, 1993.)

	Top 25%		Bottom 25%	
	1992	1993	1992	1993
Whole farm gross margin	127446	141900	85296	93177
Overhead costs	66596	67277	81986	86053
Profit before depreciation	60850	74623	3310	7124
Depreciation	11681	12856	10582	10925
Profit/(deficit) after depreciation	49169	61767	(7271)	(3801)
Unpaid family labour (UPFL)	34490	34190	23852	24243
Profit/(deficit) after UPFL	14679	27577	(31124)	(28044)
Total cash available	58679	78585	10584	21455
Total cash spent	61418	69664	35119	32307
Cash surplus/(deficit)	(2739)	8921	(24535)	(10852)

the worst 25% herds have very much higher fixed costs across almost all categories, especially interest costs (£23763 for the worst 25% in comparison with £7690 for the top 25%). These poorer herds are 'locked in' to their financial circumstances, and, while making a profit, are in a worsening cash flow position with their loans and overdrafts increasing. The better farms can afford double the capital expenditure, half as much again of private drawings, and pay four times as much tax, yet still have enough cash to be able to reduce their borrowings.

The limiting factor in dairy farming is not only land, which affects economies of scale, but also capital, which limits the use of mechanisation which is one of the main factors affecting growth. Normally, labour remains the most important single factor as the skills of stockmanship in dairying are the fundamental element. Attending to husbandry and keeping control of the financial details are often the responsibility of the same person. It should be appreciated that farmers do not farm normally to maximise their margins, but to attain a quality of life and a sense of achievement in the community. However, to survive there is a need to satisfy creditors above all, whatever the modesty of their own consumption.

Lenders will look at the strength of the balance sheet, checking that assets exceed liabilities in volume and type. Dairy farmers should ensure that money is invested in productive assets like dairy cows, and not so much in depreciating assets like machinery. While lenders like to see a strong set of assets, such as land, they aim to find a 'charge' against which to set their loan, rather than to simply congratulate the farmer. The return on capital in land is not as good as the return in well-run dairy stock. Tenant farmers may make a better return on total capital, but they have little capital growth (unless they own sufficient quantities of quota) and a small net worth on which to retire.

Bank managers like to see plenty of liquid assets, such as youngstock on the farm, whereas the farmer with limited resources will find these animals give a poor return compared with milking as many cows as possible and buying in replacements. Most dairy farmers have twice too many youngstock on their farms.

The main index of financial viability, apart from profit and cash flow, is growth. This is the rate at which the assets-less-liabilities position, known as the 'net worth' on the balance sheet, is increasing, and comes about when the profits are large enough to leave something over when private drawings, taxes and interest have all been paid.

Key indices

Unless the farm is using one of the more sophisticated computerised accounting schemes, it is not possible to keep producing full year-end accounts at the end of each month. Farmers are able to join one of a range of costing schemes that use 15 or so pieces of information each month to produce a wide range of physical and financial performance indices. These can be for the month in question, the same month last year, the cumulative position compared since the beginning of the financial year or the rolling 12-month position. Better schemes also allow the comparison of performance with budget. The better schemes show how the farm is performing in relation to quota. The most useful indices are those that relate closest to the farm profit. As the data entered only at best consist of milk, calf, cull sales and the costs of feed and fertiliser, the margin will only be a crude index of performance.

The first indices to look at are the margin over feed and fertiliser per litre, hectare and per cow (see Table 11.15). These take account of the main limiting factors: quota, stocking rate and cow numbers. However, on most dairy farms, the fixed costs remain fairly set for a year in any case, and the non-food variable costs for the herd, such as AI, veterinary and medicines, recording, bedding and dairy sundries, are fairly static.

These can all be added up and act as a target for the herd margin of milk sales less all purchased feed and fertiliser costs to beat. With an adjustment for calf sales, cull income less heifer costs, and cow valuation changes, this index of MOFF (margin over feed and fertiliser costs) for a year for a herd is most useful. The other indices to graph and monitor are the margin over feed and fertiliser costs per litre (to show efficiency by one of the limiting factors, quota), the same per hectare (to show it by another, land). All other indices are subordinate to these three. Some of the other useful figures to track are yield versus quota, and milk quality (particularly butterfat and somatic cell count), as well as herd calf income.

Targets and indices of performance in herd fertility (see Chapter 5)

A number of targets for the main fertility and health performance indicators have been drawn up. These targets are the ideal standards in that particular factor. While there are plenty of farmers who have achieved the target for *each* of these individual indices, very few achieve them in *all*. This may not be important, as, to achieve ideal herd fertility performance (an average herd calving interval of around 1 year and a culling rate below 20%), it requires a lower standard in the

Table 11.15 An example of a DAISY margins report.

Farm number 1 Farm name FARM LATEST FARM SUMMARY			MARGINS M1 DATE 2SEP96
	Mar 96	Cumulative from Apr	Rolling 12 months to end Mar 96
STOCK			
Cows/heifers in herd	177	183	183 herd
Cows/heifers in milk	177	154	154 milking
Number calved	0	194 (total)	194 calved
dry	0	15	15% dry
Annual replacement rate	—	—	25% replaced
Annual depreciation rate	—	—	19390 depreciation
Calf sales £ (number)	0 (0)	12267 (132)	12267 (132) calf income
Cull sales £ (number)	0 (0)	19390 (57)	19390 (57) cull income
MILK			
Total yield (litres sold)	127336	1222040	1222040 litres
Value of milk sold (£)	34332	315112 (total)	315112 £ total
Milk prices (p/litre)	26.962	25.740	25.740 p/litre
Yield per cow in milk (litres/day)	23.2	21.3	21.3 litre/cow/day
Yield per cow from forage (litres/day)	−2.8	2.8	1033.3 forage litres
Yield per cow in herd (litres/month)	720	6693	6693 litre/cow/year
Weight of fat + protein (kg/cow)	57	505	505 kg F + P
White cell count ('000s)	—	—	183 thousands

Contd.

Table 11.15 *Contd.*

	Mar 96	Cumulative from Apr	Rolling 12 months to end Mar 96
FEED AND FERTILISER			
kg Concs per cow per day	5.19	1.44 (tonne/cow)	1.44 tonne/cow/year
kg Concs per litre milk	0.22	0.22	0.22 kg/litre
Concs price (£/tonne)	198.3	178.2	178.2 £/tonne
Other purchased feeds (£ total)	4618	26769 (total)	26769 £ total OPF
Fertiliser costs total (£)	3708	7734 (total)	7734 £ total fert
Fertiliser kg N applied/ha	60	171	171 kg/ha N
MARGINS over			
Concentrates per cow (MOC/cow £)	162.1	1466.5	1466.5 MOC/cow
All purchased feed per cow (MOAPF/cow £)	136.0	1320.2	1320.2 MOAPF/cow
All purchased feed for herd (MOAPF £)	24070	241478	241478 MOAPF/herd
Feeds and fertilisers for herd (MOFF £)	20362	233744	233744 MOFF/herd
Feeds and fertilisers per ha (MOFF/ha £)	199.6	2291.6	2291.6 MOFF/ha
Feeds and fertilisers per cow (MOFF/cow £)	115.0	1277.9	1277.9 MOFF/cow
Feeds and fertilisers per litre (MOFF/litre p)	15.968	19.093	19.093 MOFF/litre
OTHER			
UME GJ per ha from forage	2.7	52.4 (total)	52.4 total GJ
Estimated DM per ha (tonnes)	0.3	5.5 (total)	5.5 total tonnes DM
Stocking rate	—	—	1.79 cows/ha
Forage hectares	102	102	102 hectares
Gross output (£)	—	—	346769 £ Gross output

Table 11.16 Fertility target, Interference and Alarm Levels (1992–1993 calving season). Data are sorted for each parameter on its own. (From Kossaibati and Esslemont, 1995; Table 2.1.)

	Target (top 25%)	Interference Level (2nd 25%)	Alarm Level (bottom 25%)
% Served of calved	>95	<92	<86
First service 24-day submission rate (%)	>67	<58	<43
% Served <40 days postpartum	<1	>2	>9
% Served >100 days postpartum	<2	>5	>15
First service pregnancy rate (%)	>58	<50	<36
All service pregnancy rate (%)	>54	<49	<37
Services per conception	<1.8	>2	>2.6
% Conceived of served	>94	<91	<85
% Conceived of calved	>88	<84	<75
Failure to conceive culling rate (%)	<5	>8	>14
Total culling rate (%)	<14	>19	>29
Mean calving to first service interval (days)	<60	>66	>80
Mean calving to conception interval (days)	<87	>95	>115
Mean calving interval (days)	<368	>375	>395
Days open	<110	>120	>150

main indices, provided the standards are achieved in all these 'crucial' main indices. The targets for the individual factors are given in Table 11.16.

Interference Levels are the levels of performance where it is worth taking action, as the herd will, if performing at this level, be losing significant sums of money. For instance, in comparison with target performance, the cost of sub-optimum achievements in the main fertility indices (number of services per conception at £20 per service, calving interval at £3 for each extra day, and failure to conceive culling rate at £770 per extra cull cow) is estimated at £4810 per 100 cows. In extreme situations (the worst 25% of dairy units), where the herd fertility status is at the Alarm Level (see Table 11.16), the annual loss in profit could be over £16 630 per 100 cows. These estimations are based on the new DAISY approach in costing herd fertility, as shown in the DAISY study (Report No. 4) by Kossaibati and Esslemont (1995).

Next, one must consider what are the 'crucial' indices that guide the performance of the herd in the financially sensitive areas such as calving interval and culling rate, and what level of performance has to be achieved in *each* to attain the ideal result. The five 'crucial' factors are given in Table 11.17. Such a combination will deliver a calving interval of less than 375 days, with culling for failure to conceive of less than 8%. Of 90 herds studied (Kossaibati and Esslemont, 1995), only 13 achieved the above double target. Other financially important indices of performance in terms of disease are shown in Table 11.18.

Costs of infertility and disease (see also p. 134 onwards)

To produce milk economically, the farmer has to organise the cows to deliver their milk and calves at the correct time, and in the correct quantities. There are

Table 11.17 Crucial indices that affect herd fertility performance (1992–1993 calving season). Based on financial performance of the top 25% of dairy units in terms of FERTEX (cost of fertility and culling). (From Kossaibati and Esslemont, 1995; Table 2.8.)

Parameters*	Target
Per cent served after calving	>93
AND	
Average heat detection rate (%)	>62
AND	
Calving to first service interval (days)	<66
AND	
Pregnancy rate (%)	>49
AND	
Total culling rate (%)	<16
Cost of fertility and culling (per 100 cows per year)	<£2800

* All the parameter targets should be met, not just one parameter on its own.

Table 11.18 Health indices of financial importance in dairy herd management (1992–1993 calving season). Targets are based on financial performance of top 25% and second 25% of dairy units for the interference level in terms of HEALEX (an index of the cost of production diseases). (From Kossaibati and Esslemont, 1995; Table 4.27.)

	Average herd	Target	Interference Level
Twinning (cases/100 cows)	4	<4	>5
Calf mortality (cases/100 calves born)	8	<8	>9
Aid at calving (cases/100 cows)	8	<5	>9
Retained afterbirth (% of herd affected)	4	<3	>4
Milk fever (% of herd affected)	8	<5	>8
Vulval discharge (cases/100 cows)	24	<14	>23
Oestrus-not-observed (treatments/100 cows)	50	<45	>56
Mastitis (cases/100 cows)	37	<13	>26
Lameness (cases/100 cows)	25	<10	>17
Cost of health (per 100 cows per year)	£6300	<£2300	>£4800

certain fertility and health parameters that can be used to keep the business proceeding in the right direction and at the correct pace and efficiency. Many of these factors can be derived from simple recording schemes, but today it is more efficient for a manager to have these records processed on a microcomputer. Without analysis, the records are relatively useless.

The fertility indices revolve around the need for heifers to calve at 2 years of age, for the herd to have an average calving interval of 368 days, and a total culling rate of less than 20% (5–8% sold for failure to conceive). Many of the delays in conception, and the extra losses of culls, will be due to the incidence of disease, such as endometritis, lameness and mastitis. However, the largest proportion of the problems arise from poor husbandry, such as heat detection and timing of insemination.

Pregnancy rates are under 50% on average, and inadequate feeding levels may be partly to blame for this. The costs of some of the more common health problems are outlined. They are not all mutually exclusive. Nevertheless, the cost of average achievement (in terms of incidence of production diseases) compared to the performance of a farm in the top 25% is worth £4000 in a 100-cow herd.

Delay in the calving interval has complex effects, and it is not easy to measure in financial terms. Broadly speaking, it leads to a loss of about £2.14 per day of delay as a net loss in milk return (see Table 11.8). To this can be added the cost of about 33 p a day in terms of reduced calf income (if a calf was worth, say, £120). Also the farmer will lose about 53 p as a result of a slightly longer dry period. This adds up to £3.00 per extra day on the calving interval.

Herds with poor fertility management often have to resort to selling about 10 more culls per 100 cows for failing to conceive within the farmer's target 'window' of time. Each extra cull costs about £525 of extra herd depreciation and the lower margin from the heifer's lactation (Table 11.19). The total cost of an extra cull cow is estimated at £770.

Disease is also expensive for the farmer, especially if the cow has to be culled. For example, a case of severe mastitis can cost more than £360. Based on the prevalence rate of each type of this disease (Blowey, 1986), an average case of mastitis has a direct cost of about £119 with a total cost of £183, assuming 70% of the cases are mild, 29% severe and 1% end up in fatality. Details of the costs of each different case are shown in Tables 11.20a–c, (see Chapter 8) respectively.

Lameness, which often leads to reduced fertility in addition to other effects, costs £93 per case on average. This estimate is based on the assumption that 47% of lameness cases are digital, 22% interdigital and 31% sole ulcer (Collick *et al.*, 1989). However, the cost can be much higher (especially if the cow has to be culled) and the total cost is calculated at £246 per single case. The costs of the three types of lameness are shown in Tables 11.21a–c, respectively (see p. 149).

Where cow health affects milk yield or quality, there are major financial implications. Each litre below quota costs the farmer the margin of the milk price per litre less the major variable costs. This may amount to 18–20 p/litre, so being 10 000 litres under quota may cost £1800.

Reduced milk quality costs a considerable amount, as there are usually no quota implications. Disease may reduce butterfat and protein percentages. If

Table 11.19 Cost of an extra cull cow. (From Kossaibati and Esslemont, 1995.)

	Unit	Cost (£)	Total (£)
Return from a cull sale (£/cow) (A)			450
Losses due to culling:			
Cost of replacement (£/heifer)			975
Lower margin from a heifer			
lower yield (litre)	1000		
margin (litre)		0.20	200
Lower calf value			45
Total losses (B)			1220
Total cost for each extra cull cow (B − A)			770

Table 11.20 Cost of clinical mastitis. *These items have been included in the calculation of the direct cost. (from Kossaibati and Esslemont, 1995.)

(a) Cost (in £) of a mild cow-case of clinical mastitis.

Drugs (*a*)	10.50*
Herdsman's time (15 minutes @ £5/hour) (*b*)	1.25*
Discarded milk (80 litres @ £0.24/litre) (*c*)	19.20*
Reduced milk yield (247 litres @ £0.20/litre)	49.40*
Direct cost of a single cow-case of mild mastitis	*80.35*
Cost of 0.6 repeat case [(*a* + *b* + *c*) × 0.6]	18.57
Direct cost of 1.6 cases per average affected cow	98.92
Total cost of a mild cow-case	80.35
Total cost of 1.6 cases per average affected cow	98.92

(b) Cost (in £) of a severe cow-case of clinical mastitis.

Drugs (*a*)	26.50*
Vet's time (2 visits × 25 minutes each:	
£54.17 routine work + £8.50 turnout) (*b*)	62.67*
Discarded milk (120 litres @ £0.24/litre) (*c*)	28.80*
Reduced milk yield (450 litres @ £0.20/litre)	90.00*
Increased risk of culling	
(20% @ £770 per cull cow)	154.00
Direct cost of a single cow-case of	
severe mastitis	*207.97*
Cost of 0.6 repeat case [(*a* + *b* + *c*) × 0.6]	70.78
Direct cost of 1.6 cases per average	
affected cow	278.75
Total cost of a severe cow-case	361.97
Total cost of 1.6 cases per average affected cow	432.75

(c) Cost (in £) of a fatal case of mastitis.

Treatments	36.50*
Vet's time (3 visits × 45 minutes each:	
£146.25 routine work + £17.00 turnout)	163.25*
Fatality	2014.60
Direct cost of a case of fatal mastitis	*199.75*
Total cost	2214.35

quality (butterfat) is 3.75% instead of 4%, the cost to the farmer is 0.62 p/litre, which, if the herd produces 500000 litres per year, is worth £3100. In a similar example concerning protein (say 3.3–3.05%), the cost at present would be 1.12 p/litre (£5600 in total).

If a farmer is producing milk in Band 3 for somatic cell count instead of Band 1, this will cost him 2.0p/litre for the months affected (say, £830 per month in the herd example above). The dairy farmer has also to face the Bactoscan penalty (now used as a replacement for total bacterial count). If the milk

Table 11.21 Cost of lameness. *These items have been included in the calculation of the direct cost. (from Kossaibati and Esslemont, 1995.)

(a) Cost (in £) of digital lameness (occurring at 50 days postpartum).

Treatments (spray, block, etc.) (*a*)	13.00*
Vet's time (15 minutes: £16.25 routine work + £3.25 turnout) (*b*)	19.50*
Herdsman's time (3 hours @ £5/hour) (*c*)	15.00*
Milk withdrawal (90 litres @ £0.24/litre) (*d*)	21.60*
Reduced milk yield (120 litres @ £0.20/litre)	24.00*
Increased risk of culling (11% @ £770 per cull cow)	84.70
Longer calving interval (9 days @ £3/day)	27.00
Extra services (0.39 @ £20 per service)	7.80
Direct cost of a single case of digital lameness	*93.10*
Cost of 0.4 repeat case [(*a* + *b* + *c* + *d*) × 0.4]	27.64
Direct cost of 1.4 cases per affected cow	120.74
Total cost of a single case	212.60
Total cost of 1.4 cases per affected cow	240.24

(b) Cost (in £) of interdigital lameness (occurring at 20 days postpartum).

Treatments (spray, injection, etc.) (*a*)	10.80*
Vet's time (12 minutes: £13 routine work + £2.60 turnout) (*b*)	15.60*
Herdsman's time (1 hour @ £5/hour) (*c*)	5.00*
Milk withdrawal (60 litres @ £0.24/litre) (*d*)	14.40*
Reduced milk yield (60 litres @ £0.20/litre)	12.00*
Longer calving interval (17 days @ £3/day)	51.00
Extra services (0.2 @ £20 per service)	4.00
Direct cost of a single case of interdigital lameness	*57.80*
Cost of 0.4 repeat case [(*a* + *b* + *c* + *d*) × 0.4]	18.32
Direct cost of 1.4 cases per affected cow	76.12
Total cost of a single case	112.80
Total cost of 1.4 cases per affected cow	131.12

(c) Cost (in £) of sole ulcer lameness (occurring at 75 days postpartum).

Treatments (medicine, block, etc.) (*a*)	15.00*
Vet's time (20 minutes: £21.67 routine work + £4.33 turnout) (*b*)	26.00*
Herdsman's time (5 hours @ £5/hour) (*c*)	25.00*
Milk withdrawal (70 litres @ £0.24/litre) (*d*)	16.80*
Reduced milk yield (180 litres @ £0.20/litre)	36.00*
Increased risk of culling (18% @ £770 per cull cow)	138.60
Longer calving interval (40 days @ £3/day)	120.00
Extra services (0.72 @ £20 per service)	14.40
Direct cost of a single case of sole ulcer	*118.80*
Cost of 0.4 repeat case [(*a* + *b* + *c* + *d*) × 0.4]	33.12
Direct cost of 1.4 cases per affected cow	151.92
Total cost of a single case	391.80
Total cost of 1.4 cases per affected cow	424.92

produced is in Band C instead of Band A, then that farmer will lose another £830 per month.

It is estimated that each case of milk fever costs £220 in reduced profit and each case of vulval discharge £162, mostly due to the extended calving interval and higher culling rate in the affected stock (Kossaibati and Esslemont, 1995). A case of hypomagnesaemia costs about £160 (Chamberlain, 1989).

Another factor is the cost of an extra day to rear from birth to calving (beyond 2 years), which is about £1.65 (Kossaibati and Esslemont, 1997), and each animal lost costs about £100 to £650 depending on when and how they go (£375 on average).

Benefits of herd health and fertility improvement in practice

There are considerable benefits to be gained from improving herd health and fertility. Case study material shows that when preventive medicine routines are installed, the cost benefit ratio comes out very favourably.

Collick (1982) found that farm margins for ten herds on DAISY went up by over £200 in today's terms when compared with ten herds not on the scheme. Eddy (1982) showed that better heat detection and more timely intervention by the veterinarian, using techniques like injections of prostaglandin to synchronise service, took 12 days off the calving interval for 1800 cows in ten herds. In a 200-cow herd studied by ICI and the University of Reading, the margin went up by £200 a cow when the fertility management of the cows and youngstock was improved (Esslemont *et al.*, 1985).

There are several case studies of herds using information systems to improve fertility management, by being able to install and operate the use of the milk progesterone test as part of the routine. Provided the test is kept up and heat detection rates and accuracy improve through the use of heat detectors or tail paint, then calving intervals and culling rates are improved, with herd margins rising by over £125 per cow (Williams and Esslemont, 1993).

A farmer with 77 cows, who went onto DAISY and used the reports properly, and who adopted a planned approach to management, saw his farm profits improve by a real increase of £13 000 in 2 years. It was estimated that £6000 of this came from improved fertility management alone.

Another farmer working with DAISY improved his heat detection rates and pregnancy rates to near model levels. The culling rate for failing to conceive in his 127 cows was cut from 16 or so, to 1 or 2 per year. The farmer achieved this through his own enthusiastic efforts, using tail paint on the cows highlighted by DAISY to help him with heat detection. He cut his veterinary costs by some £1000 per year, as there were very few cows put forward for the vet for oestrus-not-observed or for pregnancy diagnosis. In addition, the farmer improved his margin per cow through shorter and more timely calving intervals and a lower culling rate.

It should be made clear that these improvements came about through the efforts of the *people*; the computers are simply tools in their hands and are not in any sense 'magic'.

In one interesting case of ten herds being monitored by a veterinarian, the benefits from improved fertility accrued for 5 years as the preventive medicine scheme was being applied by the skilled extension specialist that he was. When the work was handed over to a less appropriate colleague, even though the herds were still on the scheme, the fertility indices all slipped back to their original position, with a consequent reduction in margin. When this was recognised, and the work put into the hands of a more successful (from the point of view of extension skills) partner, the improved performance returned, and has been maintained.

On another farm, the new manager who arrived in 1987 got to grips with fertility management, particularly by using milk progesterone tests. So, by 1990 the failure to conceive (FTC) culling rate dropped to 7% and the calving to conception interval was kept at around 95 days. In 1991 this farm manager left and a new manager was appointed who used DAISY and milk progesterone tests to a lesser extent. The Fertility Factor slipped from a very high level of 40 to 25 (which is average). Culling for FTC is now 14% and calving to conception interval is over 100 days (see Fig. 11.5).

'Herd Health Schemes' take many forms and are more often than not simply visits to carry out pregnancy diagnosis. If the pregnancy diagnosis is carried out

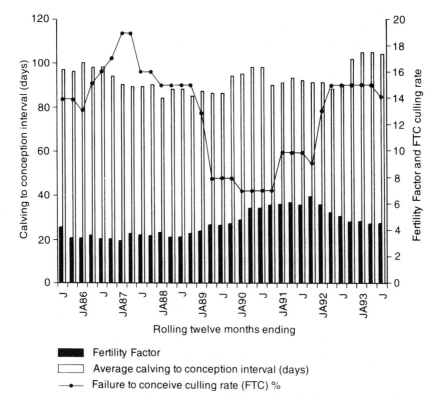

Fig. 11.5   Rolling 12-month (every 3 months) Fertility Factor, calving to conception interval and failure to conceive (FTC) culling rate on an example farm. (J, July.)

at about 65 days and is 100% accurate, then the benefits to the farmer of having the negative cases treated lead to net *benefits* of only £9.74 per cow (Esslemont, 1995). Clearly, a more intensive system would be attractive to farmers. If the pregnancy diagnosis at this stage is only 95% accurate, and if prostaglandin is used on cows actually pregnant but diagnosed negative, then, in terms of extended calving intervals, extra culls, more services, etc., this process in a herd *costs* the farmer £15 per cow in the herd.

Improved cost effectiveness accrues to the farmer if the pregnancy diagnoses are accurate and if they are carried out earlier. The use of the milk progesterone tests at 19 days post service, with the negative animals treated with tail paint, coupled with an accurate manual pregnancy diagnosis on the positives at 50–65 days (then using prostaglandin on the negatives) plus ultrasound scanning leads to cost-effective use of modern technology (over £50 benefit per cow per year).

Recording

Today there is no escape from keeping reliable records on dairy farms. There are now a number of statutory requirements covering the identification and movements of cattle. In addition, the use of all drugs and medicines has to be rigorously logged, treatment by treatment. Passports are now issued for all cattle, with the need for logging the farms where the animal is kept throughout its life.

There is increasing pressure from milk buyers for quality assured production systems which means that much fuller (if not complete) animal and facility recording is needed. Some of the schemes from the dairy companies include elaborate checklists, but no-one has come up with a means or system of recording the status of all the elements.

To comply with modern requirements the dairy farmer probably needs to consider the following recording schemes:

- Individual field records, including: gateways; tracks; staff records; buildings; bedding; passageways.
- Records of milking machine maintenance.
- Feed store records, including: stock control (sources, dates of purchases, transfers, opening and closing stock); quality control (pests, vermin, etc.).
- Milk sales, including: bulk tank quantity and quality; disease tests.
- Individual animal records, including: pedigree; full identification; birth through to calving; lactation by lactation in detail; disease, preventive medicine; blood tests; treatments; insemination; pregnancy diagnosis; milk yield; drying off; culling (date, reason and destination); calf I.D.; passport records.

While these records can be kept on paper, there is increasing sense in using computerised systems. Unfortunately, no one system covers all the requirements so a combination is needed. There is no absolute need for the computer to be on the farm (although this can be justified on practically any sized herd) as bureau services (post in–post out) are available. It is likely that the greatest coverage of records comes from schemes offered by NMR (an organisation which also offers milk recording PC-based systems such as Herdsman and DAISY), but the software from firms such as SUM-IT, Orchid and the parlour manufacturers also need examining.

There is a need for more and more details so the more elaborate systems are worth seeking out and considering. It is important to identify schemes that are well supported and that are being constantly updated. Veterinary practitioners can offer a recording and data processing scheme that enhances their professional services to farmers. It may be sensible to operate a weekly service with data faxed to and fro where it is needed quickly. Action lists can be sent out to the farmer this way in a same-day turnaround service. The essential action lists include a 'Veterinary Visit List', which in turn includes cows calved; cows not seen in heat; pregnancy diagnosis; repeat services; cows suffering mastitis, lameness and yield variation; cows to dry off; recheck; revisit; etc.

Properly managed computer-based schemes can also help in dealing with decisions on feeding, culling, heifer rearing and breeding. It is crucial that such schemes are devised to reduce repetition and errors. At the same time reminders need to be produced to ensure the farmer complies with up-to-date recording requirements.

References

ADAS (1996) *Heifer Management.* ADAS Information Notes for Dairy Consultants. ADAS Bridgets, Martyr Worthy, Winchester, Hants, SO21 1AP.

Anon (1995) *Dairy Facts and Figures.* The England and Wales Residuary and Milk Marketing Board, Thames Ditton, Surrey.

Blowey, R. W. (1986) An assessment of the economic benefits of a mastitis control scheme. *Veterinary Record* **119**, 551–3.

Chamberlain, A. T. (1989) *Dairy Herd Management for Profit.* Notes for University of Reading Course, March 1989.

Collick, D. (1982) *Use of computerised herd health and fertility recording schemes.* Proceedings of the 12th World Association of Buiatrics, Amsterdam, September 1982.

Collick, D. W., Ward, R. & Dobson, H. (1989) Association between different types of lameness and fertility. *Veterinary Record* **125**, 103–106.

Drew B. (1998) Targets for rearing dairy heifers, weaning to calving. *In Practice*, **20**, Part 1, 35–9.

Eddy, R. G. (1982) *Data quality in herd health schemes.* Proceedings of the 12th World Association of Buiatrics, Amsterdam, September 1982.

Esslemont, R. J. (1995) Economic appraisal of herd health schemes. *The Veterinary Annual* **35**, 243–80.

Esslemont, R. J., Bailie, J. H. & Cooper, M. J. (1985) *Fertility Management in Dairy Cattle.* Collins, London.

Esslemont, R. J. & Marsh, W. E. (1987) *The economic importance of fertility in terms of dairy herd growth and productivity; the use of models on micro-computers.* European Association of Animal Production Conference, Lisbon, Portugal, July 1987.

Furniss, S. J., Stroud, A., Barrington, H., Kirby, S. P. J., Wray, J. P. & Dakin, P. (1986) *The effect of dam's parity on the performance of dairy heifers.* Abstract. BSAP Winter Meeting, Scarborough, March 1986.

Gartner, J. A. (1980) *Replacement in dairy herds.* PhD thesis, University of Reading.

GENUS Management (1993) *An Analysis of Genus Management – Costed Dairy Farms, 1992–1993.* Report no. 79, P. Tomlinson & A. Perry, Genus Management, 3 Grove Road, Wrexham, Clwyd, LL11 1DY.

Hocking, P. (1984) *Cross breeding in Canada.* Proceedings of the British Cattle Breeders Club, Cambridge, January 1984.

Kossaibati, M. A. & Esslemont, R. J. (1995) *Wastage in Dairy Herds.* Report no. 4, DAISY – The Dairy Information System. University of Reading.

Kossaibati, M. A. & Esslemont, R. J. (1997) *Understanding the Rearing of Dairy Heifers. A Stockman's Guide.* NMR/DAISY, University of Reading.

McGuirk, B. (1992) *The development of the GENUS MOET dairy breeding programme.* Proceedings of the British Cattle Breeders Club, Cambridge, January 1992.

Peeler, E. J. (1992) *A study of factors affecting the rebreeding success of dairy cows.* MSc thesis, University of Reading.

Solbu, H. (1978) *Breeding for improved disease resistance, with special emphasis on a practical method of collecting data.* Proceedings of the 29th Annual Meeting of the European Association for Animal Production. Stockholm, 5–7 June.

Van Arendonk, J. A. M. (1985) *Studies on the replacement policies on dairy cattle.* PhD thesis, Departments of Animal Breeding and Farm Management, Wageningen University, The Netherlands.

Williams, M. E. & Esslemont, R. J. (1993) A decision support system using milk progesterone tests to improve fertility in commercial dairy herds. *Veterinary Record* **132**, 503–506.

Chapter 12
Disease Security

Laurence A. S. Gibson and Anthony H. Andrews

Introduction

Most significant infectious diseases of cattle are brought into the herd by adding a 'carrier' animal to the herd or adding one that is incubating a frank disease. Although there are important exceptions to this statement (e.g. airborne transmission of foot-and-mouth disease; feed contaminated with *Salmonella* or BSE), it is true that simple quarantine measures for animals introduced into a herd can protect it from costly disease outbreaks. Viewed from the ivory tower of the veterinary idealist, a 'closed' herd surrounded by arable farms should be quite easy to keep free from new infections. In reality, however, such herds scarcely exist under British conditions. The challenge facing practising veterinary surgeons is to persuade their clients that every animal added to their herds is a potential Trojan horse.

In Great Britain at present this challenge is possibly more important than ever. When the Single European Market came into operation in January 1993, it became easier to import cattle from other member states and from elsewhere (see page 336). Until 1998, farmers who bought cattle at auction, market or via dealers may have been quite unaware as to whether or not their purchases were recent imports. Indeed, many farmers thought they were buying British cattle when in fact they were buying European animals after retagging in Britain. On occasions cattle imported from one country were in fact born and reared in another country before being exported to the country from which the export to Britain was made. This was perfectly acceptable under EU regulations provided that the normal veterinary conditions were met and the correct documentary procedures followed. In 1998 the British Cattle Movement Service came into operation. This should mean that, in future, the farmer should know the origin and movement of the animal from its passport. In addition, the requirement for double tagging of all cattle and the use of replacement with the same number if one is lost will be other safeguards.

Historically, many diseases have entered Britain from the importation of cattle, thus enzootic bovine leukosis (EBL) and probably *Mycoplasma bovis* were introduced into Great Britain by imported cattle. Most of the cases of EBL identified soon after introduction originated in Canada, or had contact with Canadian

The information used and opinions made in this chapter are entirely those of the authors and do not necessarily represent those of any organisation for which they work or with which they are associated.

imports, but a few cases appear to have been imported from Europe. The out-breaks of infectious bovine rhinotracheitis (IBR) which spread through Europe in the late 1970s and early 1980s are widely thought to have originated in North America, but may have entered Great Britain via Europe.

International health certification cannot cover every eventuality. For example, a severe haemorrhagic strain of bovine virus diarrhoea (BVD) Type II has appeared in North America in the last few years, and import health certificates for animals moving to the EU may not give adequate guarantees concerning this disease. Recent work by the Veterinary Laboratories Agency (VLA) shows no evidence of BVD Type II in Britain, although Type II strains are present in other parts of the EU. Animals imported into the EU from elsewhere must either be vaccinated or, if not vaccinated, they must be seronegative using an SNT. However, there is no requirement under EU law for a virus negative test, and so there is no protection against persistently infected (PI) animals (Commission Decision 83/494 Annex A, para v.7 vii). Thus, there is a significant risk that this variant virus will be introduced into Europe in the future. Purchasers of imported cattle would be well advised to ask for additional private certification from the vendor over and beyond that on the international health certificate, or to take additional precautions after the animal has arrived. Thus, in the case of BVD a request should be made for an antigen test to be made on blood. In addition, once imported, the animals should be isolated and re-tested.

Although British farmers have traditionally supposed that British cattle are healthier than those from elsewhere, there is no reason to suppose that only imported cattle pose a health risk. It is true that eradication programmes for tuber-culosis and brucellosis began earlier in Britain than in many other countries, and Britain gained significant export advantages owing to its freedom from foot-and-mouth disease – and the prohibition on vaccination – at a time when the disease and vaccination were widespread elsewhere. Nevertheless, purchased cattle of British origin may carry IBR, Johne's disease, leptospirosis, BVD, campylobacter or other diseases just as well as imported cattle. Besides, a British-born animal may well have an imported dam or originate from a herd containing many imported animals. Although EBL was certainly initially an imported disease, in recent years the EBL reactors revealed in a national testing programme in Great Britain have been mainly commercial cattle of 'domestic' origin.

Furthermore, outbreaks of tuberculosis continue to occur in certain parts of Great Britain, mainly attributed to infection in badgers. Cattle sold out of infected herds in the period before the disease is discovered can spread the disease. In 1997 fresh outbreaks of tuberculosis were confirmed in 523 herds in Great Britain. It has been estimated that about 20 animals are traced out of each herd in which TB is confirmed. This suggests that in 1997 around 10500 potentially tuberculous animals were traded. Of the new outbreaks, only 34 were attributed to the purchase of an infected animal. Statistically, therefore, the chance of buying an animal infected with tuberculosis is very small: but it is not totally negligible, and the consequences of introducing TB into a herd can be very severe.

The primary frontier for disease control must be the farm boundary, and it is up to the farmer to decide what precautions he can afford to take or not to take. A farmer can only make rational decisions to protect the health of his herd if properly advised by a veterinary surgeon. The veterinary surgeon in turn can only give sound advice if he or she knows what diseases are already present in the herd, and what diseases are likely to be present in the herd of origin of the purchased animal. At the moment there is no simple means by which the latter can be ascertained. Unless the industry can be persuaded to adopt a system of voluntary health declarations for traded cattle, the only way a farmer can reduce the risks inherent in bringing animals into the herd is a system of quarantine. This is very different to the pig and poultry industry where almost all farmers, be they breeders or commercial units, would never entertain the principle of introducing new stock without a period of quarantine and often a time of acclimatisation. Animals added to a herd should be isolated and subjected to a comprehensive screening programme agreed between the farmer and the veterinary surgeon.

Principles of herd security

The main principles of protecting herd security have been described by Duncan (1990). They can be summarised as follows:

- Maintain a closed herd.
- Isolate animals added to the herd and test for relevant diseases.
- Ensure feed and water are free from contamination.
- Control visitors.
- Control rodents and birds.
- Define and monitor the health status of the herd.
- Establish an agreed disease control programme.

There is evidence that visitors or their vehicles can introduce pathogens, in particular *Salmonella*. However, in practical terms, it is often regarded as of less importance for cattle than it is for pigs, although perceptions are likely to change during a foot-and-mouth disease emergency. Regular visitors and contractors should be asked whether they have a disinfection policy, and their vehicles and clothing should be inspected to ensure that they are satisfactorily clean. Wherever possible, livestock lorries, feed merchants' lorries etc. should be kept away from cattle. Significant outbreaks of disease can be caused by contamination of feed (for example and especially by *Salmonella*), either at source or by birds, vermin or cats on the farm. Pasture may be contaminated by drainage (e.g. anthrax downstream of old tanneries) or by manure or pasture dressings (e.g. botulism introduced in poultry waste). Forage may be contaminated (e.g. outbreaks of listeriosis from excessive soil contamination of poor-quality silage), as may grain (e.g. by lead shot after a clay shoot over unharvested grain!) Apart from the example of *Salmonella*, feed is generally much less important than the carrier animal as a vehicle for diseases of cattle. This chapter will therefore concentrate on the problem of the 'added animal'.

Practical limitations of the closed herd

The totally closed herd is a comparative rarity in Great Britain. Even when most female replacements are home bred, a few heifers may have to be brought in occasionally from other sources to replace unplanned culls (e.g. through an outbreak of mastitis or lameness) or if yields are below quota because of unexpected feed problems. A purchased young (maiden) bull probably represents a similar risk to any other animal, but a hired, shared, loaned or purchased bull previously used on other premises requires particular care (Anon, 1995).

While many farmers believe that they operate a closed herd policy, close investigation shows that in most cases this is not true. During a 10-year study period (1978–1987) involving 88 dairy farmers from the Reading area, only four farmers had not purchased stock (Hartley and Richards, 1988). In fact, 69% had purchased female cattle, 74% had purchased bulls and 22% had hired bulls.

The purchase of cattle via a market or dealer's premises poses a particular problem. There will be an increased risk of contact with other cattle and the mixing and movement of the animals to the market or dealer's premises may decrease their resistance to disease, thereby making the animals more likely to contract infection. In addition, symptomless carriers (as with IBR) may provide a source of disease. Scudamore (1988) reported results of a study of an outbreak of brucellosis in which a dealer sold freshly calved cows following the purchase of animals in late pregnancy from farms from all over the country. The animals were allowed to calve before being sold on again, and were thus more likely to spread infection to other animals on the premises. It was found that any cow on the holding could, at any time, be in contact with up to 100 other cattle. These animals might then be sold direct to another farm or via special sales and markets, compounding even further the problems of disease spread.

Artificial insemination and embryo transfer are often considered together, but the hazards associated with each are rather different. The health precautions followed in the production of semen are quite stringent, and for practical purposes AI in Britain can be considered safe. Nevertheless, the potential remains for the widespread dissemination of a pathogen from a single infected stud bull. Embryo transfer itself is also potentially very safe, since most pathogens can be removed from the embryo by the usual washing procedures. Besides, the number of potentially infected embryos produced by any donor is limited. However, embryos are commonly implanted into recipient animals bought specifically for the purpose: these represent a much greater danger than the embryos themselves. It should also not be forgotten that the media used in collecting, washing and preserving embryos may contain components of animal origin which may be contaminated, particularly with BVD virus.

Animals that return to the herd after coming into contact with stock on other premises pose a risk. Clearly, the longer the animals have been on other premises, the greater the risk. At one extreme, home-bred heifers may be reared under contract on other premises, where they may remain for a year or more. During this time they may mix with animals from a variety of sources and with a very different disease status. At the other extreme, the risk in attending a local one-day agricultural show held outdoors is generally very slight.

The dangers of agricultural shows are difficult to quantify but should not be ignored. For instance, the conditions under which cattle are washed at large shows would appear to provide good conditions for the transmission of *Leptospira hardjo*. The operation of the former Cattle Health Scheme provided some evidence of the transmission of IBR at agricultural shows. Cattle from IBR-monitored herds were required to be tested in isolation after attendance at shows, and some animals from herds that had previously been wholly seronegative for IBR were found to be seropositive at the end of a show season. This was rarely accompanied by any evidence of clinical disease, either at the shows or in the animals in isolation after returning home. Experience from Germany also suggests that IBR can spread at shows – and in at least one instance, a cluster of clinical outbreaks occurred in animals that had attended the same large indoor event.

A herd cannot be considered to be closed if the cattle share common grazing with animals from other herds, or if the farm boundaries do not prevent contact with livestock on adjacent premises. Again, experience from the Cattle Health Scheme suggests this is more than a theoretical risk. Investigation of some cases in which IBR-free herds became infected revealed good circumstantial evidence that the first group of animals to seroconvert had been grazing fields where they could make physical contact with cattle on adjacent farms across defective boundary fences or hedges. Where adjacent farms have livestock and hedges are inadequate, then double fencing with a 3-m (10-ft) gap between fences will reduce the possibility of infection spreading.

Contact with livestock species other than cattle may also pose a risk. Under British conditions cattle commonly have contact with sheep, but usually have little direct contact with other species. Free-range poultry may provide a possible exception, and could in theory transmit *Salmonella*. Deer and cattle may be present on the same farm, but are generally kept apart. Deer share some diseases with cattle (Johne's disease, malignant catarrhal fever), but there is little information on the epidemiological significance of this.

Sheep are susceptible to many diseases that also affect cattle, but whether or not sheep will transmit these diseases to cattle under field conditions is in most instances unclear. For instance, Johne's disease can cause severe problems in sheep (although the consensus now is that sheep strains probably do not affect cattle); *Coxiella burnetti* (the organism of Q-fever) is quite widespread in sheep and can occasionally cause disease in cattle; chlamydial (enzootic) abortion of sheep can cause disease in cattle; cattle herds are more likely to be infected with *Leptospira interrogans* serovar *hardjo* if sheep are present; calves can be affected with the nematode *Nematodirus battus* which is normally a parasite of lambs. The parasite *Trichostrongylus axei* has a wide range of ruminant hosts in which it is pathogenic, and can in principle spread between species, although clinical disease in either sheep or cattle is rare. It is probable that most sheep are asymptomatically infected with the virus of malignant catarrhal fever (MCF), which can cause devastating outbreaks of disease in cattle as well as the more usual sporadic cases. Until more is understood about the circumstances that enable diseases to pass from sheep to cattle, it would seem prudent to keep cattle well away from sheep – at least at lambing time.

There are instances where experimental evidence suggests a risk which may or may not be significant in practice. For example, the sheep scab mite *Psoroptes ovis* can be transmitted experimentally to cattle and will cause psoroptic mange in them: but despite a long history of scabby sheep mixing with cattle in the field, transmission of scab to cattle does not seem to occur. The evidence is less clear with pestivirus infections. Although the 'type strains' of border disease virus and bovine virus diarrhoea (BVD) can be distinguished by serological means, both viruses will spread between sheep and cattle under close confinement but without any other intervention. If sheep or cattle become infected with either virus while pregnant, the offspring may develop persistent infection. Calves born persistently infected with pestivirus are likely to develop mucosal disease later in life; persistently infected lambs are at risk of border disease. Many isolates from clinical border disease in sheep in Great Britain prove to be of a BVD (or 'cattle') type rather than border disease (or 'sheep') type; there is a report from Australia of a bull persistently infected with a typical border disease strain. Recent work by the VLA suggests that, in the field, cattle more commonly transmit viral infections to sheep, but only rarely does the reverse occur.

Wildlife species do not seem to be significant reservoirs of cattle diseases in Britain, apart from the clear link between badgers and tuberculosis. Wild birds or rodents may contaminate feed or pasture with *Salmonella*; rodents may be responsible for sporadic cases of infection with *Leptospira icterohaemorrhagiae* (although carriage by rats may be less widespread than has generally been thought). Intriguingly, rabbits are experimentally susceptible to IBR, but there is no evidence that they become infected in the field or can act as a reservoir for cattle. However, *Mycobacterium paratuberculosis* has been recovered from lesions in rabbits on farms with a problem with Johne's disease. Although it might seem more likely that the rabbits picked up the infection from cattle than vice-versa, it is not yet clear whether they can transmit the infection to livestock.

Dealing with the added animal

It is not easy to persuade most farmers to keep purchased animals in isolation for even a short time before they are added to the herd, let alone for the 4 weeks or so that have been recommended. There are real practical problems to face relating to the way that trade in cattle is normally organised. Dairy cattle are commonly sold as freshly calved animals or as pregnant heifers, and many farms will not have suitable arrangements for milking animals in isolation. An acceptable compromise is to milk the 'isolated' animals last, after the remainder of the herd has been removed from the vicinity of the milking parlour. The parlour should then be properly cleaned and disinfected before the next milking.

A further problem comes from the common practice of running pregnant animals with the milking herd for the latter part of pregnancy so as to habituate them to milking parlour routines, and to establish their position in the social hierarchy of the herd. This is clearly sound on behavioural and practical grounds, but equally clearly it is incompatible with the isolation of purchased pregnant animals. One conclusion from this might be that it is preferable to buy bulling heifers rather than pregnant heifers or freshly calved animals – but this would represent a considerable change in established practice.

The timing of a bull sale may be such that the purchaser wants to make use of the bull as soon as possible, and is unwilling to isolate him for the recommended period. All the veterinary surgeon can do in these circumstances is to point out the risks, suggest a programme of blood tests and treatments anyway, and advise either a greater period of forethought the next time a bull is to be bought or a rearrangement of the herd's breeding pattern. Neither piece of advice is likely to be readily accepted! It may be possible to limit the exposure of a bull to a small group of females in the first instance and in effect to isolate these animals as well, pending the bull's test results: but few farmers would be willing to sacrifice the whole group, or even to prolong the isolation period, in the case of adverse results.

There is no satisfactory way of introducing new animals to a dairy herd. However, if they do have to be purchased they should come from a herd with a known health status. Ideally, as mentioned above, if cattle have to be bought the best time to buy is often at about the bulling heifer stage or before a bull is used. If bought between 1 and 2 years old most of the diseases that affect young cattle will be over and, provided the animals have not been run with the adult herd, infections from that source will be reduced. A possible protocol for new entrants to a herd is given below:

- Buy from a known source.
- Know the disease problems on other farms so that animals can be bought from farms with similar disease problems as on the farm buying the animals, i.e. the same disease profile.
- Carry out blood tests on the original farm to ascertain the presence or absence of diseases.
- If practicable, vaccinate for any disease on the farm before the introduction of new animals.
- Use an anthelmintic and an ectoparasiticide before entry.
- Clinically examine all animals for problems including those of the skin, alimentary system, mammary glands, respiratory and muscular systems, feet, etc. Reject animals if there are any problems.
- Strictly quarantine the animals for a month. The building should be separate and there should be a no-contact gap between the entrants and animals on the farm of at least 4 m (14 ft).
- A different person should look after the new animals, or the new animals should be handled last on the farm. Separate clothing and footwear should be used with the new animals, as should a foot dip.
- Watch all cattle, both home bred and the new animals, for signs of disease.
- Once the new animals are settled they should be treated with an anthelmintic and an ectoparasiticide.

- Once the new animals are settled a disease test should be carried out to retest for the presence or absence of diseases on the farm.
- Antibiotics should be used to remove latent diseases, e.g. leptospirosis.
- Vaccinate for diseases if appropriate.
- Treat with a second ectoparasiticide after 2 weeks.
- Treat with a second anthelmintic after a month.
- After a further month, mix in some cull cows into the new entrants and watch for signs of disease.
- Foot bath at least twice in the quarantine period.

For a hired bull it should normally be possible to arrange the hiring long enough in advance for ensure a full quarantine. Such animals should be tested for venereal diseases.

Having agreed that a quarantine period is necessary, the farmer and the veterinary surgeon must then decide where to isolate the animals and what tests or treatments to carry out during the isolation period. The isolation requirements for animals imported from Canada are given in Schedule 2 of the Animals (Post Import Control) Order 1995 (see Appendix 12.1). These set a standard which should be aimed at wherever possible. Compromises and adaptations can be made in the light of the practical conditions on the farm; for instance, a well-isolated paddock can be ideal for animals obtained during the grazing season. The basic minimum for the isolation accommodation is that the isolated animals should not be able to make nose-to-nose contact with the rest of the herd, and should be separated by as great a distance as is practical; the isolated animals should not share an enclosed air space with other members of the herd, and the drainage from the isolation area should not be accessible to the herd.

The testing and treatment programme will depend upon what infections are known to be present in the herd already, and what is known about the health status of the herd of origin. For instance, if the purchasing herd is thought to be free from *Leptospira hardjo*, the purchased animals should be treated with two doses of streptomycin/dihydrostreptomycin at a dose rate of 25 mg/kg body weight – whatever the results of any blood tests. This dose rate is established in the literature and in international certification, but is without the data sheet recommendations for the product. Milk from treated animals must therefore not be used for human consumption for at least 7 days after treatment, and treated animals must not be slaughtered for human consumption within 28 days of treatment. Other antibiotics such as amoxycillin are active against leptospirosis *in vitro*, attain high concentrations in urine and have been used at data sheet doses for prophylactic treatment of leptospirosis, but data are lacking as to whether they will remove all infection from the kidneys of carrier animals. However, if the herd is known to be endemically infected with *L. hardjo*, or if the farmer regularly vaccinates against the disease, then the introduced animal should be vaccinated before joining the herd. Similarly, a 'naive' animal entering a herd in which IBR is endemic may itself be at risk of disease, whereas a seropositive animal may carry the risk of introducing disease into a previously uninfected herd.

A practical guide to dealing with added animals is given by Pritchard (1996). Tables 12.1 and 12.2 are modified from his paper and with kind permission from *Cattle Practice* journal.

It should be recognised that there are many infections for which no test is routinely available but which can be introduced by carrier animals. *Mycoplasma bovis*, *Haemophilus somnus* and infectious keratitis (New Forest eye) are examples. Even if a test is available, it may not be very useful. For instance, whereas some cows may be seronegative to the microscopic agglutination test (MAT) for *Leptospira hardjo* and yet be excreting live bacteria in the urine, others may remain serologically positive for some time after the infection has been eliminated. The MAT is thus of little use in attempting to classify the *L. hardjo* status of individual animals of unknown origin – which is what one is attempting to do with a quarantine test. This is also true of tests currently available for Johne's disease: testing individual animals is far less accurate than testing the whole group or herd.

Besides diagnostic tests in isolation, there is a place for treatment for certain conditions. Treatment for *L. hardjo* has already been mentioned. Cattle imported from other member states of the EU are required to be treated for warble fly on arrival, which incidentally also gives useful protection against psoroptic mange caused by *Psoroptes natalensis*. This species of mite is common and troublesome in some parts of Europe but has never become established in Great Britain. Prophylactic foot bathing in formalin may prevent the introduction of *Fusobacteria* which cause 'superfoul', although close clinical examination of the (clean!) feet, together with local treatment where necessary probably gives better control over digital dermatitis. Antibiotic sheath lavage as prophylaxis against *Campylobacter* spp. should be given to any bull added to the herd unless it can be guaranteed that he has never served.

Cattle imported into Great Britain

The establishment of the Single Market after the end of 1992 does not mean that cattle trade is now a free-for-all, and nor was it associated with the drastic reduction in the requirements for health certification which some seemed to fear. The health certificate for breeding cattle throughout the EU is exactly the same now as it was in 1992. What changed was the administrative procedures required before and after the movement – but the purely veterinary standards did not change. It must be remembered that in the years that the EU has been operating the overall health status of cattle in the whole Community has steadily risen. Thus many diseases are the problems of yesteryear. However, foot-and-mouth disease remains a potential threat, with infection still present in the Magreb and in Asiatic Turkey where new strains of the virus have appeared in recent years.

Perhaps of more significance was the abolition of quarantine. Until 1992 cattle imported into Great Britain from 'mainland' Europe were kept in quarantine with sentinel British cattle. This was as a precaution against the introduction of

Table 12.1 Main bacterial and viral conditions likely to be introduced by added animals. (From Pritchard, 1996.)

Disease/infection	Preventive measures			Vaccination option	Comments
	Clinical examination	Prophylactic treatment	Laboratory tests		
BVD	(+)	—	+	Yes	It is essential to test for BVD virus (up to 1.8% of cattle may be virus positive); serology also useful. Calve pregnant females in isolation and test calves at birth for virus if dam seropositive.
IBR	(+)	—	+	Yes	Significance of adding seropositive (potentially infectious) animals depends on virus strain, existing herd status and possible implications for sale of cattle, semen and embryos.
Leptospira hardjo	(+)	+	+	Yes	25 mg dihydrostreptomycin/kg given twice within 14 days reduces risk of excretion. Could repeat if added animals are seropositive and entering a naive herd, but may still need to vaccinate latter. Zoonotic.
Salmonella	(+)	(+)	+	Yes	Although not validated, culture of 50 g pooled faeces after 3 weeks' isolation should help to detect carriers. Positive SAT titre for *S. dublin/S. typhimurium* on serum may indicate recent exposure. Zoonotic.
Johne's disease	(+)	—	(+)	Yes	Individual animal screening to detect subclinical infection is hampered by lack of suitable tests, all of which can produce false positive and false negative results. Tests such as adsorbed ELISA may be useful on a group basis. Request certification of clinical freedom. If scour develops in isolation check CFT titre on serum and examine faeces for acidfasts; culture if suspicious.
Streptococcus agalactiae	(+)	(+)	+	No	Should be readily preventable by using CMT, culturing positive quarters and treating where appropriate.
Staphylococcus aureus	(+)	(+)	+	No	

SAT, serum agglutination test; CFT, complement fixation test; CMT, California mastitis test.
+ Indicated; (+) possible benefit; — not indicated.

Table 12.2 Miscellaneous conditions likely to be introduced by added animals. (From Pritchard, 1996.)

Disease/infection	Preventive measures			Vaccination option	Comments
	Clinical examination	Prophylactic treatment •	Laboratory tests		
Digital dermatitis	+	(+)	—	No	Good clinical examination essential. If in doubt use prophylactic antibiotic spray/footbath or footbath as appropriate.
'Superfoul'	+	(+)	—	No	
Ringworm	+	(+)	(+)	Yes	Can cause quite serious problems in naive herds, particularly amongst adult animals. Zoonotic.
Miscellaneous udder/skin conditions (pseudo-cowpox, warts, etc.)	+	(+)	(+)	No	Troublesome and best avoided.
Ectoparasites	+	(+)	(+)	No	Use appropriate prophylactic or curative treatment.
Liver fluke	—	+	(+)	No	Use carefully selected, appropriate anthelmintics.
Lungworm	—	+	(+)	No	
Campylobacteriosis	(+)	+	(+)	No	Prophylactic treatment probably more cost-effective than laboratory testing.
Trichomoniasis	(+)	—	(+)	No	Not present in UK, but check imported bulls.
Neospora caninum	—	?	(+)	No	Problematical, epidemiology unclear. Consider not retaining calves from seropositive cows because of risk of congenital infection.

+ Indicated; (+) possible benefit; — not indicated.

foot-and-mouth disease (FMD), since other EU states practised FMD vaccination. Although only unvaccinated cattle were (and are) permitted to be imported, it was feared that virulent virus might be carried asymptomatically by the vaccinated stock and passed to the imported (unvaccinated) stock shortly before shipment. As the other member states of the EU abandoned FMD vaccination, their cattle were allowed into Britain without quarantine. This change led to a significant increase in the number of cattle imported from Europe. In 1991, a total of 6830 cattle were imported; in 1992 this rose to 15316. The establishment of the Single Market in 1993 did not result in any further increase, and in 1995 cattle imports had reduced to around 9000. Although no uncontained disease outbreaks have resulted from this major influx of animals, cases of warble fly have been confirmed in imported cattle, necessitating treatment and movement restrictions (warble fly having been eradicated from Britain). An incident of brucellosis in 1993 also appears to be linked to importation. Imported animals may well carry strains of certain diseases which differ from those already present. For instance, strains of IBR or Johne's disease elsewhere in Europe may have different characteristics from those already established in Britain.

In the first few years after the abolition of quarantine, comparatively large numbers of cattle were imported from the Netherlands and significant consignments from Eastern Europe via the EU. By 1995, most of the trade originated in Northern Ireland and Eire, with significant contributions from the Netherlands and France, and a few cattle (including some water buffalo) from Romania. The interest in cattle from Canada remains, and around 400–500 cattle from there have been imported each year.

Although it is not possible at the time of writing to judge the long-term effect of changes in BSE policy on cattle movements into Britain, at least one can expect that trade will become more diverse as the Single Market develops. The effect of the Single Market has not yet been to flood British auctions with foreign cattle, but any increase in the exchange of cattle between *and within* countries is bound to increase the exchange of pathogens carried by them.

Legislative requirements

Importers of all livestock must make sure that they know the conditions relating to both health and welfare under which the animals may be imported. It is the importer's responsibility to ensure that the imported cattle fully comply with these conditions. Advice should therefore be obtained from the local Animal Health Office well before the intended importation.

When cattle or bovine semen or embryos are to be imported from other members states of the EU, the importer is required by the Animals and Animal Products (Import and Export) Regulations 1995 to notify the local Animal Health Office at least 24 hours in advance, giving details of what animals or genetic materials are to be imported, the intended destination, and the date of arrival.

When an export health certificate is signed in any EU state, the veterinary surgeon who signs it must confirm the details of the consignment (including destination) to the local veterinary authorities in the country of origin. They then transmit these details by means of an 'ANIMO' (Animal Movement) message to the veterinary authority responsible for the place of destination, either by a computer link or by fax.

The Divisional Veterinary Manager (DVM) in Great Britain should thus be informed from two sources of the impending arrival of cattle from the EU – directly from the importer, and from the exporting Veterinary Authorities by the ANIMO message. If only one notification is received, or if the details on the two notifications do not match, then immediate investigations can be made.

When the cattle have arrived, the importer (that is, the person to whom the animals are consigned, as shown on the health certificate) is required to check that the animals are accompanied by the necessary documents – especially the health certificate and the journey plan as appropriate. If the animals appear unwell, or if the documents are incomplete or incorrect (e.g. if the identification of the animals does not match that on the certificates, or if there are more or fewer animals in the consignment than on the certificate), the importer is responsible for informing the DVM.

The arrival of the cattle must be entered into the farm's movement records, and if the animals are subsequently moved off the premises, the destination must be recorded. The cattle must be treated with an approved treatment for warble fly within 24 hours of arrival, and the DVM must be notified of the treatment within 5 days.

Consignments of cattle arriving from the EU are thus not routinely inspected by the British veterinary authorities. Although under Community law the veterinary authorities of member states may not impose routine health checks other than those described above, they may make random, non-discriminatory spot checks, or carry out extra tests in response to particular risks. If alerted to a problem by the veterinary authorities in the exporting state, they may also intercept consignments or make other conditions. Incoming ANIMO messages are routinely subject to 'risk analysis', and if particular risks are associated with the area of origin of the animals the DVM responsible for the premises of destination is given appropriate instructions.

Cattle imported directly from countries not in the EU (known as 'third countries') may only be landed at specified ports or airports known as Border Inspection Posts (BIP). At least one working day before the cattle arrive, the importer is required to notify the official veterinary surgeon (OVS) responsible for the BIP at which the animals will be landed. The precise requirements for veterinary certification vary according to the country of origin, and health tests before consignment, etc. are stipulated in individual European Directives or Commission Decisions. Documentary checks and any necessary blood tests or treatments are made by the Official Veterinary Surgeon (OVS), who also registers their arrival on a computer system known as SHIFT. In the case of cattle from Canada and certain other sources the animals may then be moved under licence to a specified destination for them to undergo on-farm isolation as specified in the Animals and Animal Products (Imports and Exports) Regulations 1995 (see Appendix 12.1). In other cases, the cattle may be released into the country.

Once accepted into any EU-state, cattle imported from outside the Union may subsequently be traded as if they were of EU origin. Thus, cattle imported from, for example, the Netherlands may in fact have originated in, say, Poland. However, if cattle are refused entry into the EU for any reason, the SHIFT system alerts the OVS at all other BIPs so that the intending importer cannot try his luck elsewhere.

The health certificate for EU trade in breeding cattle requires the animals to be free from clinical signs of disease (including mastitis). They must not have been vaccinated against FMD, and must not be animals that are due to be destroyed under any eradication programme. The herd of origin must be free from tuberculosis, brucellosis and enzootic bovine leukosis, and in some circumstances the animals must be tested for some or all of these three diseases before export. If a member state has an EU-approved eradication programme for either IBR or Johne's disease, then the state may add extra health conditions relating to these diseases to the health certificate for animals brought into the country. Denmark has eradicated IBR and thus requires what are known as 'additional guarantees' for IBR.

Apart from this, the health certificate makes no provision for statements concerning, or tests for, any other disease. Under Community law, national authorities are not permitted to ask for other tests or veterinary certification as a condition of import. *However, the purchaser in a private capacity may ask the vendor for whatever assurances he or she may choose.* Many cattle breeders in France and Germany can provide evidence that their herds are free from IBR; many in the Netherlands can provide evidence (based on tests carried out on bulk milk samples) that *Leptospira hardjo* is not active in their herds; Sweden is attempting BVD eradication and has a pool of BVD-free herds. These examples all rest on officially supported testing programmes: but a purchaser can just as well ask for private certification from the vendor's veterinary surgeon that, for instance, Johne's disease has not been diagnosed in the herd.

Guidance as to the sort of certification that might be suitable for various diseases can be found in the International Animal Health Code, which is produced by the Office Internationale d'Epidemiologie (OIE) and intended as a basis for certification for international trade. Appendix 12.2 summarises the diseases covered by the code.

Herd accreditation schemes

In this context, an accredited herd is one in which the cattle have been tested for a particular disease to the extent that assurances can be given that the disease is absent. The aim is to establish a pool of herds with the relevant disease-free status, so that cattle can be bought and sold without risk of transmitting the disease. Purchasers of accredited cattle will then, in theory, pay a better price for them.

Both the tuberculosis and brucellosis eradication campaigns in Britain began with voluntary accreditation programmes organised by the State Veterinary

Service of the Ministry of Agriculture Fisheries and Food (MAFF). The testing costs were met by the State. Once a significant pool of voluntarily accredited herds had been established, testing became compulsory so that in time all herds in the country became accredited. A similar voluntary non-chargeable accreditation scheme for enzootic bovine leukosis was launched in Great Britain in 1982.

In 1987 the voluntary EBL scheme became chargeable, and additional schemes for IBR and *L. hardjo* were launched. Although the IBR scheme was technically successful, neither additional scheme ever achieved a large membership, and in 1996 they were handed over to the private sector to operate.

There is no reason in principle why industry-run voluntary accreditation schemes could not be made to succeed for a variety of diseases. In considering why the MAFF schemes had such a small uptake, it may be instructive to consider the features necessary for success.

- The disease in question should be capable of causing significant economic losses to infected herds.
- The infection can be transmitted by apparently healthy animals, i.e. there is a subclinical carrier state.
- Sensitive and specific laboratory tests must be available to detect the carrier state with a high degree of reliability.
- It must be practical to eliminate the disease from the herd by a 'test and cull' programme.
- It must be practical to prevent the reintroduction of the infection.
- The benefits of membership of the programme must exceed the costs of operating it.

It is evident that leptospirosis does not meet many of these criteria. The available tests do not reliably indicate the status of individual animals; the disease cannot be eliminated by 'test and cull'; although it is possible to guard against introducing infection it requires considerable attention to detail and is impractical in many herds; the costs of testing and the necessary veterinary advice were high, and there was no market premium for cattle from herds in the scheme; the costs of testing exceeded the cost of controlling the disease by vaccination. This does not mean that an alternative type of scheme may not be successful: Dutch experience suggests that a herd with a history of negative ELISA tests on bulk milk samples has no active disease, and that animals purchased from such a herd are unlikely to transmit infection.

By contrast, when judged against these principles, an IBR accreditation scheme should have a better chance of success. The MAFF scheme failed mainly on the cost–benefit analysis: again, there was usually no market premium for cattle from IBR-free herds to offset the considerable costs of routine testing. There was an exception: before the export of breeding stock to the EU was banned because of BSE, considerable numbers of Highland cattle were exported to Germany. Voluntary IBR programmes are widespread in Germany, and exporters gained a significant market advantage from membership of the IBR scheme.

On the criteria cited, Johne's disease seems an unpromising candidate for an accreditation scheme. However, its potential long-term economic impact means that (at least for some breeds of cattle) a practical scheme might be very attractive. Older testing methods (complement fixation test; skin testing with purified protein derivative from either *M. avium* or *M. paratuberculosis*) have not been sufficiently sensitive or specific. Faeces culture, if repeated at regular intervals over a long period, could form the basis of a herd accreditation programme, and a series of wholly negative results could give useful assurance that the herd was free from infection. However, faecal culture is too slow and expensive for such a voluntary scheme to be financially viable without exterior funding (i.e. in practice from the State). Test methods developed more recently (ELISA and gamma-interferon assays) have been claimed to have useful advantages. A polymerase chain reaction assay is also available. This can detect bacterial DNA in faeces samples within a few days (rather than the months required for faecal culture), but its usefulness in practical conditions is not yet clear.

Despite these technical difficulties, voluntary accreditation schemes for Johne's disease are available in Australia, parts of France and some parts of the USA. A compulsory accreditation/eradication programme is also under development in the Netherlands.

Any future development of voluntary accreditation programmes depends critically upon the balance between the costs and the benefits of membership. Cattle from accredited herds will only fetch a market premium if the purchaser is convinced that accredited cattle will save him money or trouble – in other words, if he is aware of the disease risks associated with cattle of unknown health status, and is confident of the disease-free status of the accredited cattle. If the demand for accredited cattle is high enough, then the costs of membership may be less important – but unless demand is strong, testing costs may be prohibitive. It may be possible to reduce testing costs if very sensitive tests become available: but any reduction in the rigour of a testing programme may reduce the level of assurance given by accredited status, and thus reduce the value of the status.

Nevertheless, the Dutch leptospirosis testing scheme mentioned above suggests that, provided the testing programme is cheap enough, there is a place for a scheme that offers less than an implied guarantee that the herd is totally free from evidence of infection. It can be argued that the cattle industry has been given the wrong message over a succession of accreditation schemes, from the original voluntary TB scheme onwards. Buying from an accredited herd has been seen as a sufficient precaution against introducing the disease in question. Perhaps if it were the normal practice to quarantine all added animals, herd testing schemes could be perceived as a means of reducing the risk of detecting a 'reactor' during quarantine – not as a substitute for quarantine. Viewed in this light, buying from a 'monitored' herd – in which only a proportion of the herd had been tested – would for most purposes be as good as buying from a herd in which all animals had been tested. For instance, in a herd of 100 cows, a negative test on 27 animals randomly chosen will give 95% confidence that fewer than 5% of the herd members are infected. In practice, this may be good enough – and testing 27 animals is much cheaper than testing 100!

Private veterinary certification for cattle movements

As discussed above, *official veterinary certification for international trade should only be considered as a starting point,* and importers should be advised and encouraged to ask for supplementary health information – using the Office International d'Epidemiologie (OIE) code as a useful reference. The logical extension of this is to encourage purchasers of cattle from 'domestic' sources to ask for comparable assurances or certification. Since this is not the current practice, and since there is no agreed standard for any such certification, this may seem a utopian prescription at present. One can imagine the incredulity that would face individual farmers asking for such certification, and the indifference greeting anyone who supplied it unasked to a purchaser.

However, there are two groups of people in key positions in the industry who could make a significant impact – the breed societies, and the organisers of major agricultural shows. As a condition of entry to a Breed Society show and sale, or as a condition of entry to a county or regional show, exhibitors could be required to present a certificate from their veterinary surgeon. When first introduced, the conditions on the certificate would need to be fairly easy to fulfil, e.g. that the cattle had been inspected by the veterinary surgeon; that no contagious diseases had been diagnosed in the herd in the previous, say, 14 days. Certain breed societies could benefit from specific declarations concerning Johne's disease: e.g. that no cases had been diagnosed in the herd in the previous 5 years.

Once the idea of veterinary inspection before the event had been accepted, the conditions could be made more stringent. They could include some of the tests discussed earlier in the section 'Dealing with the added animal' on p. 333. The next stage would be to persuade auctioneers to encourage vendors to provide similar certification for commercial (as opposed to pedigree) auctions, so that the 'culture' of herd security could be extended to all sectors of the industry.

As an example of the sort of certification which could be adapted for this purpose, the Tb Declaration cards used in New Zealand are worth consideration (Appendix 12.3). It is relevant to note that in New Zealand (unlike in Britain) animals which pass a tuberculin test may, in certain circumstances and subject to further controls, be permitted to move from herds which are classified as infected. All cattle and deer populations in New Zealand are given a Tb status by the veterinary authorities. Vendors are required to provide a declaration which includes details of this status, whether the animals are home bred, and their recent test history, for example. The declaration thus provides a means for the purchaser to identify the level of security he requires and is prepared to pay for. A similar mechanism could, in principle, be adopted by the cattle industry for other diseases without any involvement from the veterinary authorities.

However fanciful this may seem, private veterinary certificates are already required for entry to some major shows in other European states. Once the BSE crisis has passed, if the British cattle industry wishes to compete in the developing Single Market, it will have to match the highest health standards accepted by any of the European industries. If the British veterinary profession and cattle breeders cannot rise to this challenge, then Britain is likely to become a nation of cow-keepers buying genetics from abroad, rather than regaining any reputation as a stockyard.

Private health and preventive medicine schemes

Disease testing

The following is concerned mainly with Great Britain, although private health and preventive medicine schemes of a similar nature are available throughout the world. Some will have different features and procedures will alter. They all have the aim of identifying dairy herds that have been monitored for specific diseases and to see if members of the scheme are of known superior health status to other herds. The schemes all cost money to join and to have regular testing and so are mainly undertaken by those with pedigree herds, presumably with an eye to sell stock to other farmers in the same country or for export.

In the 1990s the government decided that the MAFF-run Cattle Health Scheme should be privatised except for the statutory disease component. Thus in 1996 Cattle Health 2000 took over the management of the other components, i.e. the monitoring of IBR and *Leptospira hardjo*. Since then the scheme has also incorporated BVD and Johne's disease. In 1998 the Premium Cattle Scheme was set up by the Scottish Agricultural College with the objective of monitoring BVD, IBR and Johne's disease. The schemes are based on blood testing and strict recording.

Many European countries already have eradication schemes for BVD and IBR, including Sweden, Denmark, Finland, Estonia, northern Germany and the Netherlands. Many of the IBR schemes involve the use of a live gene-depleted marker vaccine to reduce the level of IBR in the herd. There is also a *Leptospira hardjo* eradication scheme in the Netherlands. The possibility of eradicating Johne's disease is being considered in Sweden, but this will be much more difficult because the test cross reacts in response to other disease organisms, and because many other species can harbour the disease and act as a reservoir.

Monitoring herds for disease via milk sampling has also been undertaken. Originally testing was done on individual cows and this is still important for indicating exposure to infection and when attempting control and eradication. Almost all the testing involves determination of an immune response. However, as testing has become more sophisticated it is now possible to examine bulk milk samples to determine the antibody level and thus determine the proportion of the herd that has been exposed to infection and is immune.

Production testing

Production testing has been available for many years to enable the veterinary surgeon, farmer and nutritionist to assess the herd's production and relate this to such factors as feed levels, disease and reproductive performance. It is mentioned in more detail in Chapter 4. Testing mainly involves blood sampling, but more recently milk has been used. While the latter is easier to obtain and may be useful to evaluate certain parameters, it may be difficult to assess others. In addition, there has been less research in the use of milk in such testing programmes.

It is probable that in the next few years many other tests will become available for assessing both disease and production status. This will mean that by routine monitoring of herds, a profile of their disease status and management proficiency will be compiled. This will, in turn, allow management decisions to be made on the basis of knowledge rather than assumption.

References

Anon (1995) *Bull Hiring*. British Cattle Veterinary Association, Frampton-on-Severn.
Duncan, A. L. (1990) Herd security in cattle herds. *In Practice* **12** (1), 29–32.
Hartley, P. E. & Richards, M. S. (1988) A study of the transmission of bovine viral diarrhoea between and within cattle herds. *Acta Veterinaria Scandinavica* **84**, 164–6.
Pritchard, G. C. (1996) Added animals: the challenge to preventative medicine. *Cattle Practice* **4**, 253–7.
Scudamore, J. M. (1988) Outbreaks of brucellosis in south west England during 1984–6. *The State Veterinary Journal* **42**, 68–75.

Appendix 12.1

The following is an extract from the Animals (Post Import Control) order 1995, and is reproduced with the permission of the Controller of Her Majesty's Stationery Office. SI 1995 No. 2439, Article 4.

SCHEDULE 2

Conditions applicable to post import isolation premises for cattle

1. In the case of isolation in buildings:
   (a) the building must be cleansed and disinfected prior to use;
   (b) drainage from the building must not flow into any area or onto any land accessible to other stock;
   (c) if the route of entry to the building is used by other stock it must be cleansed and disinfected both before use by imported cattle and immediately after they have been housed;
   (d) during transfer of the imported cattle to the building there must be no contact with other stock or sharing of air space; and
   (e) imported cattle must be kept in an enclosed secure building with no access to or sharing of air space with other stock.

2. In the case of field isolation:
   (a) boundary fences must prevent contact with other stock and be in the form of double fencing 3 metres apart, and
   (b) a suitable building meeting the requirements of paragraph 1 of this Schedule must also be available.

3. Animals may only be kept in group isolation if there are facilities on the premises for isolating individual animals in the event of injury or disease.

4. No animals other than imported cattle shall be moved into the isolation premises.

5. The attendant for the imported cattle will be allowed to have contact with native livestock providing:
   (a) native livestock is attended to first;
   (b) suitable protective clothing (boots, overalls and gloves) is worn while tending the imported animals; and
   (c) personal cleansing and disinfection is carried out immediately thereafter.

6. Animals from separate imported consignments may share the same isolation premises. However, in such circumstances none of the animals may be released from isolation until the latest date on which the isolation periods for the individual consignments expire, irrespective of whether the consignments initially qualify for 4, 6 or 9 months' isolation.

7. During the isolation period, no movement of imported cattle off the isolation premises is permitted unless under the authority of a licence issued by an authorised inspector, which licence may only be issued either
   (a) if the animals are to be taken directly to an abattoir for immediate slaughter, or
   (b) to another isolation premises if this is necessary for welfare reasons.

Any animal with a positive reaction to the EBL test shall be slaughtered forthwith without compensation to the importer.

8. The imported cattle shall not be vaccinated or subjected to any test without the authority of an authorised inspector.

9. Any illness in imported cattle shall be notified to the Minister. If any of the cattle die or have to be slaughtered the carcase or carcases must not be removed from the isolation premises without the authority of a licence issued by an authorised inspector.

10. A duly authorised officer of the Minister may take samples for testing for enzootic bovine leukosis (EBL)
    (a) where a 4 month isolation period applies, within 120 days of landing;
    (b) where a 6 month isolation period applies, between 70 and 74 days after landing and again between 180 and 184 days after landing; and
    (c) where a 9 month isolation period applies, between 150 and 155 days after landing and again between 270 and 275 days after landing.

11. Where cattle are imported pregnant, they must be housed separately from non-pregnant animals on the isolation premises. Details of any animal found to be pregnant without the pregnancy recorded on the certification accompanying the animal must be notified to the Minister and the animal must immediately be isolated from other animals on the isolation premises.

12.   Animals which are imported as pregnant shall be isolated from other cattle when calving is imminent.

13.   Arrangements for milking imported cattle, should this be necessary, must be agreed with an authorised inspector.

14.   Contacts with reactors to an EBL test shall remain in isolation for 120 days after the positive test after which they shall be given a further EBL test, but they may be licensed by an authorised inspector to isolation at other premises or direct to a slaughterhouse.

15.   After the isolation period, the animals shall not be permitted to leave the isolation premises unless authorised by an authorised inspector in writing, which authorisation shall not be given until all imported animals on the isolation premises have passed the final EBL test; except that where pregnant animals calve more than 120 days after importation, release of other imported animals in the isolation premises is at the discretion of an authorised inspector. Any animals which have calved in the isolation premises may be released at the discretion of an authorised inspector when all the animals in isolation premises have met the EBL testing requirements.

16.   Embryos may be collected from animals in isolation providing prior approval has been obtained from an authorised inspector.

17.   Artificial insemination of imported cattle may be allowed subject to the approval of an authorised inspector.

18.   Natural service of imported cattle is permitted only in the case of imported bulls running in the same isolation as the imported heifers or cows.

19.   An imported bull not intended for direct entry to a semen collection centre may be examined and tested to establish whether or not it is fit to be used for the purposes of artificial insemination. In the case of bulls undergoing 4 months' isolation this examination and testing may be undertaken immediately upon entry into isolation and in the case of bulls undergoing 6 months' isolation it may be undertaken following confirmation of a negative result to the EBL test carried out between 70 and 74 days after landing. If it is found that the bulls are suitable, semen may be collected and stored at an approved centre. Semen may not be used until the bull and any other imported cattle in contact with it have, in the case of animals subject to 4 months' isolation, passed the single post-importation EBL test carried out within 120 days of landing or, in the case of animals subject to 6 months' isolation, have passed the final post-importation EBL test between 180 and 184 days after landing. If any imported animal on the same isolation premises as the donor bull fails the EBL test the semen must remain in isolation until all animals on that premises are released from isolation.

20.   Semen may be collected from a bull imported for direct entry to a semen collection centre and subject to 9 months' isolation. Such semen may only be collected after confirmation of a negative result to the EBL test carried out between 150 and 155 days after landing and must be stored at an approved centre. It may not be used until the bull and any other imported cattle in contact with it have passed the final post-importation EBL test between 270 and 275 days after landing. If any imported animal on the same isolation premises as the donor bull fails the EBL test the semen must remain in isolation until all animals on that premises are released from isolation.

21. Teasers may be used for the collection of semen but must be steers, over 18 months of age, tested and found negative to the EBL test. The movement of teasers into the isolation premises will only be allowed under the authority of a licence issued by an authorised inspector.

22. The use of female teasers is prohibited.

23. Teasers shall be held in separate approved isolation to the bulls and only taken to the bull for the collection of semen. After collection of semen the teasers shall be returned to their isolation section.

24. After final collection is completed the teasers shall remain in isolation until the bull has been tested for EBL and found clear, after which time the teaser may be released. Alternatively the teaser may be sent for slaughter.

Appendix 12.2

Summary of 'List B' diseases for which the International Animal Health Code contains recommendations for certification for international trade in cattle

Anthrax
Leptospirosis
Rabies
Johne's disease
Heartwater
Screw-worm
Brucellosis
Campylobacter (genital)
Tuberculosis
Enzootic bovine leukosis
Infectious bovine rhinotracheitis
Anaplasmosis
Babesiosis
Dermatophilosis
Theileriosis
Haemorrhagic septicaemia (*Pasteurella multocida* serotypes 6B and 6E)
Bovine spongiform encephalopathy

Taken from Office Internationale d'Epidemiologie (1992) *International Animal Health Code (Mammals, Birds and Bees)*, 6th edn. Office Internationale d'Epidemiologie, Paris.

Appendix 12.3   Tb declaration

This card must accompany cattle and deer one month of age and over

Owner / Manager / Grazier	
Farm / Station Name	
Farm Location	
Postal Address	

I declare that :

Number

Description

Identification	YES	NO
1. Are Owner Bred		
2. These animals have been tested while in my ownership		
3. The last Tb test for these animals was / / 19		
The last Tb test date for the herd was / / 19		
Was Tb detected at either of these tests?		
4. The Tb status of these animals is (see definitions)		
5. Is the herd under movement control? (If YES a permit is required)		
6. These animals are being moved from a property within a		
Declared Movement Controlled area.		
IF YES		
Have they been tested within 60 days prior to this movement?		

7. These animals are going to sale   Agent : ....

These animals are going to slaughter   Works : ....

These animals are going to   Other : ....

Certified true and correct :   When required, I authorise duplication of this declaration.

Signed : _____   Date :   /   / 19

THIS COPY SHOULD ACCOMPANY THE MOVEMENT OF ST CK

Purchasers / Graziers / Slaughter premises : When receiving stock, retain this Tb Declaration Card for minimum of three months.

Index